STRUCTURE AND FUNCTIONS OF THE HUMAN PREFRONTAL CORTEX

ANNALS OF THE NEW YORK ACADEMY OF SCIENCES
Volume 769

STRUCTURE AND FUNCTIONS OF THE HUMAN PREFRONTAL CORTEX

Edited by Jordan Grafman, Keith J. Holyoak,
and François Boller

The New York Academy of Sciences
New York, New York
1995

Cover: The illustration on the soft cover edition of this book shows a human head in profile with a band around the head labeling areas of the brain that are vital to the memory, imagination, cognition, and the senses. This image is from: LeLièvre, Guillaume, Ars memorativa Gulielmi Leporei Avallonensis. *[Paris], Vaenundatur in chalcographia Jodoci Badii Ascensii [ca. 1520]. It is reproduced here through the courtesy of the National Library of Medicine. The PET scans on the right show frontal lobes activated during grammatical processing.*

Library of Congress Cataloging-in-Publication Data

Structure and functions of the human prefrontal cortex / editors,
    Jordon Grafman, Keith J. Holyoak, François Boller.
        p.   cm.—(Annals of the New York Academy of Sciences ; vol.
    769)
        Includes bibliographical references and index.
        ISBN 0-89766-991-6 (cloth : alk. paper).—ISBN 0-89766-992-4
    (pbk. : alk. paper)
        1. Prefrontal cortex—Congresses. I. Grafman, Jordan.
    II. Holyoak, Keith James, 1950– . III. Boller, François.
    IV. Series.
    Q11.N5   vol. 769
    [QP383.17]
    500 s—dc20
    [612.8'25]   95-39938
                                                                    CIP

MC/PCP
Printed in the United States of America
ISBN 0-89766-991-6 (cloth)
ISBN 0-89766-992-4 (paper)
ISSN 0077-8923

ANNALS OF THE NEW YORK ACADEMY OF SCIENCES

Volume 769

December 15, 1995

STRUCTURE AND FUNCTIONS OF THE HUMAN PREFRONTAL CORTEX[a]

Editors and Conference Organizers

JORDAN GRAFMAN, KEITH J. HOLYOAK, AND FRANÇOIS BOLLER

CONTENTS

[a] This volume contains papers presented at a workshop entitled Structure and Functions of the Human Prefrontal Cortex, which was sponsored by the New York Academy of Sciences and held on March 2–4, 1995 in New York City.

Financial assistance was received from:

Major Funder
    • NATIONAL INSTITUTE OF NEUROLOGICAL DISORDERS AND STROKE

Contributors
    • THE ALZHEIMER'S ASSOCIATION
    • THE COCA-COLA FOUNDATION
    • NATIONAL INSTITUTE ON AGING
    • PFIZER CENTRAL RESEARCH
    • THE UPJOHN COMPANY
    • ZENECA PHARMACEUTICALS

Preface

JORDAN GRAFMAN,[a] KEITH J. HOLYOAK,[b]
AND FRANÇOIS BOLLER[c]

[a]Cognitive Neuroscience Section/Medical Neurology Branch
National Institute of Neurological Disorders and Stroke
National Institutes of Health
Bethesda, Maryland 20892

[b]Department of Psychology and Brain Research Institute
University of California, Los Angeles
Los Angeles, California 90095

[c]Unité 324
Institut National de la Santé et de la Recherche Médicale
2ter, rue d'Alésia
75014 Paris, France

Prefrontal cortex occupies approximately one-third of all human cortex. This proportion of cortical space occupied by the prefrontal cortex in humans is not approached in any other species. Since the reports by Harlow on his patient, Gage, who suffered a penetrating missile wound to the frontal lobes, clinicians and researchers have reported a variety of deficits following frontal lobe brain injury in humans including problems in concept formation, reasoning, social conduct, temporal ordering, planning, working memory, mood state, and creativity among others. These central themes have resulted in unidimensional frameworks that attempt to explain the workings of the prefrontal cortex. Given the size of human prefrontal cortex, its connections with widely dispersed regions of the brain, the sometimes dramatic but often elusive deficits that follow lesions to the frontal cortex, and the lack of "rich" testable theories of human prefrontal cortical functions, we believed that a meeting focusing on the clarification and development of theoretical models of prefrontal cortical functions would be both timely and exciting. The proceedings of the workshop entitled Structure and Functions of the Human Prefrontal Cortex, held March 2–4, 1995 at the New York Academy of Sciences, make up the content of this *Annals*.

Papers in this volume review the lastest neuroscientific knowledge on the normal neuroanatomy, neurochemistry, development, and aging of the human prefrontal cortex. Brief reviews of the neuropsychological findings in a number of cognitive domains following human prefrontal lobe damage or dysfunction are also included. Finally, several papers are devoted to discussing a number of competing, and potentially convergent, theoretical approaches that could help account for the cognitive and social deficits that are associated with prefrontal dysfunction.

We hope that this volume of the *Annals* both informs and inspires researchers interested in human cognition, social psychology, and the cognitive neuroscience of the human prefrontal cortex. While we acknowledge the crucial work of our scientific predecessors throughout this book (after all, a dwarf on a giant's shoulder sees the further of the two), much more work is necessary before we can confidently describe the cognitive architecture of the human prefrontal cortex.

Anatomic and Behavioral Aspects of Frontal-Subcortical Circuits[a]

JEFFREY L. CUMMINGS[b]

Departments of Neurology and Psychiatry
& Biobehavioral Sciences
UCLA School of Medicine
and
Behavioral Neuroscience Section
Psychiatry Service
West Los Angeles Veterans Affairs Medical Center
Los Angeles, California 90073

Five parallel circuits connect discrete regions of the frontal lobes with specific subregions of the striatum, globus pallidus, and thalamus. One circuit mediates motor function, another eye movements, and three of the circuits mediate cognitive, emotional, and motivational processes. The circuits serve as organizational axes integrating related information from widespread areas of the brain and mediating diverse behaviors. This review describes the anatomy of the circuits and the major transmitters present within the circuits. Circuit-specific behaviors (those that appear to be mediated exclusively by circuit structures) and circuit-related behaviors (those that involve both circuit and noncircuit structures) are discussed. Drugs that alter behavior through effects on the circuits are presented. The three circuits that are most relevant to understanding behavior are emphasized.

ANATOMY AND BIOCHEMISTRY OF FRONTAL-SUBCORTICAL CIRCUITS

Circuit Anatomy

Each of the frontal-subcortical circuits shares a common structure and a common biochemistry.[1-3] Each circuit includes the frontal lobe, striatum, globus pallidus/substantia nigra, thalamus, and connecting links between these structures. There is a projection from the frontal lobe to the striatum, either the caudate nucleus, the putamen, or the nucleus accumbens. Two pathways emanate from the striatum: (1) a direct projection to the globus pallidus interna and substantia nigra, and (2) an indirect projection from the striatum to the globus pallidus externa that in turn connects to the subthalamic nucleus, which projects back to the globus pallidus interna and substantia nigra. Globus pallidus interna and nigral neurons

[a] This project was supported by the United States Department of Veterans Affairs and a National Institute on Aging Alzheimer's Disease Core Center grant (AG 10123).

[b] Address correspondence to Jeffrey L. Cummings, M.D., Reed Neurological Research Center, UCLA School of Medicine, 710 Westwood Plaza, Los Angeles, California 90024.

1

have connections to the medial dorsal nucleus of the thalamus. Thalamic nuclei complete the circuits by projecting back to the frontal lobes.[4-6]

The circuits are parallel but discrete, and each circuit projects to a distinct area within the member structures comprising the circuit.[1,7] The *motor circuit* begins in the supplementary motor area, which projects to the putamen. This structure connects with specific regions of the globus pallidus and substantia nigra, which in turn project to the ventrolateral nucleus of the thalamus, and the thalamus connects to the frontal lobe. The *oculomotor circuit* begins in the frontal eye field. This cortical area projects to the putamen, the putamen connects with discrete areas of the globus pallidus and substantia nigra, and these areas project to the ventral anterior and medial dorsal nucleus of the thalamus. The thalamic nuclei send fibers to the frontal lobe. The *dorsolateral prefrontal circuit* begins on the lateral convexity of the frontal lobe anterior to the premotor area. The related circuit structures include the dorsolateral portion of the caudate nucleus, distinct areas of the globus pallidus and substantia nigra, and ventral anterior and medial dorsal nuclei of the thalamus. The lateral *orbitofrontal circuit* begins in the orbital cortex on the inferior surface of the frontal lobe anterior to the premotor cortex. The orbitofrontal circuit includes the ventral portion of the caudate nucleus, the globus pallidus and substantia nigra, and the ventral anterior and dorsal medial nuclei of the thalamus. The *medial frontal circuit* begins in the cortex of the anterior cingulate cortex; the circuit includes the nucleus accumbens (ventromedial striatum), globus pallidus and substantia nigra, and medial dorsal nucleus of the thalamus.

Circuit Efferents and Afferents

Circuit structures receive afferent input from noncircuit sources and provide efferent connections to structures and cortical regions outside of the circuits. The "open loop" connections are functionally related to the principal functions of each of the circuits. The *dorsolateral prefrontal cortex* has reciprocal connections with cortical and subcortical regions (TABLE 1). This circuit originates in the association cortex of the frontal lobe, and it receives input from and provides efferent output to posterior temporal, parietal, and occipital association areas.[8] Posterior cortical input reaches the frontal lobe via the superior longitudinal fasciculus from the parietal lobe and via the inferior longitudinal fasciculus or inferior occipitofrontal bundle from the occipital lobe.[8]

Nearly the entire cerebral cortex also projects to the caudate nucleus.[9] The medial parietal cortex, the caudal portion of the inferior parietal lobule, and caudal portion of the parietal operculum project to the dorsal caudate nucleus.[10] Superior temporal regions project to the ventral portion of the caudate.[11] Cortical projections to striatum are largely unidirectional, creating a funneling effect in which the dorsolateral prefrontal subcortical circuit serves as a conduit through which information derived from multiple cortical areas is projected to the caudate, processed through the circuit, and projected on to the dorsolateral prefrontal cortex.

There are projections from cortex to subcortical circuit structures in addition to the caudate nucleus as well as connections between subcortical structures.

TABLE 1. Open-Loop Afferents and Efferents of the Dorsolateral Prefrontal-Subcortical Circuit

Circuit Structures	Afferents	Efferents
Dorsolateral prefrontal cortex	Orbitofrontal cortex	Orbitofrontal cortex
	Parietal association cortex	Parietal association cortex
	Auditory association cortex	Auditory association cortex
	Visual association cortex	Visual association cortex
	Cingulate gyrus	Cingulate gyrus
	Retrosplenial cortex	Retrosplenial cortex
	Parahippocampal gyrus	Parahippocampal gyrus
	Presubiculum	Presubiculum
Dorsal caudate	Parietal cortex	
	Temporal cortex	
	Occipital cortex	
	Substantia nigra	
	MD thalamus	
Subthalamic nucleus	Frontal association cortex	
VA and MD thalamus	Frontal cortex	
	Caudate nucleus	

MD, medial dorsal nucleus of the thalamus; VA, ventral anterior nucleus of the thalamus.

Among these are projections to subthalamic nucleus that originate essentially exclusively from frontal cortex and are unidirectional.[12] The caudate receives a robust projection from the substantial nigra,[13] and the caudate projects directly to the subthalamic nucleus.[12] Subthalamic nucleus projects to thalamus, and the thalamus has direct input from the frontal lobe.[9]

The *orbitofrontal-subcortical circuit* projects from orbitofrontal cortex to the ventral portion of the caudate nucleus (TABLE 2). The orbital cortex receives projections from the dorsolateral prefrontal regions, and the ventral caudate re-

TABLE 2. Open-Loop Afferents and Efferents of the Orbitofrontal-Subcortical Circuit

Circuit Structures	Afferents	Efferents
Orbitofrontal cortex	Dorsolateral prefrontal cortex	Dorsolateral prefrontal cortex
	Temporal pole	Temporal pole
	Amygdala	Amygdala
Ventral caudate	Amygdala	
	Ventral tegmental area	
	Substantia nigra	
	Midbrain raphe nuclei	
	MD thalamus	
	Superior temporal lobe	
Medial GP/SN	Amygdala	
	Ventral tegmental area	
VA and MD thalamus	Amygdala	Amygdala
	Prefrontal cortex	

MD, medial dorsal nucleus of the thalamus; GP, globus pallidus; SN, substantia nigra; VA, ventral anterior nucleus of the thalamus.

TABLE 3. Open-Loop Afferents and Efferents of the Medial Frontal-Subcortical Circuit

Circuit Structures	Afferents	Efferents
Anterior cingulate	Dorsolateral prefrontal cortex Amygdala Ventral tegmental area	Dorsolateral prefrontal cortex Amygdala
Nucleus accumbens	Medial orbitofrontal cortex Posterior insula Hippocampal subiculum Lateral hypothalamus Ventral tegmental area Perirhinal and entorhinal cortex Amygdala Substantia nigra MD thalamus Dorsal raphe nucleus	Septum Nucleus of stria terminalis Periaqueductal gray matter Medial hypothalamus Ventral tegmental area
Ventral GP/SN	Anterior insular cortex Anteroventral temporal cortex Cingulate cortex Hypothalamus Amygdala Ventral tegmental area Raphe nuclei Lateral habenula	Ventral striatum Lateral habenula Cingulate cortex Lateral hypothalamus Amygdala Ventral tegmental area Pedunculopontine nucleus
MD thalamus	Amygdala Nucleus accumbens	Amygdala

MD, medial dorsal nucleus of the thalamus; GP, globus pallidus; SN, substantia nigra.

ceives projections from the amygdala[8,14] as well as from the substantia nigra, midbrain raphe nuclei, midbrain tegmentum, and intralaminar, ventrolateral, mediodorsal thalamic nuclei, and temporal lobe.[11,15] The ventral caudate has circuit connections to the medial globus pallidus, which receives open-loop afferents from the amygdala and ventral tegmental area. The circuit pathway then projects to the mediodorsal thalamus which has afferent and efferent open-loop connections with the amygdala as well as closed loop connections with frontal lobe.

The *medial frontal-subcortical circuit* begins in the anterior cingulate cortex and projects to the nucleus accumbens, also known as the ventral or limbic striatum (TABLE 3). The anterior cingulate has short association connections with the dorsolateral prefrontal cortex. The nucleus accumbens/ventral striatum has amygdaloid input[8,14] and also receives afferents from the ventral tegmental area, substantia nigra, dorsal raphe nucleus,[8,16] and mediodorsal nucleus of the thalamus.

Nucleus accumbens has circuit linkages to the ventral pallidum. The ventral pallidum receives afferent projections from the anterior insular cortex, anteroventral temporal regions, cingulate, hypothalamus, amygdala, raphe nuclei, and lateral habenula. Extra-loop projections from the ventral pallidum include efferents to the ventral striatum, lateral hypothalamic area, cingulate cortex, amygdala, lateral habenula, and ventral tegmental area.[17-19] Ventral pallidum connects through the circuit with the mediodorsal thalamus. The extra-loop projections of the thalamus include the amygdala and nucleus accumbens.[20]

The amygdala projects to all four members structures of both the medial frontal and the orbitofrontal circuits. The medial frontal circuit receives projections from the caudal basolateral amygdaloid nucleus; the orbitofrontal circuit receives input from the rostral basolateral amygdaloid nucleus.[3] Thus, the amygdala is in register with the frontal-subcortical circuits that mediate major limbic system functions.

The cingulum and the superior occipitofrontal bundle connect the frontal lobe with the cingulate gyrus, retrosplenial cortex, parahippocampal area, and the presubiculum.[8] Short association fibers link the orbitofrontal cortex with the dorsolateral prefrontal area. Thus, the three prefrontal regions giving rise to frontal-subcortical circuits are linked to each other at the level of the frontal lobes; they do not exhibit cross connections with each other at subcortical levels. The dorsolateral prefrontal cortex is poised to serve as the principal organ for integrating information from the three circuits. Through these and related pathways it receives information from the outside environment, the internal milieu, and the emotional state of the organism. This information can be acted upon through the executive, motor, and oculomotor circuitry.

Circuit Transmitters

Direct-acting and modulatory transmitters are present in the frontal-subcortical circuitry.[21] Corticostriatal and thalamocortical connections use excitatory glutamatergic projections. In the direct pathway, striatopallidal and pallidothalamic connections employ gamma-aminobutyric acid (GABA). The indirect pathway utilizes GABA for the links between striatum and pallidum externa and between globus pallidus externa and subthalamic nucleus; there is a glutamate projection from subthalamic nucleus to the globus pallidus interna. Intrinsic cholinergic neurons also are present within the striatum. Peptidergic transmitters of the circuit include substance P in the direct pathway and enkephalin in the indirect pathway.

The direct and indirect pathways through the circuits exert opposing influences. The direct pathway with two consecutive inhibitory GABA-ergic neurons tends to disinhibit the thalamus. The indirect pathway with an excitatory glutamatergic neuron as well as two inhibitory GABA-ergic neurons exerts an inhibitory influence on the thalamus, balancing the disinhibiting (excitatory) effects of the direct pathway.[2]

CIRCUIT-SPECIFIC AND CIRCUIT-RELATED BEHAVIORS

Circuit-specific Behaviors

Each prefrontal-subcortical circuit mediates at least one principal behavior and is associated with a distinctive marker behavior when disturbed by a neuropathological process.[22] The *dorsolateral prefrontal-subcortical circuit* mediates executive behavior, and disruption of the circuit produces executive impairment. This syndrome is characterized by a retrieval deficit syndrome (poor recall, intact recognition), reduced verbal and nonverbal fluency (word-list generation, design generation) perseveration, difficulty shifting set, reduced mental control, poor abstraction, and impaired response inhibition. Instrumental functions such as language, memory storage, perception, and calculation are preserved. A variety of diseases can affect the dorsolateral prefrontal cortex including stroke, frontotemporal dementias, infections of the central nervous system, gliomas, and convexity meningiomas. Diseases of the white matter affecting the underlying myelinated fibers can produce executive dysfunction. Schizophrenia and depression have also been found to be associated with executive disorders and dorsolateral prefrontal dysfunction.[23,24] In addition to diseases of the dorsolateral prefrontal convexity, the dysexecutive syndrome can be produced by disorders of the other member structures of the dorsolateral prefrontal-subcortical circuit. Diseases of the caudate including Huntington's disease,[25] neuroacanthocytosis,[26] and stroke[27] have produced cognitive disorders similar to those observed with cortical dysfunction. A few patients with disease of the globus pallidus have been assessed and found to exhibit executive disorders.[28] Diseases of the thalamus produce executive dysfunction as well as memory impairment.[29]

The *orbitofrontal-subcortical circuit* mediates socially modulated civil behavior, and disruption of this circuit results in disinhibited, tactless, and impulsive behavior. Few neuropsychological deficits are associated with orbitofrontal dysfunction, although patients may have difficulty with set shifting on the Wisconsin Card Sorting Test.[30] The orbitofrontal cortex is subject to injury from closed head trauma, rupture of anterior communicating artery aneurysms, and subfrontal meningiomas. This region of cortex can also be affected in frontotemporal dementias, and the fibers emanating from the area may be affected by demyelinating disorders such as multiple sclerosis. Orbitofrontal cortex is occasionally affected in viral infections including herpes encephalitis or prion infections such as Creutzfeldt-Jakob disease. Disinhibition has also been observed with disorders of the subcortical structures of the orbitofrontal-subcortical circuit including Huntington's disease, neuroacanthocytosis, postencephalitic Parkinson's disease, and thalamic lesions.[22,25,31]

The *medial frontal-subcortical circuit* mediates motivation; medial frontal-subcortical circuit disorders feature apathy with reduced interest, motivation, engagement, and activity maintenance. Few neuropsychological deficits occur in patients with medial frontal lobe lesions. Impaired inhibition of responses in the go-no go test have been observed.[32] The most common cause of the syndrome is infarction in the territory of the anterior cerebral artery; it has also occurred with falcine meningiomas, gliomas, multiple sclerosis, brain infections, and frontotemporal dementias.[22,33] Apathy is common with lesions of the subcortical structures including degenerative, neoplastic, infectious, and vascular diseases affecting the medial frontal-subcortical circuit (nucleus accumbens, globus pallidus, and thalamus).[34–36]

Obsessive-compulsive disorder (OCD) is also a circuit-specific behavior of the orbitofrontal-subcortical circuit. Idiopathic OCD is associated with increased metabolism of the orbitofrontal cortex.[37] Acquired OCD occurs in degenerative, infectious, and vascular diseases of the caudate nucleus and globus pallidus.[38,39] Obsessive-compulsive disorder is rarely observed with lesions outside the orbitofrontal circuit.

TABLE 4. Evidence of Environmental Dependency in Behaviors Associated with Prefrontal Dysfunction

Behavioral Domain	Behavioral Abnormality (Self-generated)	Preserved Behavior (Environmentally Dependent)
Memory		
Recent memory	Poor recall	Intact recognition
Remote memory	Poor recall	Intact recognition
Language		
Transcortical motor aphasia	Decreased spontaneous speech	Intact repetition, echolalia
Naming	Poor word list generation	Intact confrontation naming
Behavior		
Social	Disinhibition	Learn instructions
Spontaneous	Apathy	Follow instructions
Motor	Akinesia	Catatonia
Interpersonal	Impaired spontaneous behavior	Imitation behavior, echopraxia
Object use	Impaired planned use	Utilization behavior
Perseveration		
Alternating programs	Follows model	Perseverates beyond copy
Multiple loops	Follows model	Perseverates beyond copy
Executive function		
Wisconsin Card Sorting Test	May achieve set	Cannot change set (perseverates)
Proverb abstraction	Cannot abstract (cannot derive inapparent meaning)	Concrete interpretation (apparent meaning)
Mental control	Cannot reverse normal order (spelling, reciting months of year)	Recite normal order
Response inhibition	Cannot inhibit the usual response (Stroop test)	Provide the usual response

Shared Features of Disorders of Prefrontal-Subcortical Circuits

Description of the frontal-subcortical circuits has led to the identification of behaviors unique or characteristic of each circuit. At the same time, study of the behaviors associated with dysfunction of the circuits provides insight into behavioral changes that are common to all prefrontal disorders. One theme that characterizes many behavioral changes observed with prefrontal dysfunction is environmental dependency (TABLE 4). Behaviors that are mediated by the *dorsolateral prefrontal cortex* and that exhibit environmental dependency include alternating programs and multiple loops (patients copy the model successfully and perseverate when generating the program themselves), recent memory (patients fail to recall information but can recognize it), naming (patients cannot perform word generation tasks but are accurate on confrontation naming), Wisconsin Card Sort Test (patients may achieve set but perseverate when required to change set), abstraction (patients give a concrete interpretation by responding to the manifest content and cannot derive an abstract response requiring a metaphorical interpretation), mental control (patients cannot reverse a learned sequence but can recite a stereotyped sequence), and response inhibition (patients cannot inhibit a conventional response and provide a novel answer but can provide a traditional response). Patients with the *orbitofrontal syndrome* also exhibit environmental dependency. They are tactless and disinhibited in their behavior, responding to the environment on impulse. They are able to learn instructions. They have limited personal direction of their behavior, but imitate the actions of others (imitation behavior) or are drawn to use objects in the environment (utilization behavior).[40] Similarly, the *medial frontal syndrome* has features of environmental dependency. Patients with this lesion are apathetic but can respond to instruction. They may manifest catatonia with reduced spontaneous behavior but maintain induced postures. Left medial frontal lesions produce transcortical motor aphasia, a syndrome characterized by reduced spontaneous output but retained ability to repeat what is heard in the environment.

Environmental dependency may reflect disruption of aspects of working memory, a fundamental function of prefrontal cortex.[41] Working memory is the type of memory active and relevant only for short periods of time (usually seconds). The central executive aspect of working memory confers the ability to guide behavior through representations of the world rather than by immediate stimulation and thus frees the individual from environmental dependency. The central executive is an attention supervisor that requires conscious control via the internal state of the individual. Failure or disturbance of the central executive component of working memory may contribute to enslavement to the environment.

Circuit-related Behaviors

In addition to behavioral syndromes that occur exclusively with lesions of the frontal-subcortical circuits, several behavioral disorders are produced by lesions of circuit structures and with lesions in other brain regions. Noncircuit lesions associated with these circuit-related behaviors are located in open-loop structures closely affiliated with the frontal-subcortical circuits.

Depression has been linked to two structures of the frontal-subcortical circuits, the frontal lobes and the caudate nucleus. Studies of idiopathic depression reveal decreased metabolism of the dorsolateral prefrontal cortex and the caudate nucleus;[23] studies of depression in Parkinson's disease, Huntington's disease, and complex partial seizures demonstrate reduced metabolic activity in the orbitofrontal cortex and caudate nucleus.[42-44] Focal lesions of the dorsolateral prefrontal cortex and caudate nucleus as well as degenerative processes affecting these areas are associated with depression.[25,45-48] Depression is also closely linked with lesions of the temporal lobes, however, and thus the disorder is not circuit-specific.[49-51] As noted above, the temporal cortex is closely linked with the frontal lobes and caudate nucleus and thus with the frontal-subcortical circuits.

Mania is also a circuit-related but not a circuit-bound behavior. Secondary mania occurs with lesions or degenerative disorders affecting the orbitofrontal cortex, caudate nucleus, and perithalamic areas.[48,52-55] These structures are all encompassed within the orbitofrontal-subcortical circuit. Lesions of the temporobasal regions including the amygdala and temporal stem, however, also produce mania, and these lesions are not obligatory members of the orbitofrontal-subcortical circuit.[55-57] The intimate association of the amygdala and the limbic-related circuits was noted above. Subcortical lesions affecting the caudate nucleus and thalamus tend to produce a bipolar type of mood disorder with alternating periods of mania and depression, whereas lesions of the cortex that produce mania are not typically followed by a cyclic mood disorder.[58] Nearly all focal lesions producing secondary mania have involved the right hemisphere.

Psychosis is also a circuit-related behavior. Caudate dysfunction in Huntington's disease and idiopathic basal ganglia calcification is associated with psychosis,[25,59] but most lesions producing delusional syndromes have involved the temporal lobe, particularly medial temporal-limbic structures.[60]

NEUROCHEMISTRY, PHARMACOLOGY, AND CIRCUIT-MEDIATED BEHAVIORS

The two principal fast-acting transmitters of the frontal-subcortical circuits are GABA and glutamate. GABA is the most ubiquitous inhibitory transmitter in the nervous system, and glutamate is the most abundant excitatory transmitter. Sedative-hypnotic agents, such as the benzodiazepines, ethanol, and the barbiturates, exert their actions on the central nervous system through their effects on GABA receptors. These agents augment the inhibitory properties of GABA.[61] All actions of the benzodiazepines including anxiolytic effects, anticonvulsant actions, and sedative-hypnotic activity are mediated through GABA$_A$ benzodiazepine receptors. GABA receptors are widely distributed in the brain, and it is uncertain which of these effects might be mediated through frontal-subcortical circuits.

Glutamate exerts its effects primarily via N-methyl-D-aspartate (NMDA) receptors, and drugs acting at these sites have profound behavioral consequences. Phencyclidine (PCP), a well-known psychotogen for example, is an NMDA channel blocker.[62] Receptors affected by PCP are preferentially distributed in the medial striatum and lateral thalamus, and the former participates in frontal-subcortical circuits. Thus, the psychotogenic action of PCP may be at least partially dependent on blockade of glutamate activity within frontal-subcortical circuitry.

Dopamine, serotonin, and acetylcholine have modulatory roles in the frontal-subcortical circuits. Nigrostriatal dopaminergic projections originate in the substantia nigra and project to the caudate nucleus and putamen. Connections from the ventral tegmental area (VTA) project to the amygdala, nucleus accumbens, septum, medial temporal regions, and medial frontal areas including the anterior cingulate cortex.[63] Thus, several structures of the medial frontal-subcortical circuit and the orbitofrontal-subcortical circuit receive dopaminergic innervation. Although the circuits are discrete throughout their subcortical course, they are modulated by dopaminergic input that applies to all the circuits. Dopaminergic therapy has a panoply of motoric and behavioral effects that can be understood as resulting from effects on multiple frontal-subcortical circuits. Dopamine receptor agonists (e.g., pergolide, bromocriptine) ameliorate the apathy exhibited by some patients with akinetic mutism.[64,65] Side effects from dopaminergic therapy in Parkinson's disease include psychosis, euphoria, mania, and anxiety as well as chorea and tics;[66] these behaviors reflect dysfunction of the frontal-subcortical circuits.

Serotonin also modulates the frontal-subcortical circuits. Ascending serotonin pathways originate in the median and dorsal raphe nuclei and project to hippocampus, striatum, amygdala, nucleus accumbens, substantia nigra, hypothalamus, and broad areas of the cortex.[67] Two principal types of serotonin receptors exist in the basal ganglia: 5-HT$_3$ receptors predominate in the ventral striatum (part of the medial prefrontal-subcortical circuit), and 5-HT$_1$ receptors are the most abundant receptors in other basal ganglionic regions.[68] Selective serotonin reuptake inhibitors are powerful antidepressants and may exert their effects through stimulation of circuit-related receptors.

Cholinergic input to the frontal-subcortical circuits originates from two sources: the pedunculopontine cholinergic projection to the thalamus and the nucleus basalis projection to the cortex and the amygdala.[63] Involvement of the pedunculopontine nucleus in progressive supranuclear palsy may contribute to the observed cognitive dysfunction and apathy, and involvement of the nucleus basalis in Alzheimer's disease contributes to the characteristic memory dysfunction, indifference, anxiety, and psychosis.[69]

SUMMARY

Frontal-subcortical circuits provide a comprehensive framework for understanding the anatomy, biochemistry, and pharmacology of behavior. The three principal behaviorally relevant circuits originate in the dorsolateral prefrontal cortex, orbitofrontal cortex, and anterior cingulate cortex, respectively. Circuit-specific marker behaviors associated with each circuit are executive dysfunction (dorsolateral prefrontal-subcortical circuit), disinhibition and OCD (orbitofrontal-subcortical circuit), and apathy (medial frontal-subcortical circuit). Environmental dependency is common to all prefrontal-subcortical syndromes and may reflect disruption of working memory. Depression, mania, and psychosis are mediated by structures involved in prefrontal-subcortical circuits and are circuit-related but not circuit-specific behaviors. The actions of PCP, LSD, serotonergic antidepressants, anxiolytics, sedative-hypnotics, antipsychotic agents, and ethanol may all be partially or primarily mediated through transmitter systems and receptor effects expressed through frontal-subcortical circuits.

REFERENCES

1. ALEXANDER, G. E., M. R. DeLONG & P. L. STRICK. 1986. Parallel organization of functionally segregated circuits linking basal ganglia and cortex. Ann. Rev. Neurosci. 9: 357–381.
2. ALEXANDER, G. E., M. D. CRUTCHER & M. R. DeLONG. 1990. Basal ganglia-thalamocortical circuits: Parallel substrates for motor, oculomotor, "prefrontal" and "limbic" functions. In Progress in Brain Research. Vol. 85. H. B. M. Uylings, C. G. Van Eden, J. P. C. De Bruin, M. A. Corner & M. G. P. Feenstra, Eds.: 119–146. Elsevier Science Publishers. New York.
3. GROENEWEGEN, H. J., H. W. BERENDSE, J. G. WOLTERS & A. H. M. LOHMAN. 1990.

The anatomical relationship of the prefrontal cortex with the striatopallidal system, the thalamus, and the amygdala: Evidence for a parallel organization. *In* Progress in Brain Research. Vol. 85. H. B. M. Uylings, C. G. Van Eden, J. P. C. De Bruin, M. A. Corner & M. G. P. Feenstra, Eds.: 95–118. Elsevier Science Publishers. New York.

4. GOLDMAN-RAKIC, R. S. & L. J. PORRINO. 1985. The primate mediodorsal (MD) nucleus and its projection to the frontal lobe. J. Comp. Neurol. **242:** 535–560.

5. ILINSKY, I. A., M. L. JOUANDET & P. S. GOLDMAN-RAKIC. 1985. Organization of the nigrothalamocortical system in the rhesus monkey. J. Comp. Neurol. **236:** 315–330.

6. VOGT, B. A., D. N. PANDYA & D. L. ROSENE. 1987. Cingulate gyrus of the rhesus monkey: I. Cytoarchitecture and thalamic afferents. J. Comp. Neurol. **262:** 256–270.

7. YETERIAN, E. H. & D. N. PANDYA. 1991. Prefrontal striatal connections in relation to cortical architectonic organization in rhesus monkeys. J. Comp. Neurol. **312:** 43–67.

8. NIEUWENHUYS, R., J. VOOGD & C. VAN HUIJZEN. 1988. The Human Central Nervous System, 3rd rev. edit. Springer-Verlag. New York.

9. ALEXANDER, G. E. & M. D. CRUTCHER. 1990. Functional architecture of basal ganglia circuits: Neural substrates of parallel processing. Trends Neurosci. **13:** 266–271.

10. YETERIAN, E. H. & D. N. PANDYA. 1993. Striatal connections of the parietal association cortices in rhesus monkeys. J. Comp. Neurol. **332:** 175–197.

11. SELEMON, L. D. & P. S. GOLDMAN-RAKIC. 1985. Longitudinal topography and interdigitation of corticostriatal projections in the rhesus monkey. J. Neurosci. **5:** 776–794.

12. AFSHARPOUR, S. 1985. Topographical projections of the cerebral cortex to the subthalamic nucleus. J. Comp. Neurol. **236:** 14–28.

13. HEDREEN, J. C. & M. R. DeLONG. 1991. Organization of striatopallidal, striatonigral, and nigrostriatal projections in the macaque. J. Comp. Neurol. **304:** 569–595.

14. RUSSCHEN, F. T., I. BAKST, D. G. AMARAL & J. L. PRICE. 1985. The amygdalostriatal projections in the monkey. An anterograde tracing study. Brain Res. **329:** 241–257.

15. PARENT, A., A. MACKEY & L. DE BELLEFEUILLE. 1983. The subcortical afferents to caudate nucleus and putamen in primate: A fluorescence retrograde double labeling study. Neuroscience **10:** 1137–1150.

16. GROENEWEGEN, H. J., N. E. H. M. BECKER & A. H. M. LOHMAN. 1980. Subcortical afferents of the nucleus accumbens septi in the cat, studied with retrograde axonal transport of horseradish peroxidase and bisdenzimid. Neuroscience **5:** 1903–1916.

17. GROENEWEGEN, H. J., H. W. BERENDSE & S. N. HABER. 1993. Organization of the output of the ventral striatopallidal system in the rat: Ventral pallidal efferents. Neuroscience **57:** 113–142.

18. HABER, S. N., H. J. GROENEWEGEN, E. A. GROVE & W. J. H. NAUTA. 1985. Efferent connections of the ventral pallidum: Evidence of a dual striatopallidofugal pathway. J. Comp. Neurol. **235:** 322–335.

19. HABER, S. N., E. LYND-BALTA & S. J. MICHELL. 1993. The organization of the descending ventral pallidal projections in the monkey. J. Comp. Neurol. **329:** 111–128.

20. RAGSDALE, C. W., JR. & A. M. GRAYBIEL. 1991. Compartmental organization of the thalamostriatal connection of the cat. J. Comp. Neurol. **311:** 134–167.

21. GRABIEL, A. M. 1990. Neurotransmitters and neuromodulators in the basal ganglia. Trends Neurosci. **13:** 244–254.

22. CUMMINGS, J. L. 1993. Frontal-subcortical circuits and human behavior. Arch. Neurol. **50:** 873–880.

23. BAXTER, L. R., J. M. SCHWARTZ, M. E. PHELPS, J. C. MAZZIOTTA, B. H. GUZE, C. E. SELIN, R. H. GERNER & R. M. SUMIDA. 1989. Reduction of prefrontal cortex glucose metabolism common to three types of depression. Arch. Gen. Psychiatry **46:** 243–250.

24. HOLCOMB, H. H., J. LINKS, C. SMITH & D. WONG. 1989. Positron emission tomography: Measuring the metabolic and neurochemical characteristics of the living human nervous system. *In* Brain Imaging: Applications in Psychiatry. N. C. Andreasen, Ed.: 235–370. American Psychiatric Association. Washington, D.C.

25. FOLSTEIN, S. E. 1989. Huntington's Disease. A Disorder of Families. Johns Hopkins University Press. Baltimore, MD.

26. DELECLUSE, F., J., DELEVAL, J-M. GERARD, A. MICHOTTE & D. Z. DE BEYL. 1991. Frontal impairment and hypoperfusion in neuroacanthocytosis. Arch. Neurol. **48:** 232–234.
27. MENDEZ, M. F., N. L. ADAMS & K. S. LEWANKOWSKI. 1989. Neurobehavioral changes associated with caudate lesions. Neurology **39:** 349–354.
28. STRUB, R. L. 1989. Frontal lobe syndrome in a patient with bilateral globus pallidus lesions. Arch. Neurol. **46:** 1024–1027.
29. STUSS, D. T., A. GUBERMAN, R. NELSON & S. LAROCHELLE. 1988. The neuropsychology of paramedian thalamic infarction. Brain & Cognition **8:** 348–378.
30. GRATTAN, L. M., R. H. BLOOMER, F. X. ARCHAMBAULT & P. J. ESLINGER. 1994. Cognitive flexibility and empathy after frontal lobe lesion. Neuropsychiatr. Neuropsychol. Behav. Neurol. **7:** 251–259.
31. WYSZYNSKI B, A. MERRIAM, A. MEDALIA & C. LAWRENCE. 1989. Choreoacanthocytosis. Report of a case with psychiatric features. Neuropsychiatr. Neuropsychol. Behav. Neurol. **2:** 137–144.
32. DREWE, E. A. 1975. Go–no go learning after frontal lobe lesions in humans. Cortex **11:** 8–16.
33. BOGOUSSLAVSKY, J. & F. REGLI. 1990. Anterior cerebral artery infarction in the Lausanne Stroke Registry. Arch. Neurol. **47:** 144–150.
34. GENTILINI, M., E. DE RENZI & G. CRISI. 1987. Bilateral paramedian thalamic artery infarcts: Report of eight cases. J. Neurol. Neurosurg. Psychiatry **50:** 900–909.
35. PHILLIPS, S., V. SANGALANG & G. STERN. 1987. Basal forebrain infarction: A clinicopathologic correlation. Arch. Neurol. **44:** 1134–1138.
36. LAPLANE, D., M. BAULAC, D. WIDLOCHER & B. DUBOIS. 1984. Pure akinesia with bilateral lesions of basal ganglia. J. Neurol. Neurosurg. Psychiatry **47:** 377–385.
37. BAXTER, L. R., M. E. PHELPS, J. C. MAZZIOTTA, B. H. GUZE, J. M. SCHWARTZ & C. E. SELIN. 1987. Local cerebral glucose metabolic rates in obsessive-compulsive disorder. Arch. Gen. Psychiatry **44:** 211–218.
38. CUMMINGS, J. L. & K. CUNNINGHAM. 1992. Obsessive-compulsive disorder in Huntington's disease. Biol. Psychiatry **31:** 263–270.
39. SWEDO, S. E., J. L. RAPOPORT, D. L. CHESLOW, H. L. LEONARD, E. M. AYOUB, D. M. HOSIER & E. R. WALD. 1989. High prevalence of obsessive-compulsive symptoms in patients with Sydenham's chorea. Am. J. Psychiatry **146:** 246–249.
40. LHERMITTE, F., B. PILLON & M. SERDARU. 1986. Human autonomy and the frontal lobes. Part I. Imitation and utilization behavior: A neuropsychological study of 75 patients. Ann. Neurol. **19:** 326–334.
41. BROMFIELD, E. B., L. ALTSHULER, D. B. LEIDERMAN, M. BALISH, T. A. KETTER, O. DEVINSKY, R. M. POST & W. H. THEODORE. 1992. Cerebral metabolism and depression in patients with complex partial seizures. Arch. Neurol. **49:** 617–623.
42. GOLDMAN-RAKIC, P. S. 1994. Working memory dysfunction in schizophrenia. J. Neuropsychiatry Clin. Neurosci. **6:** 348–357.
43. MAYBERG, H. S., S. E. STARKSTEIN, C. E. PEYSER, J. BRANDT, R. F. DANNALS & S. E. FOLSTEIN. 1992. Paralimbic frontal lobe hypometabolism in depression associated with Huntington's disease. Neurology **42:** 1791–1797.
44. MAYBERG, H. S., S. E. STARKSTEIN, B. SADZOT, T. PREZIOSI, P. I. ANDREZEJEWSKI, R. F. DANNALS, H. N. WAGNER, JR. & R. G. ROBINSON. 1990. Selective hypometabolism in inferior frontal lobe in depressed patients with Parkinson's disease. Ann. Neurol. **28:** 57–64.
45. CUMMINGS, J. L. 1992. Depression and Parkinson's disease: A review. Am. J. Psychiatry **149:** 443–454.
46. JORGE, R. E., R. G. ROBINSON, S. V. ARNDT, A. W. FORRESTER, F. GEISLER & S. E. STARKSTEIN. 1993. Comparison between acute- and delayed onset depression following traumatic brain injury. J. Neuropsychiatry Clin. Neurosci. **5:** 43–49.
47. STARKSTEIN, S. E., R. G. ROBINSON & T. R. PRICE. 1987. Comparison of cortical and subcortical lesions in the production of poststroke mood disorders. Brain **110:** 1045–1059.

48. TRAUTNER, R. J., J. L. CUMMINGS, S. L. READ & D. F. BENSON. 1988. Idiopathic basal ganglia calcification and organic mood disorder. Am. J. Psychiatry 145: 350–353.
49. CUMMINGS, J. L. 1993. The neuroanatomy of depression. J. Clin. Psychiatry 54 (Suppl.) 14–20.
50. IRLE, E., M. PEPER, B. WOWRA & S. KUNZE. 1994. Mood changes after surgery for tumors of the cerebral cortex. Arch. Neurol. 51: 164–174.
51. MAYBERG, H. S. 1994. Frontal lobe dysfunction in secondary depression. J. Neuropsychiatry Clin. Neurosci. 6: 428–442.
52. BOGOUSSLAVSKY, J., M. FERRAZZINI, F. REGLI, G. ASSAL, H. TANABE & A. DELALOYE-BISCHOF. 1988. Manic delirium and frontal-like syndrome with paramedian infarction of the right thalamus. J. Neurol. Neurosurg. Psychiatry 51: 116–119.
53. CUMMINGS, J. L. & M. F. MENDEZ. 1984. Secondary mania with focal cerebrovascular lesions. Am. J. Psychiatry 141: 1084–1087.
54. KULISEVSKY, J., M. L. BERTHIER & J. PUJOL. 1993. Hemiballismus and secondary mania following right thalamic infarction. Neurology 43: 1422–1424.
55. STARKSTEIN, S. E., G. D. PEARLSON, J. BOSTON & R. G. ROBINSON. 1987. Mania after brain injury. Arch. Neurol. 44: 1069–1073.
56. BERTHIER, M. L., S. E. STARKSTEIN, R. G. ROBINSON & R. LEIGUARDA. 1990. Limbic lesions in a patient with recurrent mania. J. Neuropsychiatry Clin. Neurosci. 2: 235–236.
57. LYKETSOS, C., A. M. STOLINE, P. LONGSTREET, N. G. RANEN, R. LESSER, R. FISHER & M. FOLSTEIN. 1993. Mania in temporal lobe epilepsy. Neuropsychiatr. Neuropsychol. Behav. Neurol. 6: 19–25.
58. STARKSTEIN, S. E., P. FEDEROFF, M. L. BERTHIER & R. G. ROBINSON. 1991. Manic-depressive and pure manic states after brain lesions. Biol. Psychiatry 29: 149–158.
59. CUMMINGS, J. L., L. F. GOSENFELD, J. P. HOULIHAN & T. McCAFFREY. 1983. Neuropsychiatric disturbances associated with idiopathic calcification of the basal ganglia. Biol. Psychiatry 18: 591–601.
60. GORMAN, D. G. & J. L. CUMMINGS. 1990. Organic delusional syndrome. Semin. Neurol. 10: 229–238.
61. PAUL, S. M. 1995. GABA and glycine. In Psychopharmacology: The Fourth Generation of Progress. F. E. Bloom & D. J. Kupfer, Eds.: 87–94. Raven Press. New York.
62. COTMAN, C. W., J. S. KAHLE, S. E. MILLER, J. ULAS & R. J. BRIDGES. 1995. Excitatory amino acid transmission. In Psychopharmacology: The Fourth Generation of Progress. F. E. Bloom & D. J. Kupfer, Eds.: 75–85. Raven Press. New York.
63. NIEUWENHUYS, R. 1985. Chemoarchitecture of the brain. Springer-Verlag. New York.
64. STEWART, J. T., M. LEADON & L. J. GONZALEZ-ROTHI. 1990. Treatment of a case of akinetic mutism with bromocriptine. J. Neuropsychiatry Clin. Neurosci. 2: 462–463.
65. ROSS, E. D. & J. T. STEWART. 1981. Akinetic mutism from hypothalamic damage: Successful treatment with dopamine agonists. Neurology 31: 1435–1439.
66. CUMMINGS, J. L. 1991. Behavioral complications of drug treatment of Parkinson's disease. J. Am. Geriatr. Soc. 39: 708–716.
67. MARSDEN, C. A. 1991. The neuropharmacology of serotonin in the central nervous system. In Selective Serotonin Re-uptake Inhibitors. J. P. Feighner & W. F. Boyer, Eds.: 11–35. John Wiley & Sons. New York.
68. LAVOIE, B. & A. PARENT. 1990. Immunohistochemical study of the serotoninergic innervation of the basal ganglia of the squirrel monkey. J. Comp. Neurol. 299: 1–16.
69. CUMMINGS, J. L. & C. E. COFFEY. 1994. Neurobiological basis of behavior. In Textbook of Geriatric Neuropsychiatry. C. E. Coffey & J. L. Cummings, Eds.: 71–96. American Psychiatric Press. Washington, D.C.

Neuropsychological Aspects of Frontotemporal Degeneration

DAVID NEARY

Department of Neurology
Manchester Royal Infirmary
Oxford Road
Manchester M13 9WL, United Kingdom

A wide variety of behavioral and cognitive disorders are subsumed under the rubric of "frontal lobe syndrome," including impairments of attention, temporal integration (perceptuomotor cycles), motility, and affect. Conventionally such skills are attributed to the frontal lobes, and the seminal importance of the prefrontal cortex has been attested to by experimental studies in animals and in man following focal cerebral lesions. However, study of the neuropsychological syndromes arising from the degenerative process of frontotemporal lobar atrophy (LA) indicates that facets of behavior and cognition traditionally ascribed to the frontal cortex appear also to arise in relation to lesions of subcortical and temporal cortical structures. The LAs are highly familial, manifest chiefly in the presenium, and share a common albeit heterogeneous histology. The distribution of the latter determines the emergence of the particular syndrome.[1] Asymmetrical involvement of the left dominant frontotemporal lobe leads to the syndrome of progressive nonfluent aphasia.[2,3] Selective involvement of the temporal lobes is associated with semantic dementia.[4,5] Predominant involvement of the frontal and temporal lobes leads to the syndrome of frontotemporal dementia (FTD), the subject of this review.

FRONTOTEMPORAL DEMENTIA

Clinical Syndrome

The clinical syndrome of FTD has been described initially by Gustafson[6] and Neary *et al.*;[7] since then further reports have appeared.[8–10] Onset is most common between 45 and 65 years. A family history of a similar disorder in a first-degree relative occurs in approximately one-half of the cases. The mean duration of illness is about 8 years, although there is wide variation, and survival of 10 to 15 years is not uncommon.

The presentation is of profound alteration in social conduct and personality, and this feature predominates throughout the course of the illness. The form of the character change is not uniform. Patients may become disinhibited, overactive and restless, with a fatuous, unconcerned affect. They may clown, pun, sing and dance, usually conforming to a restricted, stereotyped repertoire. Alternatively, patients may become apathetic and inert, lacking in drive and initiative and show-

15

ing little response to stimuli. The "disinhibited" and "inert" forms represent opposite poles of a spectrum of behavioral disorder. In the inert form there is markedly reduced orientation or engagement of attention and maintenance of attention over time. By contrast, the disinhibited patients display impairments of selective attention and are highly distractible. Patients who present with extreme overactivity and disinhibition may become increasingly apathetic and inert with disease progression. Slowing of motility in the apathetic subtype is not generalized: initiation of response is often markedly slow, but an eventual response may be carried out rapidly. In the disinhibited patients rapidity of response and distractibility are characteristic. Altered preference for sweet foods, development of food fads, and oral exploration of nonedible objects may occur. Stereotypic features, such as repeated wandering following an identical route, are common in FTD. In a minority of patients, however, the stereotypic, ritualistic nature of the patient's behavior is the dominant presenting feature. Such patients may develop elaborate rituals for dressing or toileting, will adhere to a rigid daily routine, and may be unwilling, for example, to walk on cracks in the pavement. Repetitive behaviors range from simple motor perservations to highly complex and ritualistic behaviors, which appear to run as ungoverned perceptuomotor cycles. Affect is markedly blunted in the apathetic inert form, whereas fatuousness and jocularity characterize the disinhibited form. The presence or absence of a family history does not determine the dominant behavioral pattern: familial cases occur in the disinhibited, inert, and stereotypic forms of the disorder.

In FTD there is typically marked economy of speech output, conforming to a "dynamic aphasia."[11,12] Occasionally, disinhibited patients may show a press of speech, but content is repetitive and stereotyped. Echolalia and perseveration commonly occur, until mutism supervenes. Deficits in structural aspects of language—phonology, syntax, and semantics—are not typically apparent, although a minority of patients exhibit evidence of loss of word meaning as the disease progresses. Spatial and motor skills remain strikingly well preserved throughout the illness. Memory failures are variable and appear secondary to the patients' unconcern and failure of mental effort ("frontal lobe amnesia"). Formal neuropsychological assessment reveals the most profound abnormalities on tasks sensitive to frontal lobe dysfunction which make demands on abstraction, planning, and self-regulation of behavior. Performance may, however, be impaired across a wide spectrum of tests, reflecting patients' cursory mode of responding and unconcern.

Initially there are few neurological signs, limited to the presence of primitive reflexes, but with progression, striatal signs of akinesia and rigidity emerge. In those patients in whom stereotyped, ritualistic behavior dominates, the clinical presentation of akinesia and rigidity occurs relatively early in the course of the illness. The electroencephalogram (EEG) remains substantially normal in all patients. Functional brain imaging, using 133-Xenon inhalation[13,14] and SPECT,[7,9,15] reveals abnormalities in the anterior cerebral hemispheres.

Anatomical Correlates and Histology

The gross pathological and histological changes have been described by Brun,[16,17] Mann and South,[18] and Mann et al.[19] Cases of FTD are characterized by frontotemporal cortical atrophy. In overactive, disinhibited patients the orbito-medial frontal lobe is particularly affected with relative sparing of the dorsolateral frontal convexity. In addition, there is marked temporal cortical atrophy. Inert, apathetic patients, in contrast, have severe atrophy extending into the dorsolateral frontal cortex and also into subcortical structures (striatum, thalamus, hippocampi, amygdala).

In a minority of patients the brunt of the pathology is borne by the striatum with usually severe temporal involvement, but variable frontal cortical and nigral involvement. This subgroup with predominant striatotemporal pathology conforms to those patients in whom striatal neurological signs developed early, and stereotypic behavior was dominant in the disease course. The pathological distinction between predominant cortical and striatal pathology is in keeping with findings reported by Knopman et al.[20,21]

Two characteristic histologies underlie frontotemporal cortical atrophy. The most common histological change is loss of large cortical nerve cells (chiefly from layers III and V) and a spongiform degeneration or microvacuolation of the superficial neuropil (layer II); gliosis is minimal and restricted to subpial regions; layers II and V show no gliosis. No distinctive changes (swellings or inclusions) within remaining nerve cells are seen. The limbic system and the striatum are affected, but to a much lesser extent.

The second and less common histological process is characterized by a loss of large cortical nerve cells with widespread and abundant gliosis, but minimal or no spongiform change or microvacuolation. Swollen neurons or inclusions that are both tau and ubiquitin positive are present in some cases, and the limbic system and striatum are more seriously damaged. The two differing histologies nevertheless share a similar distribution within the frontal and temporal cortex, and cannot be distinguished on the basis of the behavioral disorder or the familial incidence.

Cases with predominant striatotemporal pathology appear to share features of both histological types.

FRONTOTEMPORAL DEMENTIA AND MOTOR NEURON DISEASE

Clinical Syndrome

An association between dementia and motor neuron disease (MND) has been well recognized,[22,23] although until recently there has been a lack of systematic study of the form of dementia. Neary et al.,[24] in a prospective study of five patients, reported a circumscribed frontal lobe syndrome indistinguishable from FTD. It would seem likely that other cases of amyotrophic lateral sclerosis (ALS) dementia have a similar psychological disorder. In reviewing the extensive Japanese literature, Morita et al.[25] noted that the dementia was of the "anterior" type. It is noteworthy, too, that in the clinical and pathological series of patients with FTD reported by Gustafson[6,26] and Brun,[16,17] a small proportion showed evidence of MND.

Typically, personality changes emerge first, often of the overactive, disinhibited type, although increased apathy occurs with disease progression. After some months patients develop the amyotrophic form of MND with widespread fasciculations, muscular weakness, wasting, and bulbar palsy. The latter is responsible for death which takes place within three years of onset. Extrapyramidal signs of akinesia and rigidity, reported by some authors,[23,25] emerge in patients with longer duration. Neuropsychological investigations demonstrate widespread muscular denervation, the EEG remains normal, and SPECT imaging reveals reduced tracer in the anterior hemispheres.

Anatomical and Histological Changes

Cerebral atrophy is less marked in FTD with MND than in FTD without MND—presumably reflecting the short duration of illness—and is mostly frontal involving chiefly the orbitomedial regions and also temporal lobes. There is striatal atrophy but relative sparing of thalamus, hippocampi, and amygdala, suggesting that these structures are not the primary sites of pathology in FTD. The histology in the majority of cases is characterized by loss of large cortical nerve cells, microvacuolation, and mild gliosis. Limbic involvement is slight, although nigral damage is severe with heavy loss of pigmented nerve cells and intense reactive fibrous astrocytosis. Ubiquitinated but not tau-immunoreactive inclusions are present within the frontal cortex and hippocampus (dentate gyrus). In the brain stem, the hypoglossus nucleus shows atrophy with loss of neurons. Large Betz cells of the precentral gyrus are largely preserved in number, and there is no obvious demyelination within the corticospinal tracts. Within the anterior horn cells gross loss of neurons is found at all levels, and many of the surviving anterior horn cells contain pale large ubiquitinated inclusions within the cytoplasm. No Lewy or Pick-type inclusions are observed in any cortical or subcortical neurons.

The spongiform or microvacuolar changes are highly characteristic of this syndrome, and Knopman et al.[20] refer to "dementia lacking distinctive histological features (DLDH)" to describe this nonspecific large neuronal cell loss and the spongiform appearances. Three of 14 of their patients with DLDH pathology also had MND. A familial incidence was present: in half the cases there was a family history of dementia and in one case a family history of MND.

The importance of genetic factors is also highlighted in this syndrome by Constantinidis,[27] who reported four members of two generations who developed characteristic FTD and later MND. In two autopsied cases predominant frontotemporal atrophy was found. However, the histological findings were not of microvacuolation, but of gliosis, neuronal cell loss, and ballooned neurons, in the absence of inclusion bodies. Brion et al.[28] also noted sporadic cases of FTD/MND with gliotic rather than spongiform histology in a small number of cases.

NOSOLOGY OF FRONTOTEMPORAL CEREBRAL ATROPHY

The clinical, anatomical, and histological relationships of frontotemporal cerebral atrophy have been discussed by Neary et al.[1] The clinical syndromes appear to reflect the topographical distribution of the pathology rather than the specific histological change. When the frontal and temporal lobes are bilaterally, symmetrically, and predominantly affected, the syndrome of FTD emerges, with breakdown in problem solving and regulation of conduct.

The underlying type of histology falls into three classes: microvacuolation, gliosis with or without neuronal inclusion bodies, and motor neuron disease. Confusion in the literature has occurred because of the lack of an accepted definition of the pathological criteria for Pick's disease.

In addition to confusion concerning the nosological status of Pick's disease, there have been a number of other terminological sources of misunderstanding. Brun[16] used the term frontal lobe degeneration (FLD) to refer to the spongiform histology which formed the majority of his cases. The acronym FLD then became a synonym for "frontal lobe dementia," the clinical syndrome. Neary et al.[7] used the term "dementia of frontal lobe type (DFT)" to describe the clinical syndrome without specific histological connotation. Knopman et al.[20] coined the term "dementia lacking distinctive histological features (DLDH)" to refer to dementia associated with the underlying spongiform appearances. In order to avoid terminological confusion and sterile debates about what does and does not constitute Pick's disease, it is necessary to make descriptive distinctions between clinical syndromes, anatomical distributions of atrophy, and histological changes. Accordingly, workers in Sweden and the United Kingdom have shared their clinical and pathological material and have decided on consensus criteria[29] for the clinical syndrome, designated frontotemporal dementia (FTD), and the three major histological changes. The microvacuolar or spongiform appearances have been designated frontal lobe degeneration (FLD) type. Gliosis with or without inclusion bodies and swollen neurons has been designated Pick-type histology. The amyotrophic history has been referred to as motor neuron disease (MND) type.

Currently it cannot be known whether the histologies are etiologically distinct or represent a range of pathological phenotypes. It seems likely that the issue will be decided by genetic and molecular biological studies. It would seem reasonable, therefore, on a provisional basis, to accept these descriptive pathological categories so that future clinicopathological studies can provide clear and commonly agreed clinical and pathological phenotypes, for genetic characterization.

NEUROPSYCHOLOGICAL SPECULATIONS

Lobar atrophy represents a series of natural experiments on the frontotemporal lobes and their subcortical and cortical connections and the functions of attention, the temporal organization of perceptuomotor cycle, motility, and affect.

Frontotemporal dementia is an appropriate designation because it draws attention to the contribution of the temporal lobes to this behavioral syndrome. Indeed, in the disinhibited subgroup of FTD, the temporal lobes are severely atrophied along with the orbitomedial zones of the frontal lobes. The dorsolateral convexities of the frontal lobe, conventionally attributed similar importance in the so-called frontal lobe syndrome, are severely atrophied in the apathetic subtype of FTD, but not selectively so. Indeed, widespread pathology in the dorsolateral convexities is associated with severe involvement of all frontotemporal cortex and underlying subcortical structures in keeping with the most advanced stages of the disease. That this is indeed end-stage disease is attested to by the relative sparing of the dorsolateral convexity and subcortical structures such as thalamus, amygdala, and hippocampus, in the relatively shorter duration of illness in FTD/MND. Preservation of hippocampal structures would explain the "frontal" form of amnesia in the patients who are presumably unable to engage a potentially intact limbic system. Moreover, preservation of the parietal cortex would account for the preservation of visuospatial skills. Presumably the characteristic "dynamic aphasia" reflects an intact perisylvian language area ungoverned by the frontotemporal lobes.

The basal ganglia are always involved in the disease process, but the degree of atrophy appears relatively secondary in intensity to neocortical loss. Nevertheless, when striatal atrophy is dominant and combined with temporal lobe atrophy, the stereotypic syndrome of FTD emerges in the presence of relative preservation of the frontal lobes. A link between repetitive behaviors and basal ganglia pathology has been noted.[30] Because obsessive compulsive behavior is known to be associated with orbitofrontal "hyperfrontality" on functional imaging studies[31] and because surgical section of the orbital frontal lobe redresses compulsivity, it may be that striatotemporal atrophy in LA causes release from inhibition of the orbitomedial cortex leading to the emergence of ungoverned perceptuomotor cycles. Nevertheless, the repetitive behaviors in LA range widely from simple motor acts to complex rituals, and therefore their structural and functional basis is likely to be heterogeneous.

It is likely that the secondary and later involvement of subcortical structures that initially are primarily spared in LA increases the degree of functional failure of neocortical structures because of functional deafferentation. It may be speculated that thalamic atrophy may be particularly important in such physiological deactivation, for example, in contributing to the apathetic, inert subtype of FTD in which reduced orientation of attention occurs despite relative structural sparing the parietal lobes. The affective blunting of patients with the apathetic form of FTD may relate to secondary atrophy of the amygdala, which is preserved in the disinhibited form of FTD and in FTD/MND.

The pathological findings at autopsy are frequently regarded as the touchstone of anatomical reality. However, unless neurodegenerative diseases are suspended by unrelated fatality, the inevitable secondary and nonspecific spread of primary pathology leads to a grosser and less specific distribution of lesions. Moreover, autopsy usually succeeds rapidly on the least differentiated and final stage of neuropsychological disorder. Thus, whereas broad associations can be drawn between clinical syndrome and pathological topography, more precise structural-functional relation can escape analysis. It will be apparent that some structures appear to contribute to more than one syndrome. For example, the temporal neocortex is significantly implicated in the disinhibited subgroup of FTD (orbitomedial frontotemporal atrophy) as well as the stereotypic form (striatotemporal atrophy).

In considering the implication of the temporal lobe in the differing behavioral syndromes, it might be speculated that different functional systems of the temporal lobe may be preferentially disrupted. An alternative theoretical possibility is that it is the pattern of atrophy of particular subcortical and cortical structures that is critical to the emergence of behavioral symptoms. For example, striatotemporal (stereotypic FTD type) as opposed to orbital-frontotemporal atrophy (disinhibited FTD subtype) leads to differential neuropsychological impairments. It may be that the functional relations between structures are pertinent and that the attribution of function/dysfunction to specific particular cortical and subcortical structures such as the prefrontal cortex, alone, may be an unjustified neophrenological exercise.

REFERENCES

1. NEARY, D., J. S. SNOWDEN & D. M. A. MANN. 1993. The clinical pathological correlates of lobar atrophy. A review. Dementia 4: 154–159.
2. MESULAM, M-M. 1982. Slowly progressive aphasia without generalized dementia. Ann. Neurol. 11: 592–598.
3. SNOWDEN, J. S., D. NEARY, D. M. A. MANN, et al. 1992. Progressive language disorder due to lobar atrophy. Ann. Neurol. 31: 174–183.
4. SNOWDEN, J. S., P. J. GOULDING & D. NEARY. 1989. Semantic dementia; a form of circumscribed cerebral atrophy. Behav. Neurol. 2: 167–182.
5. HODGES, J. R., K. PATTERSON, S. OXBURY, et al. 1992. Semantic dementia: Progressive fluent aphasia with temporal lobe atrophy. Brain 115: 1783–1806.
6. GUSTAFSON, L. 1987. Frontal lobe degeneration of non-Alzheimer type. II. Clinical picture and differential diagnosis. Arch. Gerontol. Geriatr. 6: 209–223.
7. NEARY, D., J. S. SNOWDEN, B. NORTHEN & P. J. GOULDING. 1988. Dementia of frontal lobe type. J. Neurol. Neurosurg. Psychiatry 51: 353–361.
8. JAGUST, W. J., B. R. REED, J. P. SEAB, et al. 1989. Clinical-physiologic correlates of Alzheimer's disease and frontal lobe dementia. Am. J. Physiol. Imaging 4: 89–96.
9. MILLER, B. L., J. L. CUMMINGS, J. VILLANUEVA-MEYER, et al. 1991. Frontal lobe degeneration: Clinical, neuropsychological and SPECT characteristics. 41: 1374–1382.
10. ORRELL, M. W. & B. SAHAKIAN. 1991. Dementia of frontal lobe type. Psychol. Med. 21: 553–556.
11. LURIA, A. R. & L. TSETSKOVA. 1978. The mechanism of dynamic aphasia. Found. Lang. 4: 296–307.
12. COSTELLO, A DE L. & E. F. WARRINGTON. 1989. Dynamic aphasia: The selective impairment of verbal planning. Cortex 25: 103–114.
13. RISBERG, J. 1987. Frontal lobe degeneration of non-Alzheimer type. III. Regional cerebral blood flow. Arch. Gerontol. Geriatr. 6: 225–233.
14. RISBERG, J. 1993. Regional cerebral blood flow in frontal lobe dementia of non-Alzheimer type. Dementia 4: 186–187.
15. NEARY, D., J. S. SNOWDEN, R. A. SHIELDS, et al. 1987. Single photon emission tomography using 99mTc-HM-PAO in the investigation of dementia. J. Neurol. Neurosurg. Psychiatry 50: 1101–1109.
16. BRUN, A. 1987. Frontal lobe degeneration of non-Alzheimer type. I. Neuropathology. Arch. Gerontol. Geriatr. 6: 193–208.
17. BRUN, A. 1993. Frontal lobe degeneration of non-Alzheimer type revisited. Dementia 4: 126–131.
18. MANN, D. M. A. & P. W. SOUTH. 1993. The topographical distribution of brain atrophy in frontal lobe dementia. Acta Neuropathol. 85: 334–340.
19. MANN, D. M. A., P. W. SOUTH, J. S. SNOWDEN & D. NEARY. 1993. Dementia of frontal lobe type; neuropathology and immunohistochemistry. J. Neurol. Neurosurg. Psychiatry 56: 605–614.
20. KNOPMAN, D. S., A. R. MASTRI, W. H. FREY, et al. 1990. Dementia lacking distinctive

histologic features: A common non-Alzheimer degenerative dementia. Neurology **40:** 251–256.

21. KNOPMAN, D. S. 1993. Overview of dementia lacking distinctive histology: Pathological designation of a progressive dementia. Dementia **4:** 132–136.

22. HUDSON, A. J. 1981. Amyotrophic lateral sclerosis and its association with dementia, parkinsonism and other neurological disorders: A review. Brain **104:** 217–247.

23. SALAZAR, A. M., C. L. MASTERS, D. C. GAJDUSEK & C. J. GIBBS. 1983. Syndromes of amyotrophic lateral sclerosis and dementia: A relation to transmissible Creutzfeldt-Jakob disease. Ann. Neurol. **14:** 17–26.

24. NEARY, D., J. S. SNOWDEN, D. M. A. MANN, et al. 1990. Frontal lobe dementia and motor neuron disease. J. Neurol. Neurosurg. Psychiatry **53:** 23–82.

25. MORITA, K., H. KAIYA, T. IKEDA, et al. 1987. Presenile dementia combined with amyotrophy: A review of 34 Japanese cases. Arch. Gerontol. Geriatr. **6:** 263–277.

26. GUSTAFSON, L. 1993. Clinical picture of frontal lobe degeneration of non-Alzheimer type. Dementia **4:** 143–148.

27. CONSTANTINIDIS, J. 1987. Syndrome familial: Association de maladie Pick et sclérose latérale amyotrophique. Encephale **13:** 285–293.

28. BRION, S., A. PSIMARAS, J. F. CHEVALIER, et al. 1980. L'association maladie de Pick et sclérose latérale amyotrophique. Etude d'un cas anatomo-clinique et revue de la littérature. Encephale **6:** 250–286.

29. BRUN, A., D. M. A. MANN, B. ENGLUND, et al. 1994. Clinical and neuropathological criteria for fronto-temporal dementia. J. Neurol. Neurosurg. Psychiatry **4:** 416–418.

30. AMES, D., J. L. CUMMINGS, W. C. WIRSHING, B. QUINN & M. MAHLER. 1994. Repetitive and compulsive behaviour in frontal lobe degenerations. J. Neuropsych. Clin. Neurosci. **6:** 100–113.

31. BAXTER, L. R., M. E. PHELPS, J. C. MAZZIOTTA, B. H. GUZE, J. M. SCHWARTZ & C. E. SELIN. 1987. Local cerebral glucose metabolic rates in obsessive-compulsive disorder. Arch. Gen. Psychiatry **44:** 211–218.

Cognitive Functioning in "Diffuse" Pathology

Role of Prefrontal and Limbic Structures

FRANÇOIS BOLLER,[a] LATCHEZAR TRAYKOV,[a-c]
MARIE-HÉLÈNE DAO-CASTELLANA,[b]
ANNE FONTAINE-DABERNARD,[b] MONICA ZILBOVICIUS,[b]
GERALD RANCUREL,[d] SABINA PAPPATÀ,[c]
AND YVES SAMSON[b,d]

[a]Unité 324
Institut National de la Santé et de la Recherche Médicale
(INSERM)
2ter rue d'Alésia
75014 Paris, France

[b]Commissariat à l'Energie Atomique
Service Hospitalier Frédéric-Joliot
Orsay, France

[c]INSERM U334
Orsay, France

[d]Hôpital de la Salpêtrière
Paris, France

The precise anatomical correlates of "executive functions" are still a matter of debate. The assessment of cognitive functions in patients with frontal lobe lesions has led to the term "frontal functions" and "frontal lobe syndrome" to characterize patients with disorders of executive functions. The very nature of executive functions implies a process of integration and the coordination of several cognitive processes. A fairly large number of tests are currently used to assess executive functions, but their specificity has not always been clearly established. These tests may at times be affected by lesions of nonfrontal areas or, paradoxically, may be spared by lesions that clearly affect the frontal lobes.[1] This does not necessarily imply that the tasks are not specific for the evaluation of executive functions, but rather that several nonfrontal structures, neural networks, and subordinate cognitive operations may participate in their performance.

The frontal lobes are not a homogeneous anatomical entity, but rather an agglomerate of structures which differ from a cytoarchitectonic viewpoint, reflecting differences in myelogenesis and ontogenesis of the human brain.[2] In addition, from the point of view of anatomy, the frontal lobe represents a "crossroads" dense with extrinsic connections that cannot always be taken into account in focal lesions studies.

Numerous studies using functional imaging and particularly positron emission tomography (PET) have attempted to define changes that occur at the level of the frontal lobes as a result of pathology, either focal or more widespread. This paper reviews clinical data and previous PET studies and combines them with some new data to show that impairments in executive functions occur in lesions not limited to the frontal lobes and that cortical structures outside the prefrontal areas may play an important role in these functions.

CLINICAL AND PET STUDIES

Executive Functions and the Frontal Lobe

Experimental data suggest that executive functions depend on the integrity of circuits involving the prefrontal cortex. However, the functional significance of the prefrontal cortex in relation to the outside world derives from the long reciprocal cortico-cortical connections with visual, auditory, and somatic sensory areas, as well as with some portions of the thalamus.[3] In addition to sensory afferents, the frontal lobe receives substantial input from the limbic and paralimbic cortex, especially the medial frontal cingulate cortex.[4]

Because of their reciprocal connections with both the telencephalic and limbic cortex, the frontal lobes seem to be centrally involved in the selection, organization, and monitoring of motor or behavioral programs that are influenced by limbic input. In an environment with changing conditions, the prefrontal cortex apparently directs activities that demand novel responses. The psychological deficits considered as "frontal" could be the result of the disruption of one or more components of the programs elaborated and directed by the frontal lobe. However, the notion that the frontal lobes are the only cortical structures involved in these processes is no longer accepted.

A fuller understanding of the role of prefrontal cortex in executive functions depends on techniques that allow measurement of cerebral functions in man, such as PET. Several studies have been performed with PET in order to investigate selectively prefrontal networks in normal subjects. The first study was that of Pardo et al.[5] They measured regional cerebral blood flow (rCBF) during Stroop performance, showing maximal activation at the level of the anterior cingulate cortex. More recently, Bench et al.[6] enlarged these findings and demonstrated the existence of activated areas in the cingulate and frontal cortex as well as areas of inhibition in the parietal cortex. The Hammersmith Hospital group[7,8] has also demonstrated participation of the frontal areas to word fluency tasks.

The PET data coming from studies with "frontal" activation paradigm confirm the crucial role of some paralimbic and dorsolateral regions. However, it is clear that executive functions are related to other cerebral areas as well, and cannot be synonymous with "frontal functions."

Focal Pathology: Pick's Disease and Frontal Lobe Dementia

It has been known for almost a century that Pick's disease produces lobar atrophy affecting the frontal and temporal lobes. Recent clinical-pathological studies have attracted our attention to pathology affecting particularly the frontal lobes. As discussed by Neary (this volume), frontal lobe dementia (FLD) and the accompanying atrophy of the orbital part of the prefrontal cortex are characterized by a disorder of attention and of the strategic regulation of sequential acts, together with a deterioration of personality and, in about half of the cases, utilization behavior.[9] Neuropsychological test deficits are found with the Wisconsin Card Sorting Test (WCST), Trail Making Test (TMT), maze, and verbal fluency tests.[10,11] Visuoperceptive and memory functions are relatively spared. FLD is, among all pathologies encountered in current clinical practice, one of the conditions that best fits the classical clinical-pathological association.

The data obtained by SPECT and PET in Pick's or FLD have shown reduction in rCBF in the frontal areas of both hemispheres that clearly accompanies frontal pathophysiology.[12,13] The rCBF patterns of frontal lobe degeneration with and without Pick bodies have shown similar characteristics,[12] but several significant differences exist between FLD and Alzheimer's disease as well as between FLD and Huntington's disease.[14,15] On the other hand, the functional neuroimaging investigations provide very useful information about diagnosis in the early stage of disease.[16] In six of the eight patients in this last study, magnetic resonance imaging (MRI) did not localize the frontal dysfunction that was suspected clinically, whereas reduced rCBF in both the basal-medial and dorsolateral frontal cortices was shown.

"Diffuse" Brain Disorders and Normal Aging

Closed Head Injury

According to most authors, many of the cognitive and behavioral disorders observed in closed head injury (CHI) are due to a disorder of frontal cortex that is affected either directly or indirectly through its many connections. This conclusion is based on clinical as well as on pathological data (the focal contusions represent 43% of the primary lesions—all in frontal and temporal regions, whereas diffuse axonal injury in the same areas reaches 48%).[17,18] From a behavioral standpoint, patients with CHI tend to have disorders involving programming, planning, elaboration of concepts and action plans, and mental flexibility with difficulty in shifting mental set. These aspects of behavior are assessed by "classical" frontal tests such as verbal fluency, the WCST, the Tower test (be it of London, Hanoi or Toronto), the TMT, and the Stroop test.[19]

Recent progress in neuroimaging has correlated cerebral lesions with cognitive and behavioral sequels in CHI. Despite an abundant literature, clear-cut results so far are rather limited. The lesions seen in severe CHI may be more focal (cerebral contusion) or more widespread (diffuse axonal injury). However, the CT and MRI assess only some of these pathological alterations.[20] The relation between structural damage, established by means of morphological brain imaging, and behavioral sequelae of CHI are often disputable and unconvincing.[21]

Functional imaging reveals a more complete picture of the distribution and extent of brain dysfunction in CHI. SPECT using [^{99m}Tc]hexamethyl-propyleneamineoxime ([^{99m}Tc]HMPAO) has proved to be a useful tool in determining the distribution of rCBF. Several authors[22,23] have shown defective perfusion even in areas that appear intact on CT or MRI. In addition, Oder et al.[23] showed a significant correlation between behavioral disorders in CHI and decreased frontal blood flow. The first PET studies, even though they were carried out on small samples, showed clear correlations between the regions of hypometabolism and the neuropsychological results.[24,25]

Marchiafava-Bignami Disease

Marchiafava-Bignami disease (MBD) is a rare complication of chronic severe alcoholism. Its pathological hallmark is damage of the corpus callosum (CC). The advent of computerized tomography (CT) and MRI has allowed a better delineation of more benign clinical presentations of MBD because the classic form had been considered lethal.

In some cases, the diagnosis is suggested by signs of interhemispheric disconnection. These include left visual and tactile anomia, left-hand agraphia, left-sided apraxia, left auditory extinction, and bimanual asynergy.[26,27]

The course of the "benign" form is often marked by progressive dementia with frontal lobe symptomatology evolving over several years superimposed on "classic" disconnection syndrome.[28,29] The patient in the study of Pappatà et al.[29] presented the neuropsychological pattern of "cortical dementia" including major frontal lobe dysfunction, memory impairment, and disturbances of language and visuospatial abilities. Symptoms in MBD may also include motor and mental slowness, apathy, abulia, muteness, grasping and sucking reflexes. Many of these symptoms may occur in any severe chronic alcoholic. They may improve with abstinence from alcohol, although more often the dementia persists.[30]

Progress in neuroradiological imaging techniques in the last years provides the possibility to diagnose the MBD more readily in life. On CT the lesions of demyelination and necrosis are seen as large symmetrical bilateral hypodense areas in the hemispheric white matter or in the CC, especially the genu and splenium.[31,32] However, on axial CT the small lesions in the body of the CC may not be visible. MRI is better than CT for the diagnosis in the chronic stage of the disease.[33] In this stage, MRI clearly shows diffuse atrophy and focal necrosis of the CC. In the acute phase, demyelination and edema are represented by diffuse ventricular enlargement with hypointensity on T1 and hyperintensity on T2 weighted image.[33]

There is good evidence that blood flow and metabolism imaging can be a valuable clinical tool for the characterization and the prognosis of patients with MBD as well as for the evaluation of functional changes. The rCBF was monitored with SPECT in a patient suffering from an acute form of MBD.[34] The SPECT examination showed biparietal hypofixation and distinct hypofixation of gray matter in the left paracentral lobule. The brain metabolism was recently evaluated in one MBD patient presenting the protracted dementia of acute onset with only partial subsequent improvement.[29] PET studies performed one and three months after onset showed a conspicuous metabolic depression that was global but prefer-

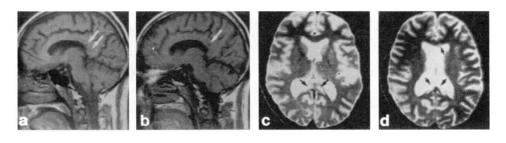

18F - FDG

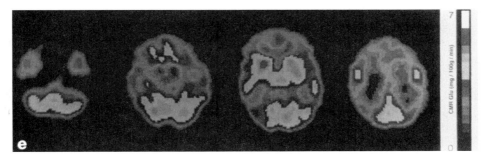

FIGURE 1. MRI and parametric PET images of the cerebral metabolic rate of glucose in a patient with Marchiafava-Bignami disease obtained one month after onset of dementia. (**a–d**) Sagittal and axial MRI views showing lesions in splenium and the genu of the corpus callosum (*arrows*). (**e**) PET images show a bilateral cortical hypometabolism more marked in association cortex than in primary areas. 18F-FDG, [18F]fluoro-2-deoxy-D-glucose. (From Pappatà *et al.*[29] Reproduced, with permission, from the *Journal of Neural Transmission*.)

entially affected the association neocortex bilaterally, relative to primary cortex and subcortical structures (FIG. 1). This striking distribution of hypometabolism is quite consistent with the observed neuropsychological pattern of "cortical dementia."

Chronic Alcoholism

Chronic alcoholics without obvious neurological complications may demonstrate cognitive disorders with appropriate neuropsychological tests. In addition to memory impairment, there can be poor performance at the TMT and other subtests of the Halstead battery. Their performance tends to be worse than that of control subjects, but also of patients with frontal lobe pathology.[35,36] Other impairments affect complex psychomotor tasks involving problem solving and manipulation of abstract concepts.[37,38]

In 1986 Samson *et al.*[39] studied six chronic alcoholics without neurological disorder compared to six healthy controls. Global glucose consumption was lower in alcoholics, but the difference did not reach significance. There was, however, a significant loss in the mediofrontal regions, suggesting an anterior cingulate dysfunction. More recently, a study carried out on 14 chronic alcoholics confirmed this mediofrontal hypometabolism.[40]

Several authors[41] have suggested links between aging and long-term effects of alcohol. Both groups have difficulty in tasks requiring short-term memory, problem solving, and organization of new information.

Normal Aging

Both cross-sectional and longitudinal studies of cognitive performance in normal aging generally demonstrate declines with aging. However, declines do not develop uniformly, either within or across cognitive domains. The areas of cognition that are more affected are memory (particularly episodic memory) and executive functions.[42] The latter are demonstrated by impaired performance on the WCST,[43,44] verbal fluency,[45] and graphic fluency.[44] Changes are also found in the performance of the Porteus maze and of the Stroop test.[44,45]

The MRI investigations in the elderly show significant MRI evidence of shrinkage in white matter especially in the region of the basal forebrain and high correlation between the cognitive decline and the percent of white matter.[46] This suggests that structural or functional alterations in the brain, apart from cortical neuronal loss, are likely to be primarily responsible for the significant age-related changes that are observed in cognitive functions. This suggestion has been confirmed in studies of rCBF with high-resolution PET in normal volunteers.[47] The authors demonstrate an age-related decrease in adjusted rCBF in the cingulate, parahippocampal, superior temporal, medial and posterior frontal cortex. The affected areas were all limbic, or association, cortices.

EXPERIMENTAL PET DATA

The executive dysfunctions reported in many diffuse brain disorders are usually explained by the high-level hierarchical organization of the prefrontal cortex because prefrontal performance depends on the input of various remote areas. Normal prefrontal cortex functions require the integrity of "lower level" cortical areas such as the frontobasal area, and of cortico-cortical connections. Alternatively, even in diffuse brain disorders, the "dysexecutive syndrome" may be due to specific impairments of prefrontal structures.

These hypotheses have been recently tested at the Service Hospitalier Frédéric-Joliot in Orsay in a variety of disorders such as severe CHI, MBD, and chronic alcoholism. The MRI and PET procedures for the first two studies are briefly explained below.

MRI and PET Procedures

MRI studies. MRI was performed the same day as the PET study. Contiguous T1-weighted 3-mm-thick axial slices were obtained throughout the entire brain, using a 0.5 Tesla MR imager (MRMAX, General Electric, Milwaukee, WI).

PET studies. All PET studies were performed using a [^{18}F]fluoro-2-deoxy-D-glucose ([^{18}F]FDG) and a high-resolution tomograph (ECAT-Siemens 953B, CTI, Knoxville, TN) that collects simultaneously 31 5-mm-thick planes, with an in-plane resolution of 6 mm. A head holder molded to each subject was used to maintain a good head position. For all PET studies, the correction for tissue attenuation of 511 keV gamma radiation was measured with an external source of ^{68}Ge (germanium), giving a 31-slice transmission image. Plasma [^{18}F]FDG curves were obtained from 24 arterial blood samples collected from the radial artery over the course of one hour after the intravenous injection of 6 mCi of the radiotracer.

Image analysis. We used a newly developed method based on the anatomical images acquired by MRI to determine the PET regions of interests (ROIs).[48] This method uses both transmission and dynamic PET images that define the surfaces of the head and the brain, respectively. These surfaces are matched in 3D to the surfaces of the head and the brain obtained by MRI. The ROIs are first defined on the MRI for each subject.

Circular ROIs (diameter = 15 mm) were placed over the cortical structures, thalamus, striatum, caudate, hippocampus, and the cerebellum on the contiguous MRI slices where these structures could be visualized. The data from cortical ROIs were subsequently averaged according to a limited number of anatomical-functional brain areas. The ROIs were then copied onto the corresponding PET images. This method allows an accurate and reliable positioning of the ROIs on the structures of interest across PET examinations. In addition, the absolute cerebral metabolic rate of glucose (CMRGlu) values so obtained were normalized for the occipital cortex in the study of patients with MBD and for the whole cortex in CHI.

Severe Closed Head Injury

As previously mentioned, severe CHI is often associated with neuropsychological impairments involving memory, attention, and executive functions. These in turn affect performance and socioprofessional outcome. The underlying neurobehavioral disturbances are poorly correlated with MRI lesions and vary from focal lesions to diffuse axonal injury. They may involve alterations of specific neural networks, which may be more detectable by FDG-PET. A series of CMRGlu PET studies was conducted on head-injured patients to examine the regional pattern of metabolic values accompanying the post traumatic period, and to examine the changes in these patterns in subjects showing neurobehavioral difficulties in their socioprofessional life.

Nine patients with severe CHI (initial coma > 24 h; Glasgow coma score, 6.1 ± 1.2) were investigated 6 ± 4 months later with FDG-PET on a high-resolution tomograph. Four patients had good socioprofessional outcome; five remained dependent and unable to work because of behavioral and memory disturbances (Glasgow outcome scale, moderate-to-severe disabilities). Frontal function was assessed by the Stroop test, WCST, Tower of London, and verbal fluency tests.

Mean cortical CMRGlu was significantly ($p < .01$) and similarly decreased compared to controls in patients with poor (-27%) and with good outcome

(-26%). Poor outcome was associated with lower metabolic values than good outcome in the following regions: right medial cingulate ($p < .02$), right and left anterior cingulate ($p < .02$), left medial prefrontal cortex ($p < .01$), and right temporal pole ($p < .02$). The same areas showed no MRI evidence of lesions (FIG. 2).

The Stroop test and the verbal fluency tests were significantly altered in the poor recovery group. We studied the correlation between the hypometabolic cortical patterns and neuropsychological abnormalities. The Stroop interference time correlated with the hypometabolism in the dorsolateral area of the left frontal lobe and in the medial prefrontal region bilaterally. The impairment in verbal fluency was correlated to left prefrontal cortex hypometabolism (FIG. 3).

One possible explanation of these results is that neurobehavioral abnormalities leading to poor outcome after severe CHI may be mainly related to the dysfunction of limbic or limbic-related frontal structures, whereas frontolimbic and dorsolateral prefrontal dysfunction may contribute to the impairment of executive functions.

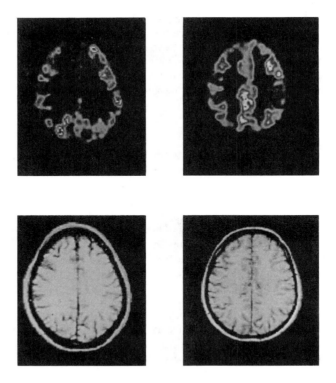

FIGURE 2. MRI and parametric PET images of the cerebral metabolic rate of glucose in patients with poor (*left*) and with good (*right*) outcome after severe closed head injury.

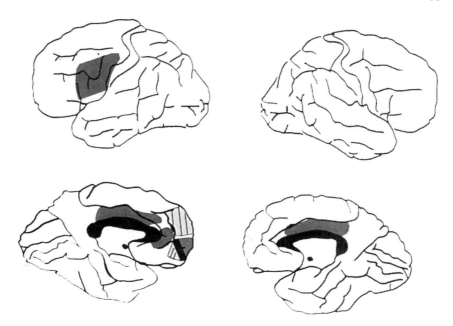

FIGURE 3. Relation between cortical hypometabolism and the performance of the neuropsychological tasks in patients with severe closed head injury. Diagram of lateral (*top*) and medial (*bottom*) views of the right and left hemispheres demonstrating the correlations between the Stroop test (in grey) and verbal fluency (striped light grey).

Marchiafava-Bignami Disease

The contrast between major cognitive impairment and lesions apparently limited to the CC, as assessed by CT or MRI, is intriguing and raises the issue of associated, but structurally undetectable, damage to cortical neurons and/or hemispheric white matter. We previously reported a profound cortical hypometabolism in a single case of MBD.[29] We subsequently attempted to analyze in more detail the metabolic regional pattern in a series of patients.

Four patients with MBD (ages, 39 ± 9 years) were studied. All had a history of severe alcoholism and cc lesions documented on MRI. Three had a rapidly progressive dementia without delirium or tremor, and one was comatose. Neurological examination showed no gaze palsy and no nystagmus. Disconnection symptoms were found in two patients. The PET scan was performed on a 31-slices ECAT camera, and data analysis was done on MRI-defined brain regions, by comparison with six controls (ages 23 ± 1 year).

Metabolism was severely decreased in the associative and medial frontal cerebral cortex (range, 54 to 45%, $p < .001$) and in all subcortical regions (range, 32 to 36%), except in the cerebellum (9%, NS). After normalization by cerebellar values, metabolism was significantly decreased in all associative and in cingulate cortices, but not in other limbic areas (hippocampus, orbitofrontal cortex, and temporal pole), primary cortical areas, or in subcortical areas.

The parametric CMRGlu images displayed a clear-cut global hypometabolism, more marked in the anterior and posterior associative and medial frontal cerebral cortices, with relative sparing of the cerebellum, the deep gray nuclei, and the primary cortex. The CMRGlu in the basal ganglia, the thalamus, and the cerebellum was in the low range but did not reach statistical significance relative to controls.

The absolute cortical metabolic values were significantly decreased for the whole cortex ($\sim$50% of controls, $p < .05$). All cortical regions were hypometabolic, with the lateral prefrontal, the medial frontal (including the anterior cingulate gyrus), and the posterior associative (i.e., parieto-temporo-occipital) cortices reaching statistically significant ($p < .01$) metabolic depression bilaterally; the sensory-motor, lateral temporal (which includes the primary auditory cortex) and the visual cortices were not significantly hypometabolic. The primary visual cortex was least reduced (65% of controls). After normalization by cerebellar values, the analysis of metabolic values revealed essentially similar findings, but with enhanced significance. Metabolism was significantly decreased in all associative and in cingulate cortices ($p < .001$), but not in other limbic areas (hippocampus, orbitofrontal cortex, and temporal pole), primary cortical areas, or in subcortical areas.

MBD is associated with a profound hypometabolism that predominates in regions with numerous callosal connections, but is probably too severe to be exclusively secondary to callosal lesions.

Chronic Alcoholism

We measured CMRGlu with PET and [^{18}F]FDG in 17 alcoholic patients. PET scans in this study were performed with the LETI TTV01 time-of-flight four-ring seven-slice camera with axial and lateral resolution of about 13 mm. The patients were selected according to DSM-III-R criteria and were studied after 1–3 weeks of alcohol withdrawal. Duration of alcoholism was 12 years. None had neurological symptoms related to their intoxication, nor psychiatric disorders. Frontal function was assessed by the Stroop test and verbal fluency tests. Using MRI studies performed at the same levels than PET images, we defined four large lobar regions (frontal, temporal, parietal, and occipital) and three smaller frontal areas (medial prefrontal, dorsolateral prefrontal, and orbitofrontal). Regional CMRGlu values were normalized to mean cortical values. Patients' values were compared to those of nine control subjects with similar age.

A significant relative hypometabolism was found in the whole frontal lobe ($p = .009$), and was marked in medial prefrontal ($p = .001$) and in dorsolateral prefrontal ($p = .03$) cortex (FIGS. 4 and 5). The degree of relative medial prefrontal hypometabolism correlated with verbal fluency performance ($r = .63$, $p = 0.02$) (FIG. 6), and with Stroop interference time ($r = -.51$, $p = .04$). The left dorsolateral prefrontal relative metabolism correlated with the number of errors on the Stroop test ($r = -.86$, $p = .001$) (FIG. 7). No other correlations were found with

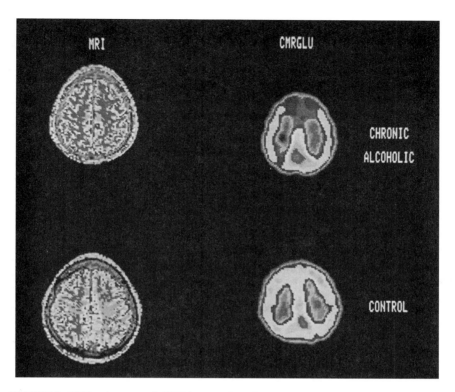

FIGURE 4. MRI and parametric PET images of cerebral metabolic rate of glucose (CMRGlu) in a chronic alcoholic patient (*top*) and a control subject (*bottom*). An important relative hypometabolism was found in the whole frontal lobe in alcoholic patients with mild cortical atrophy on the MRI image.   FIG 4-4

any other brain regions. On the MRI images, a global cortical atrophy was found, but the degree of atrophy in the frontal lobes did not correlate with frontal hypometabolism.

These data suggest that chronic alcoholism leads to cognitive and functional alterations in frontal regions. Thus, the inner face of the frontal lobe, which includes the cingulate gyrus, and the dorsolateral prefrontal cortex may be specifically impaired in chronic alcoholism.

DISCUSSION

The results reported here show that executive dysfunctions are strongly and selectively correlated with metabolic alterations distributed in specific prefrontal, premotor, and anterior cingulate regions.

The results were obtained in a group of diseases usually considered "diffuse,"

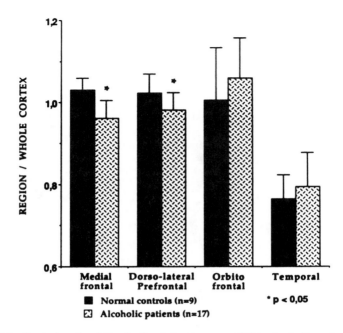

FIGURE 5. Cortical regional distribution index (mean ± SD) in alcoholic and control subjects. A significant selective decrease is found in the medial prefrontal and in the dorsolateral prefrontal cortex. Regional cerebral metabolic rate of glucose values were normalized to mean cortical values.

but where patients show significant changes in cognitive functions generally considered specific for frontal brain damage. Several conclusions can be drawn. The PET scans in each study demonstrated cerebral pathology not visualized by CT and, in some cases, not visualized by MRI either. In the three pathologies, all patients demonstrated a decrease of global cerebral glucose consumption ranging from 25 to 50%. This hypometabolism was marked in the association cortical regions and at the subcortical level. The internal frontal areas and prefrontal dorsolateral areas were especially affected. In these regions the hypometabolism demonstrated by the PET scans was generally correlated with impaired performance on "executive function" tasks. This strongly suggests that, even in "diffuse disorders," executive dysfunctions are related to functional alteration of specific frontal and frontolimbic circuits.

Yet, it is important to recall that FDG PET does not give cues about the structural changes underlying the functional alterations. In the three pathologies, all patients demonstrated a decrease of global cerebral glucose consumption ranging from 25 to 50%. This hypometabolism was marked in the association cortical regions and at the subcortical level. The internal frontal areas and prefrontal dorsolateral areas were especially affected. Hence, hypometabolism may reflect very

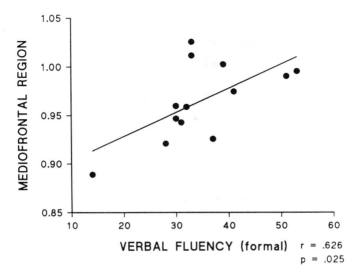

FIGURE 6. Correlation between the medial prefrontal relative metabolism and the verbal fluency performance in alcoholic patients.

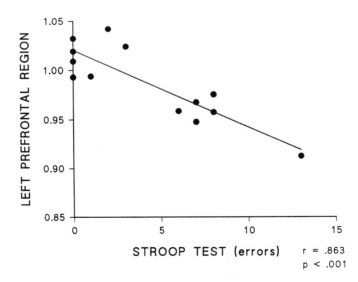

FIGURE 7. Correlation between the left dorsolateral prefrontal relative metabolism and the number of errors on the Stroop test in alcoholic patients.

different mechanisms, such as local neuronal loss or severe deafferentation. The latter phenomenon may be especially frequent in the prefrontal structures because of their high degree of cortico-cortical or subcortico-cortical connections. Thus, it is likely that both local neuronal loss and dysconnection contributed in various degrees to the frontal hypometabolism observed in the very different pathologies that were studied here, and in normal aging. For example, local neuronal loss and/or neuronal atrophy may be found in severe head injury, as well as in normal aging,[49] MBD,[28] and chronic alcoholism.[50] Yet, in each of these pathologies, disconnections of frontal structures are likely to occur, due to white matter lesions or injury to remote cortical structures. It must also be pointed out that similar metabolic changes in normal aging and in diffuse brain disorders do not imply a common pathogenic mechanism, but suggest the vulnerability of certain brain structures. *In vivo* PET neuronal markers will probably help to resolve these issues in the near future. As an example, it has already been shown that the benzodiazepine receptor ligand [^{11}C]flumazenil is able to distinguish functional from structural hypometabolism in frontal dementias.[51]

In conclusion, functional prefrontal disorders may occur without apparent structural damage probably because prefrontal performance depends on the input of various remote areas. Prefrontal functions are the common pathway for the effects of anatomically distant cerebral lesions and the cumulative results of diffuse pathology. As the most recently evolved and functionally complex cortical area, the frontal lobe may be the most vulnerable to disruption.

REFERENCES

1. TRANEL, D., S. W. ANDERSON & A. BENTON 1994. Development of the concept of "executive function" and its relationship to the frontal lobes. *In* The Frontal Lobes. Computational Modelling and Neuropsychology. Handbook of Neuropsychology. F. Boller & J. Grafman, Eds. Vol. **9:** 125–149. Elsevier. Amsterdam.
2. PETRIDES, M. & D. PANDYA. 1994. Comparative architectonic analysis of the human and macaque frontal cortex. *In* Handbook of Neuropsychology. F. Boller & J. Grafman, Eds. Vol. **9:** 17–58. Elsevier. Amsterdam.
3. NAUTA, W. J. H. 1971. The problem of the frontal lobe: A reinterpretation. J. Psychiatr. Res. **8:** 167–187.
4. PANDYA, D. N. & C. L. BARNES. 1987. Architecture and connections of the frontal lobe. *In* The Frontal Lobes Revisited. E. Perecman, Ed.: 41–72. IRBN Press. New York.
5. PARDO, J. V., P. J. PARDO, K. W. JANNER & M. E. RAICHLE. 1990. The anterior cingulate cortex mediates processing selection in the Stroop attentional conflict paradigm. Proc. Natl. Acad. Sci. USA **87:** 256–259.
6. BENCH, C. J., C. D. FRITH, P. M. GRASBY, K. J. FRISTON, E. PAULESU, R. S. J. FRACKOWIAK & R. J. DOLAN. 1993. Investigations of the functional anatomy of attention using the Stroop test. Neuropsychologia **31:** 907–922.
7. FRITH, C. D., K. J. FRISTON, P. F. LIDDLE & R. S. J. FRACKOWIAK. 1991. A PET study of word finding. Neuropsychologia **29:** 1137–1148.
8. FRISTON, K. J., C. D. FRITH, P. F. LIDDLE & R. S. J. FRACKOWIAK. 1991. Investigating a network model of word generation with positron emission tomography. Proc. R. Soc. Lond. **244:** 101–106.
9. LHERMITTE, F., B. PILLON & M. SERDARU. 1986. Human autonomy and the frontal lobes. Ann. Neurol. **19:** 326–334.

10. ELFGREN, C., U. PASSANT & J. RISBERG. 1993. Neuropsychological findings in frontal lobe dementia. Dementia **4:** 214–219.
11. KNOPMAN, D. 1993. The non-Alzheimer degenerative dementias. *In* Handbook of Neuropsychology. F. Boller & J. Grafman, Eds. Vol. **8:** 295–313. Elsevier. Amsterdam.
12. RISBERG, J. 1987. Frontal lobe degeneration of non-Alzheimer type. III. Regional cerebral blood flow. Arch. Gerontol. Geriatr. **6:** 225–233.
13. ZILBOVICIUS, M., C. RAYNAUD, G. RANCUREL, N. TZOURIO, A. ARZIMANOGLOU, S. LEDER, M. BOURGIGNON & A. SYROTA. 1989. Regional cerebral blood flow measured by SPECT in Pick's disease. J. Cereb. Blood Flow Metab. **9(Suppl. 1):** S521.
14. JAGUST, W. J., B. R. REED, J. P. SEAB, J. H. KRAMER & T. F. BUDINGER. 1989. Clinical-physiologic correlates of Alzheimer's disease and frontal lobe dementia. Am. J. Physiol. Imaging **4:** 89–96.
15. GUSTAFSON, L. 1993. Clinical picture of frontal lobe degeneration of non-Alzheimer type. Dementia **4(3–4):** 143–148.
16. MILLER, B. L., J. L. CUMMINGS, J. VILLANUEVA-MEYER, K. BOONE, C. M. MEHRINGER, I. LESSER & I. MENA. 1991. Frontal lobe degeneration: Clinical, neuropsychological, and SPECT characteristics. Neurology **41:** 1374–1382.
17. LEVIN, H. S., F. C. GOLDSTEIN, D. H. WILLIAMS & H. M. EISENBERG. 1987. The contribution of frontal lobe lesions to the neurobehavioral outcome of closed head injury. *In* Neurobehavioral recovery from head injury. H. S. Levin, J. Grafman & F. C. Goldstein, Eds.: 321–338. Oxford University Press. New York.
18. BOWEN, M. 1989. Frontal lobe function: Review essay. Brain Injury **2:** 109–128.
19. MATTSON, A. J. & H. S. LEVIN. 1990. Frontal lobe dysfunction following head injury: A review of the literature. J. Nerv. Ment. Dis. **178:** 282–291.
20. HESSELINK, J. R., C. F. DOWD, M. E. HEALY, P. HAKEK, L. L. BAKER & T. G. LUERSSEN. 1988. MR Imaging of brain contusions: A comparative study with CT. AJR **150:** 1133–1142.
21. LEVIN, H. S. & W. M. HIGH. 1989. Contributions of neuroimaging to neuropsychological research on closed head injury. Neuropsychology **3:** 243–253.
22. WIEDMANN, K. D., J. T. L. WILSON, D. WYPER, T. M. HADLEY, G. M. TEASDALE & D. BROOKS. 1989. SPECT cerebral blood flow, MR imaging, and neuropsychological findings in traumatic head injury. Neuropsychology **3:** 267–281.
23. ODER, W., G. GOLDENBERG, J. SPATT, I. PODREKA, H. BINDER & L. DEEKE. 1992. Behavioural and psychosocial sequelae of severe closed head injury and cerebral blood flow: A SPECT study. J. Neurol. Neurosurg. Psychiatry **55:** 475–480.
24. LANGFITT, T. W., W. D. OBRIST, A. ALAVI, R. GROSSMAN, R. ZIMMERMAN, J. JAGGI, B. UZELL, M. REIVICH & D. PATTON. 1987. Regional structure and function in head injured patients: Correlation of CT, MRI, PET, CBF, and neuropsychological assessment. *In* Neurobehavioral Recovery from Head Injury. H. S. Levin, J. Grafman & F. C. Goldstein, Eds.: 30–42. Oxford University Press. New York.
25. RUFF, R. M., M. S. BUCHSBAUM, A. I. TROSTER, L. F. MARSHALL, S. LOTTENBERG, L. M. SOMMERS & M. D. TOBIAS. 1989. CT, neuropsychology and PET in the evaluation of head injury. Neuropsychiatr. Neuropsychol. Behav. Neurol. **2:** 103–123.
26. LHERMITTE, F., R. MARTEAU, M. SERDARU & F. CHEDRU. 1977. Signs of interhemispheric disconection in Marchiafava-Bignami disease. Arch. Neurol. **34:** 254.
27. CANNAPLE, S., A. ROSA & J. P. MIZON. 1992. Maladie de Marchiafava-Bignami: Disconnexion interhémisphérique, évolution favorable. Aspect neuroradiologique. Rev. Neurol. **148:** 638–640.
28. ADAMS, R. D. & M. VICTOR. 1989. Diseases of the nervous system due to nutritional deficiency. Marchiafava-Bignami disease (primary degeneration of the corpus callosum). *In* Principles of Neurology. R. D. Adams & M. Victor, Eds.: 837–840. McGraw-Hill Information Services Company. New York.
29. PAPPATÀ, S., H. CHABRIAT, M. LAVASSEUR, F. LEGAULT-DEMARE & J. C. BARON. 1994. Marchiafava-Bignami disease with dementia: Severe cerebral metabolic depression revealed by PET. J. Neural Transm. **8:** 131–137.
30. RENNER, J. A. & J. C. MORRIS. 1994. Alcohol-associated dementia. *In* Handbook of

Dementing Illnesses. J. C. Morris, Eds. Vol. **22**: 393–412. Marcel Dekker, Inc. New York.

31. KAWAMURA, M., J. SHIOTA, T. YAGISHITA & K. HIRAYAMA. 1985. Marchiafava-Bignami disease: Computed tomographic scan and magnetic resonance imaging. Ann. Neurol. **18**: 103–104.

32. HEEPE, P., L. NEMETH, F. BRUNE, J. W. GRANT & P. KLEIHUES. 1988. Marchiafava-Bignami disease: A correlative computed tomography and morphological study. Eur. Arch. Psychiatr. Neurol. Sci. **237**: 74–79.

33. CHANG, K. H., S. H. CHA, M. H. HAN, S. H. PARK, D. L. NAH & J. H. HONG. 1992. Marchiafava-Bignami disease: Serial changes in corpus callosum on MRI. Neuroradiology **34**: 480–482.

34. HUMBERT, T., P. DEGUILHERMIER, C. MAKTOUF, G. GRASSET, F. M. LOPEZ & P. CHABRAND. 1992. Marchiafava-Bignami disease. A case studied by structural and functional brain imaging. Eur. Arch. Psychiatry Clin. Neurosci. **242**: 69–71.

35. SMITH, J. W., D. W. BURT & R. F. CHAPMAN. 1973. Intelligence and brain damage in alcoholics. A study in patients of middle and upper social class. Q. J. Stud. Alcohol **34**: 414–422.

36. LONG, J. A. & J. F. C. MCLACHLAN. 1984. Abstract reasoning and perceptual motor efficiency in alcoholics. Impairment and reversibility. Q. J. Stud. Alcohol **35**: 1220–1229.

37. CHELUNE, G. J. & J. B. PARKER. 1981. Neuropsychological deficits associated with chronic alcohol abuse. Clin. Psychol. Rev. **1**: 181–195.

38. TARTER, R. E. & C. M. RYAN. 1983. Neuropsychology of alcoholism etiology, phenomenology, process, and outcome. *In* Recent Developments in Alcoholism. M. Galander, Ed.: 449–469. Plenum Press. New York.

39. SAMSON, Y., J. C. BARON, A. FELINE, J. BORIES & C. CROUZEL. 1986. Local cerebral glucose utilisation in chronic alcoholics: A positron tomography study. J. Neurol. Neurosurg. Psychiatry **49**: 1165–1170.

40. GILMAN, S., K. ADAMS, R. A. KOEPPE, S. BERENT, K. J. KLUIN, J. G. MODELL, P. KROLL & J. A. BRUNBERG. 1990. Cerebellar and frontal hypometabolism in alcoholic cerebellar degeneration studied with positron emission tomography. Ann. Neurol. **28**: 775–785.

41. RYAN, C. & N. BUTTERS. 1980. Learning and memory impairment in young and old alcoholics: Evidence for the premature aging hypothesis. Alcoholism **4**: 288–293.

42. BOLLER, F., P. MARCIE & L. TRAYKOV. La neuropsychologie du vieillissement normal. *In* Neuropsychologie clinique et neurologie du comportement. M. I. Botez, Ed. Masson & Presse Universitaire du Québec. Paris and Montreal. In press.

43. GRANT, D. A. & E. A. BERG. 1948. A behavioral analysis of degree of reinforcement and ease of shifting to new response in a Weigl type card-sorting problem. J. Exp. Psychol. **38**: 404–411.

44. DAIGNEAULT, S., C. M. J. BRAUN & H. A. WHITAKER. 1992. Early effects of normal aging on perseverative and non-perseverative prefrontal measures. Dev. Neuropsychol. **8**: 99–114.

45. WHELIHAN, W. M. & E. L. LESCHER. 1985. Neuropsychological changes in frontal functions with aging. Dev. Neuropsychol. **1**: 371–380.

46. ALBERT, M. 1993. Neuropsychological and neurophysiological changes in healthy adult humans across the age range. Neurobiol. Aging **14(6)**: 623–625.

47. MARTIN, A. J., K. J. FRISTON, J. G. COLEBATCH & R. S. J. FRACKOWIAK. 1991. Decreases in regional cerebral blood flow with normal aging. J. Cereb. Blood Flow Metab. **11**: 684–689.

48. MANGIN, J. F., V. FROUIN, I. BLOCH, B. BENDRIEM & J. LOPEZ-KRAHE. 1994. Fast nonsupervised 3D registration of PET and MR images of the brain. J. Cereb. Blood Flow Metab. **14**: 749–762.

49. TERRY, R. D., R. DETERESA & L. A. HANSEN. 1987. Neocortical cell counts in normal human adult aging. Ann. Neurol. **21**: 530–539.

50. HARPER, C. & J. KRIL. 1989. Patterns of neuronal loss in the cerebral cortex in chronic alcoholic patients. J. Neurol. Sci. **92:** 81–89.

51. ZILBOVICIUS, M., G. RANCUREL, S. LEDER, C. RAYNAUD, C. LOC'H, R. WANG, C. CROUZEL, J. CAMBIER & Y. SAMSON. 1993. PET study of benzodiazepine receptors (BZR) with 11C-Flumazenil (CFLU) distinguish cortical functional abnormalities from neuronal loss in frontal type dementias. Neurology **43(Suppl. 2):** A213.

Experimental Approach to Prefrontal Functions in Humans

BRUNO DUBOIS, RICHARD LEVY, MARC VERIN,
CARLA TEIXEIRA, YVES AGID, AND BERNARD PILLON

INSERM U.289 and Fédération de Neurologie
Hôpital de la Salpêtrière
47 boulevard de l'Hôpital
75651 Paris cedex 13, France

In the human, the role of the frontal lobes remains poorly understood. Clinical observations of patients with frontal lobe lesions have not yet provided a coherent interpretation of the overall function of this cerebral structure for several reasons: (1) The cognitive deficit related to the frontal lobe dysfunction could be very subtle and not detected either by the clinical investigations or the usual neuropsychological assessment. The case of EVR[1,2] well illustrates this fact because neuropsychological tests thought to be sensitive to frontal lobe dysfunction failed to detect any alteration of the cognitive processes, even though EVR underwent the bilateral ablation of the ventromedial part of the frontal lobes. However, specific analysis showed that EVR exhibited a social adaptative deficit ("sociopathy") associated with unfitness to forecast in real life the future consequences of his choices (2) In other cases, a wide range of behavioral or cognitive modifications could be observed after frontal lobe lesions such as alterations in motor control,[3,4] language,[5] memory,[6,7] attention,[8] temporal integration,[9] problem-solving ability or planification of actions,[10] and affects and emotions.[11] Furthermore, apparently opposite disturbances (i.e., distractibility or perseverations on the same responses; hyperactivity or severe inertia) have been reported after frontal lobe lesions. Such extreme manifestations following lesions of the same structure are difficult to conciliate with a global cognitive model and may reflect a functional compartmentalization of the frontal lobe according to its cytoarchitectonic subdivision.

However, it is generally agreed today that the prefrontal cortex plays a major role in higher behavioral functions such as planning, problem-solving, and conceptualization. To better understand how these highly integrated functions are elaborated, it is important to determine what the fundamental processes are and the neuronal basis that supports these functions. Real progress in the understanding of frontal lobe functions has come from animal experiments. From those works, two major and intermingled concepts have emerged: the involvement of prefrontal lobe in working memory and its segmentation into functional subunits according to cytoarchitectonic subdivisions. Working memory is viewed here as the ability to hold the internal representations of the outside world or from the past in short-term memory and to manipulate this mnemonic information to provide a behavior based on ideas and thoughts rather than immediate stimuli[12] (see also Goldman-Rakic, this volume). In other words, working memory could be seen as a buffer space between perception and action which integrates the incoming information to elaborate the future action schemes.[13] Several studies demonstrated the preeminent involvement of the dorsolateral part of the prefrontal cortex (DLPFC) in working memory in nonhuman primates as measured by the delayed response tasks combined either with single-cell recordings or experimental and restricted lesions of this region.[12–22] Single-cell recording studies have shown that a large number of neurons of the DLPFC were activated during the delay and kept track of the stimulus that had just been previously presented.[18,19,22] The role of the DLPFC in working memory has also been confirmed in humans by employing modifications of tasks used with monkeys in combination with functional imaging techniques such as PET scan and functional MRI.[23–26]

However, the nature of the basic operations under the control of the different architectonic areas of the DLPFC remains in question (TABLE 1). Are the same working memory functions replicated in different areas that are functionally differentiated by the sensory modality they process, as proposed by Goldman-Rakic;[12] or are these different areas characterized by a distinct level of information processing? A set of electrophysiological and lesion studies in primates supports the idea of a compartmentalization of the DLPFC into working memory subunits specialized in a specific sensory domain.[15–17,27–31] The neurons located within the principal sulcus (Walker's area 46) are activated by spatial information, whereas the neurons located in the inferior convexity (Walker's area 12) respond to pattern information (form or color).[32] This segregation fits well with the anatomical evidence that area 46 receives strong input from the posterior parietal cortex (area 7) which processes spatial information, whereas the inferior convexity is mainly connected with the inferotemporal cortex (area TE) which is involved in visual discrimination.[33–34] Furthermore, single-cell recordings within the principal sulcus have shown the coexistence of a large number of "mnemonic" neurons with others neurons which appeared to participate in preparatory motor set. These findings indicate that within a given region neurons that maintain internal representations are intermingled with others that prepare a programmed response.[35–37] Functional studies in the humans have provided controversial results because they have shown that during spatial working memory tasks, the region the most activated within the DLPFC is either Brodmann's area 47, in the inferior convexity,[23] or Brodmann's area 46, which corresponds to the region of principal sulcus in monkey.[25] Another level of specialization of the DLPFC has been suggested by Petrides and colleagues in human and nonhuman primates.[24,38,39] They isolate different areas according to their functions in the processing of the information. For example, they allocate to the upper- and mid-dorsolateral part of the DLPFC (Walker's and Brodmann's area 9) the most executive part of the nonspatial working memory that requires a high level of monitoring. By contrast, when the monitoring requirements are low (such as during the delayed matching to sample), lesions of area 9 do not induce deficit, suggesting that processing nonspatial working memory with low monitoring does not depend on area 9 but mainly on areas below it (i.e., the inferior convexity). Finally, the concept of a division of the DLPFC into several functional subunits based upon a particular aspect of working memory is brought into question by works of Fuster and his collaborators.[20,40,41] They have shown that monkeys with reversible lesions of the DLPFC were im-

TABLE 1. Functions of the Different Cytoarchitectonic Areas of the Lateral Part of the Prefrontal Cortex

Role of the Lateral Prefrontal Cortex Main Theories	Nonhuman Primate Studies			Human Studies	
	Critical Regions	Tasks	Methods	Critical Regions	Methods
Sensory modality dissociation [refs. 12, 14–18, 22, 27–30, 32]					
Spatial working memory	Sulcus principalis Walker's area 46	Spatial delayed response; Spatial delayed alternation; Delayed saccade and antisaccade oculomotor tasks	Lesions and single cell recordings in area 46	Brodmann's area 46 (mid-dorsolateral PFC) or Brodmann's area 47 (inferior dorsolateral PFC)	Spatial WM task and fMRI[25]; Spatial WM task and PET scan[23]
Pattern (form, color) working memory	Inferior lateral PFC Walker's area 12	Delayed object alternation; Delayed matching to sample	Lesions and single cell recordings in area 12	Dorsolateral PFC	Nonspatial WM task and PET scan[26]
Processing dissociation [refs. 38 and 39]					
High monitoring within working memory (nonspatial information)	Dorsolateral PFC Walker's area 9	Nonspatial self-ordered tasks	Lesions in area 9	Brodmann's areas 9 and 46 (mid-dorsolateral PFC)	Nonspatial self-ordered tasks and PET scan[24]
Low monitoring within working memory	Areas under 9 (mid and inferior dorsolateral PFC)			/	/
No dissociation [refs. 20, 36, 37, 40, and 44]					
Supra-modal/cross-modal working memory	Lateral PFC (dorsal and inferior parts)	Cross-modal (visual/tactile) delayed matching to sample; Various other spatial and nonspatial WM tasks	Cooling and single cell recordings in the dorsolateral PFC	To be determined	/

PFC, prefrontal cortex; WM, working memory. Slash (/) indicates not studied.

paired in cross-modal versions of delayed matching to sample tasks and that the lesion in the DLPFC produced a deficit in somesthesic, visuospatial, and visual nonspatial working memory tasks. These data emphasize the cross- and supramodal processing of the DLPFC in working memory. Thus, although there is a general consensus attributing the neuronal basis of working memory to the DLPFC, the fundamental nature of the processes involved and the control of different subregions remains debated.

Lesions studies in the human have also shown that patients with a prefrontal dysfunction were impaired in tasks directly adapted from delayed response tasks in monkey.[42,43] However, due to the heterogeneity of the lesions exhibited by the patients included in these studies, no clear conclusion has been drawn concerning the involvement of the lateral part of the prefrontal cortex in working memory. Strict criteria of inclusion according to the location of the lesion and its etiology may provide important clues on the role of the DLPFC and render possible the investigation of the fundamental processes that are the most sensitive to DLPFC lesions.

By integrating the working memory concepts developed in nonhuman primates, we undertook two consecutive studies in patients with DLPFC lesions to verify whether DLPFC lesions produce an impairment in working memory and to assess which fundamental processes are mainly disrupted by DLPFC lesions. Indeed, working memory necessitates a set of serial-ordered operations including sensory perception, elaboration and maintenance of mental representations (storage in short-term memory), monitoring of this information ("working with memory"), and execution of a self-programmed behavior based on these mental representations. According to that theoretical segmentation of cognitive operations, one may hypothesize that one or several types of impairment could be observed after DLPFC lesions: a deficit of the selection or the encoding of relevant information; a short-term storage deficit; an executive deficit when sequencing successive information or planning self-generated responses are required. We further attempted to determine whether DLPFC lesions could reveal deficit in cognitive processes beyond the realm of working memory such as rule-finding or rule-learning deficit.

Because anatomical and behavioral data have strongly emphasized the role of the DLPFC in visuospatial working memory, we first designed a set of tasks derived from the spatial delayed response and spatial delayed alternation tasks developed in nonhuman primates.[44] Second, we designed spatial working memory tasks thought to tax separately and specifically several fundamental mechanisms that cooperate in the achievement of working memory operations.[45]

IS THERE A WORKING MEMORY DEFICIT IN PATIENTS WITH DLPFC LESIONS?

To address this issue we designed a simple task derived from the spatial delayed response task, currently used in primates to assess spatial working memory (FIG.

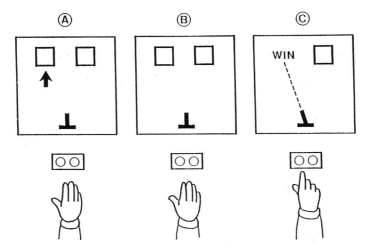

FIGURE 1. Delayed response task. Two colored squares were presented on the microcomputer screen (**A**). An explicit cue (an arrow) indicated for two seconds the correct response. Then, the two squares disappeared for 15 seconds. After this delay, the stimuli reappeared on the screen (**B**) for the selection of the response. If the choice was correct, the square disappeared, and the word "win" appeared in its place (**C**)—this was the reinforcement. If the choice was incorrect, the square did not disappear: there was no reinforcement; the subject had lost.

1). Two large squares were arranged horizontally on a microcomputer screen. An arrow appeared for two seconds under one of the squares, indicating the one the subject should choose after the beep, that is to say, after a 15-s delay. The choice was externally guided because it was indicated by an explicit cue. Thus, the requirements for the success of this task were very low: the subject only had to remember the spatial position of the arrow during the delay and to execute the correct response after the signal. As emphasized by Goldman-Rakic,[12] the delayed response task is a prototypical working memory task because it demands that the memory be updated from trial to trial. In this situation, where no rule has to be learned, normal controls met the criterion of 10 successive correct responses with no errors. They had no trouble in maintaining an internal representation of the stimulus during the delay and in responding in accordance with its trace. In contrast, a group of patients with a single, isolated, vascular ischemic lesion of the dorsolateral prefrontal cortex (right/left = 7/3) made a mean number of 2.8 errors before reaching the same criterion. The deficit seems unlikely to result from difficulty in understanding the task for patients who had no comprehension disorders and obtained scores within the normal range on a global intellectual efficiency task. The patients' performance rather suggests a severe working memory deficit for visuospatial stimuli, because the response should be planned on the basis of an internal representation. Predictably, this deficit seems to be specific for the prefrontal location of the lesions since no difficulty was observed in a group of patients with focal lesions of the post-central cortex.

Why do lesions of the dorsolateral prefrontal cortex in humans affect the handling of visuospatial representations or the selection of the correct response? A supramodal attentional deficit can alter the temporal processing of consecutive stimuli. During the successive trials, patients with prefrontal lesions might have difficulty inhibiting nonpertinent internal cues,[11,46] that is, traces of previous stimuli, because of an abnormal sensitivity to proactive interference. This type of disorder has also been described in humans as a deficit in judging recency.[47] A specific deficit in the processing of visuospatial information within working memory is an alternative hypothesis inasmuch as it has been shown that lesions of area 46 impaired the monitoring of visuospatial cues in primates.[12] Finally, dysfunction of the prefrontal cortex may intervene at the level of integration needed for coupling the correct analysis of the specific requirements of the task and the selection of the appropriate response, as if patients with prefrontal damage were unable to bind a specific situational demand with a specific response set.

WHAT ARE THE FUNDAMENTAL WORKING MEMORY PROCESSES MOST IMPAIRED IN DLPFC LESIONS?

To delineate at which particular cognitive steps the deficit observed in the spatial delayed response tasks after the DLPFC lesions corresponds, we designed a specific visuospatial working memory task, the temporospatial recall task, consisting again of three successive phases (FIG. 2): first, a presentation phase in which a set of blue squares turned successively into red (the "stimulus"), then a 10-s delay, and, finally, a response phase where the subject himself had to program the entire sequence of response on the touch screen by reproducing the stimulus

--→

FIGURE 2. Visuospatial working memory tasks: the temporospatial recall task and its control tasks. The general procedure consisted of three successive phases: (1) the presentation of a visuospatial stimulus, (2) a 10-s delay, and (3) the response phase. In recall tasks, the subject himself had to program the entire sequence that he saw previously. In contrast, in the recognition task, he only had to decide whether a new sequence presented was similar to or different from the one presented first. (Left panel) Temporospatial recall task: A set of 2, 3, 4, 5 or 6 blue squares turned successively into red (the "stimulus"). At the response phase, the blue squares reappeared (a). The subject had to touch the squares that formed the stimulus in their sequential order (b). (Right panel) (A) Recognition task: The stimulus was similar to that of the temporospatial task. After the delay, a second set of red squares, either similar to or different from the one shown first, was presented (a). The subject had to indicate if the second cue was similar to or different from the stimulus (b). (B) Spatial recall task: A set of blue squares (2, 3, 4, 5 or 6) turned simultaneously into red (the "stimulus"). In the response phase, the blue squares reappeared (a). The subject had to touch the squares that formed the stimulus in any order he wanted (b). (C) Temporal recall task: A set of 2, 3, 4, 5 or 6 blue squares turned successively into red (the "stimulus"). In the response phase, the set of red squares reappeared simultaneously. Thus, the spatial location of the squares that belong to the stimulus was provided to the subject before his response (a). The subject had to reproduce the temporal sequence by touching the red squares in the sequential order of the stimulus (b). The four tasks were given successively in the same session. Thirty randomly distributed trials were given for each task (six trials for each length of set; a 10-s delay was present in half of the trials).

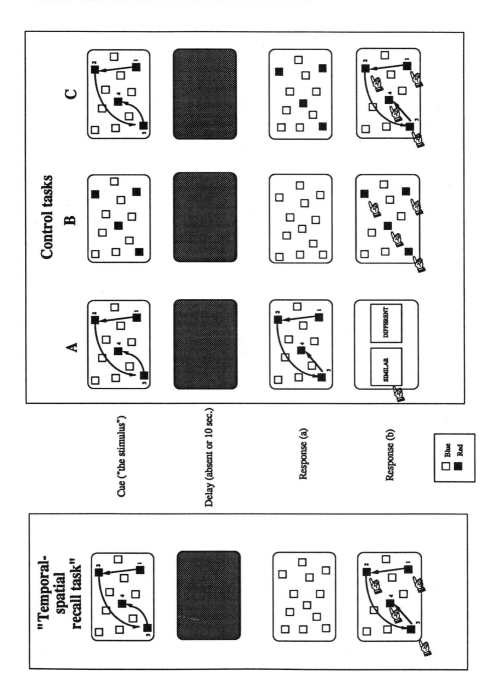

that he saw before. Response programming in this case is only based on the internal representation of the stimulus he had encoded and maintained during the delay. In half of the trials no delay was interposed. In this latter condition, the short-term representational memory requirements were dramatically reduced because response programming was generated immediately after the presentation phase. Thus, this task involved at least three different processes: encoding of the relevant visuospatial information, self-programming of a response, and, in the presence of a delay, the maintenance of the visuospatial information in a short-term representational memory.

A set of three other tasks has been proposed as control of the temporospatial recall task (FIG. 2) to analyze separately and specifically the different aspects of information processing required, which include (1) encoding (or selection) of the visuospatial information to be processed in short-term memory; (2) maintenance of this information in a short-term store; (3) the executive phase when planning of self-generated responses is required; (4) processing of the spatial component of visual information within the working memory; and (5) processing of the temporal ordering component of visual information within the working memory.

Patients with ischemic and unilateral DLPFC lesions exhibited a sharp deficit in the temporospatial recall task with delay when compared with their age- and education level–matched controls (FIG. 3). In contrast, patients with lesions of the post-central cortex, that is, the parietal and temporal regions, had performance in that task similar to that of control subjects (results not shown). Furthermore, patients with degenerative diseases of the basal ganglia (Parkinson's disease and progressive supranuclear palsy), when associated with a severe frontal lobe dysfunction, performed significantly worse in this task than a group of parkinsonian patients with no frontal lobe dysfunction. These results are in agreement with our first study and suggest that the deficit observed during this "visuospatial working memory" task is related to a frontal lobe dysfunction.

Surprisingly, the DLPFC patients were impaired even in the absence of delay (FIG. 3), suggesting that the deficit resulted, at least in part, from a dysfunction situated beyond or outside the strict realm of the short-term representational memory. Two alternative but not exclusive mechanisms can explain the severe impairment in this task even in the absence of delay: (1) patients have difficulties downstream of the short-term memory processing, at the stage of programming and executing sequential motor actions because the responses are self-generated and (2) the deficit lies, partly, upstream of the short-term memory storage, at the stage of encoding or selecting the information to be processed in working memory.

Is the Impairment a Result of the Response Programming?

To approach this issue we compared the performance of patients in the temporospatial recall task without delay to that obtained by the same patients in one of the control tasks, the temporospatial recognition task *without* delay ("ND recognition" task) (FIG. 2). In the ND recognition task, a set of blue squares turned successively into red as in the recall task. But unlike in the latter, the subject

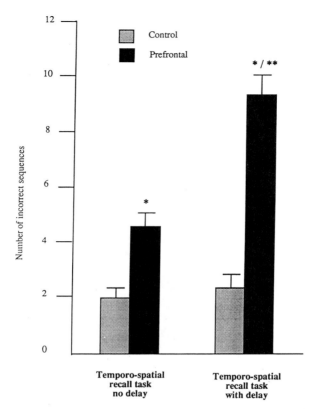

FIGURE 3. Effect of the delay in the temporospatial recall task in controls and patients with DLPFC lesions. Results are expressed as the mean number of incorrect sequences ± standard error. *$p < 0.001$, difference statistically significant when compared with the control group; **$p < 0.001$, difference statistically significant when the performance with delay was compared with the task without delay in the group of the prefrontal patients.

had to indicate, at the response phase, whether a new temporospatial sequence presented immediately after was similar to or different from the previous sequence. The difference between the temporospatial recall task without delay and the ND recognition task was the response modality: in the temporospatial recall task, the subject had to self-program and execute a sequence of motor actions, whereas in the ND recognition task no sequence programming was required. Because patients with DLPFC also exhibited a significant impairment, when compared with controls, in the ND recognition task (FIG. 4) where the motor executive aspect is by-passed, it can be concluded that a programming deficit is insufficient to explain the difficulties encountered by the patients with DLPFC in the temporospatial recall task without delay.

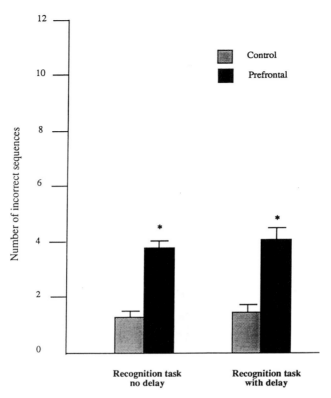

FIGURE 4. Effect of the delay in the temporospatial recognition task in controls and patients with DLPFC lesions. Results are expressed as the mean number of incorrect sequences ± standard error. *$p < 0.001$, difference statistically significant when compared with the control group.

Is This Impairment Also a Result of a Selective Attention Deficit?

The deficit exhibited in the ND recognition task suggests that an isolated executive dysfunction cannot account solely for the impairment observed in the recall task. Since in the ND recognition task programming a complex motor action and maintaining an internal representation in short-term memory are considerably minimalized, the deficit observed could rather result from a dysfunction at an early stage of the information processing, that is, at the stage of the selection of the information to be processed in working memory. Deficits of selective attention following lesions of the frontal lobe have previously been reported in animals and humans.[48–50] Altogether, these studies suggest that one of the functions of the prefrontal cortex is to select the relevant information by inhibiting irrelevant sensory information at their early stages of processing. The specific connectivity of the DLPFC provides a substrate for its effects because it projects in turn to those associative sensory areas from which it receives inputs, for example, the posterior parietal cortex.[51] It may therefore exert a control on the selection of the sensory processing of information via those reciprocal connections. Moreover, the dorsolateral prefrontal cortex is strongly connected with posterior (the posterior parietal cortex and the pulvinar) and anterior (the anterior cingulate cortex, the basal ganglia) networks that are involved in the selective attention processing.[52] Consequently, the disruption of these networks induced by the DLPFC lesion can lead to a selective attention deficit resulting in an inability to select the pertinent information. In agreement with an "encoding hypothesis" is the fact that verbal recall deficits of patients with frontal lobe lesions or dysfunction are dramatically improved when encoding is controlled.[53,54]

Is There a Short-Term Representational Memory Deficit?

First, it may be argued that the deficit in the temporospatial recall task without delay reflects a short-term representational memory deficit as well, given the time needed for the complete presentation of the stimuli, at least for the longest sequences: as each square was presented during two seconds, the presentation phase lasted 12 s for a sequence of six squares. Second, the number of errors in this recall task with delay significantly increased when compared to the task without delay (FIG. 3), in favor of a difficulty in processing the temporospatial components of visual information when this information was out of sight for several seconds and, consequently, had to be held on internal representation. In fact, this additional effect of delay was only observed in the recall tasks, where self-generated responses had to be programmed according to a mental representation of the stimulus maintained in working memory. Indeed, the delay did not worsen the performance of the DLPFC patients in the recognition task (FIG. 4). Thus, the worsening of the performance with delay is only observed when the internal representations held on line need to be manipulated to provide a self-generated pattern of actions. This suggests that (1) the short-term memory factor alone does not account for the additional deficit observed in the temporospatial recall task and (2) the increased deficit in the recall task with delay results in the compounding effect of the delay and a particular response modality. In other words, the deficit increases when the response programming necessitates the manipulation (or monitoring) of complex information held in mental representations. Thus, the critical function of the DLPFC might be to link internal representations to the selection of appropriate goal-directed actions. In contrast, when a simple decision ("similar" or "identical") is required, DLPFC lesions spare the link between this decision-making processing and the internal representations. This interpretation outwardly contradicts the fact that DLPFC lesions in monkeys produce an impairment in matching to sample tasks that are considered as recognition memory tasks. However, it may be argued that matching to sample tasks necessitates a self-generated pattern of response (i.e., to link internal representations to a self-generated decision-making process), whereas in the recognition task used in our study, external clues were given at the response phase. Moreover, lesions in monkeys involved the inferior convexity,[29,30] whereas the vascular damage in our patients spared constantly the most inferior part of the lateral prefrontal cortex. Thus, our study emphasizes that DLPFC is essential for a form of memory focused on actions that necessitates a planned program. It points out the strong link between the short-term storage and the central executive as modeled by the cognitive theory of the working memory system[55] and the role of DLPFC in this linkage as shown by neuropsychological studies in human[56–58] and nonhuman primates.[38,39]

Is the Working Memory Deficit More Dependent on Spatial Modality or on Temporal Components?

In the temporospatial recall task, the visual information presented to the subject had two attributes that could have been remembered in order to provide the correct answer: the spatial and the temporal order components. Does the deficit depend on the monitoring of a specific modality such as the spatial component of the stimulus or rather on the temporal sequencing of this specific information as pro-

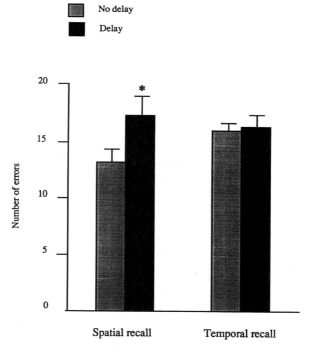

FIGURE 5. Effect of the delay in the spatial and temporal recall tasks in the patients with prefrontal lesions. Results are expressed as the mean number of errors ± standard error. *$p < 0.001$, difference statistically significant when compared with the performance without delay.

posed by Milner[56,58] and Petrides[57]? To answer this question we compared the performance of patients with DLPFC lesions in two other tasks. The first was a spatial recall task, in which, at the presentation phase, squares changed from blue to red simultaneously. At the response phase, the subject had to reproduce the pattern that he saw previously by touching the corresponding squares in any order he wanted (FIG. 2). There was no temporal sequencing in this task either at the presentation or at the response phases. The second task was a temporal recall task in which squares changed sequentially, as in the temporospatial recall task, but unlike in the latter, at the moment of the response, the complete spatial pattern was provided to the subject who only had to program the temporal sequence (FIG. 2). No recall of spatial location of the squares was needed in this task. Although DLPFC patients were impaired in both tasks without delay, the presence of a 10-s delay increased significantly the deficit only in the spatial recall (FIG. 5), suggesting that the working memory for spatial representations is more dependent on the DLPFC than temporal sequencing of visuospatial information. According to the domain-specific processing of the prefrontal cortex found in nonhuman primates,[12,32] our data suggest that DLPFC lesions produce a domain-dependent deficit rather than a temporal-ordering deficit.

To summarize, this study showed that the DLPFC lesions produced a complex working memory deficit based on the disruption of several fundamental processes: (1) an early alteration in the cognitive process needed to discriminate or select the relevant visuospatial information to be held in representational memory; (2) a difficulty in linking and manipulating these internal representations for the planning of a program of action; and (3) a preeminent difficulty in monitoring the spatial component (or more globally the sensory component) within the working memory.

DOES THE WORKING MEMORY DEFICIT ALONE ACCOUNT FOR THE DIFFICULTIES EXHIBITED BY PATIENTS WITH A DLPFC LESION?

A study on delayed alternation conducted in frontal lobe patients showed, however, that lesions of the DLPFC induce finding rule deficits that may not be explained only by a perturbation in holding on line the relevant information.[44] The general procedure was similar to the delayed response task presented previously (FIG. 1), except that in this situation no external cue was present to indicate the correct response; therefore, the patients themselves had to find the rule that governed the reinforcements. When asked to find an alternation rule (win-shift strategy), that is, to choose the square opposite to the one they chose previously, normal controls got the rule and met the criterion of success of 10 successive correct responses with an average number of three errors (FIG. 6). We further analyzed their behavior just after the first trial, which was systematically reinforced no matter which square was chosen by the subject. Interestingly, they tended to choose the same square again—that is, not to alternate—because their first choice was reinforced (unpublished data). This sorting process is a cognitive behavior, which explains why normal controls do not catch on to the alternation rule right away and require additional trials before alternating. In fact, they de-

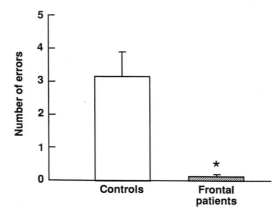

FIGURE 6. Performance of control subjects and patients with frontal lesions on the delayed alternation task. Results are expressed as the number of errors made before reaching the criterion of 10 successive correct responses.

duced the rule by means of an adaptive process, taking into account feedback from the environment, that is, the nature of the reinforcement of their last response. And indeed, the percentage of control subjects that achieved the criterion of 10 successive correct responses increased progressively during the successive trials. In the same task, the performance of patients with DLPFC was unexpected because they made significantly fewer errors (0.1 ± 0.3) than controls and patients with post-central lesions. They alternated spontaneously and their performance may be considered, at first glance, as better because they immediately found the alternation rule. In fact, a detailed analysis of performance of DLPFC patients may give some clues to their behavior (FIG. 7). They expressed the rule spontaneously from the first trial rather than deducing the rule by a learning process

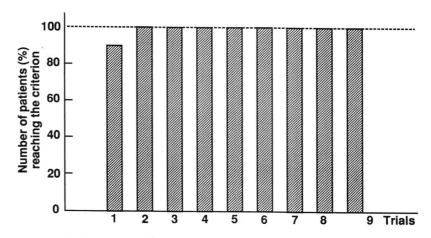

FIGURE 7. Performance of patients with frontal lobe lesions on the delayed alternation task. Results are expressed as the number of patients (%) reaching the criterion of 10 consecutive correct responses in the course of successive trials.

based on the distribution of reinforcement, as normal controls did. This tendency to alternate was opposite to the spontaneous win-stay strategy exhibited by the controls and may be considered as an abnormal schema of response. Despite this apparently good performance in the delayed-alternation task, the emergence of such a stereotyped program cannot be considered as a behavioral gain, because it overshadows the normal cognitive process leading to environmental adaptation. In contrast to normal controls, the DLPFC patients tended to maintain alternation despite changes in environmental clues, that is, when a nonalternation rule (win-stay strategy) and reversal (transfer to the other side) strategy were required. The rule-finding deficit in frontal lobe patients seems to result from the previous pattern of response as shown by their low performance on the reversal task, in which there is no rule to be elaborated.

To which processes does this spontaneous pattern of alternation correspond? Luria has already reported, clinically, automatisms in frontal lobe patients that he described as "an inability to suppress involuntarily emerging inert stereotypes."[59] Closer to our view is the statement of Fuster for whom "the frontal patient, like the frontal animal, tends to repeat old patterns of behavior even in circumstances that demand change. Repetitious routine seems to preempt what under those circumstances would be more adaptative behavior."[13]

Why alternation? A tendency to alternate after lesions of the frontal cortex was unexpected, given experimental results which invariably demonstrated a deficit in finding alternation in lesioned nonhuman primates. The major problem concerns the significance of this spontaneous tendency after lesions of the frontal cortex in humans: it may result from a utilization behavior that pushes frontal patients into using all the environmental clues; alternatively, it may be the expression of an inherent program that would correspond to a rule by default—that is, a basic process to which the cognitive experience may apply. According to this latter hypothesis, alternation might be a phylogenetic residue of an archaic behavior based on the search for novelty or exploration, which consequently imposes avoiding the last visited square. Accordingly, it may be proposed that the major function of the prefrontal cortex in humans is to inhibit old patterns of behavior and to allow elaboration of goal-related activities, based on cognitive experience (i.e., sorting behavior) and guided by feedback, which lead to environmental adaptation. These observations suggest that, besides working memory, rule-finding ability, which requires the inhibition of more automatic or archaic activities, might be another fundamental process under the control of the frontal lobes. Incidentally, the ability of frontal patients to perform a complete series of 10 successive correct alternating responses implies that they could keep their last response in mind during the delay, in contradiction to their poor DR performance, as if the working memory deficit applies for an externally driven task, but not in a situation where a spontaneous pattern of response is expressed.

As already mentioned, patients with prefrontal lesion tend to maintain a spontaneous tendency to alternate even when the distribution of reinforcements has changed and when they have to find a nonalternation rule. The persistency of alternation despite changes in environmental clues demonstrates the strength of this spontaneous behavior and the difficulty of inhibiting an already established mental set. Although feedback from the environment seems to be perceived by the patients ("Each time I choose this side I win, but every time I choose the other side I lose"), it remains inoperative as if frontal lobe dysfunction disrupted the level of integration needed for coupling the analysis of the specific requirements of the situation and the selection of the appropriate response. This knowing/doing dissociation has already been described,[6,60] but it underscores one function of the prefrontal cortex, mainly the orbitofrontal part, in stimulus-reinforcement learning and emotional responses to objects.[61] In a recent study in humans, Rolls and colleagues[62] found the same tendency in patients with damage to the ventral part of the frontal lobes to perseverate on the previously rewarded stimulus suggesting that dysfunction of the prefrontal cortex induces difficulty in modifying responses even when followed by negative consequences.

Our results revealed two closely related processes in patients with prefrontal lesions: (1) In these patients, feedback remains inoperative as if the frontal lobe dysfunction disrupted the level of integration needed for coupling the analysis of the specific requirements of the situation on the one hand, and the selection of the appropriate response on the other hand. (2) In these patients, the rule-finding process is disrupted because of the emergence of noncognitive and rigid patterns of behavior. The emergence of stereotyped programs of response and the inadequacy of feedback integration, which consequently entertains ongoing sets, overshadows the heuristic processes leading to environmental adaptation exhibited by both control subjects and patients with post-central lesions whose behavior is guided by reinforcement. These two behavioral consequences of prefrontal lesions, the emergence of elementary patterns of behavior and the predominance of previously acquired sets, are in agreement with the model developed by Shallice,[10] according to which behavioral schemas are dependent on two different systems of activation—the supervisory attentional system (SAS), postulated to be controlled by the prefrontal cortex, and the contention scheduling system (CS). When the prefrontal cortex is damaged, we may postulate that the SAS would become inoperative and that the CS would continue to function. In new situations, the CS would activate either (1) a behavioral schema that has become predominant, as seen in the alternation task, or (2) the last dominant schema, as in the nonalternation and reversal tasks. The fact that patients with striatal lesions (Huntington's disease) or with striatal dysfunction (Parkinson's disease) do not express this spontaneous tendency to alternate, although they share the same difficulty as patients with frontal lesions in learning new rules,[63] strongly suggests that the basal ganglia may be part of the anatomical substrate for pre-elaborated, overlearned or automatic routine programs that might be under an inhibiting control of the frontal cortex. Thus, in contrast with Rosvold's proposition[64] that both frontal and caudate nucleus are part of the same anatomofunctional system (the "frontal system"), suggesting that lesions located in different parts of the system may produce similar behavioral disturbances, studies in humans rather favor the hypothesis of a cooperation between the two structures at different levels of behavioral organization. It is noteworthy that both the cognitive model[10] and experimental studies are convergent to support the concept of two levels of organization, one implicated in more automatic conducts and the other being solicited when challenging situations require the elaboration of a new pattern of response.

In conclusion, the specific connectivity of the prefrontal cortex and the electrophysiological properties of its neuronal components account for the complex and multiple role of this structure in higher behavioral functions as shown by our results. Indeed, the functions of DLPFC extend further than only the short-term storage of internal representations because DLPFC also participates in the encoding of the sensory information to be maintained in short-term memory, and it intervenes in the binding of the mental representations with a specific self-generated response set. It may also be involved in the adequate understanding of the general context needed for rule finding which is the prerequisite for working memory operations to be in harmony with environmental demands.

Thus, in accordance with concepts in nonhuman primate model,[12,13] our results confirm that the dorsal part of the prefrontal cortex is a central node for the working memory function in humans, because it provides the dynamic ability to disrupt automatic stimulus-response cycles, by creating a temporal buffer between the sensory and motor systems in which information is manipulated and confronted with past experiences for elaboration of a goal-oriented ongoing schema of response.

The importance of this function, which is characteristic of the most developed species (primates and humans *a fortiori*), has to be compared with the concomitant growth of the prefrontal cortex in the course of phylogenetic evolution. And indeed, available data in rodents, in which the prefrontal cortex is "embryonic," suggest that this working memory function is organized within a network involving mainly the hippocampus.[65] It seems likely that, in the course of the evolution, there is a progressive transfer of working memory function toward the prefrontal cortex explaining the significant growth of this structure in higher-ordered species together with the development, in parallel, of more complex adaptive behaviors. This "working memory hypothesis" can account for the evolutionary and functional dynamic of the frontal lobes.

ACKNOWLEDGMENTS

We thank Patricia Goldman-Rakic and Jordan Grafman for their helpful comments in the preparation of the manuscript.

REFERENCES

1. ESLINGER, P. J. & L. M. GRATTAN. 1993. Frontal lobe and fronto-striatal substrates for different form of human cognitive flexibility. Neuropsychologia 31: 17–28.
2. SAVER, J. L. & A. R. DAMASIO. 1991. Preserved access and processing of social knowledge in a patient with acquired sociopathy due to ventromedial frontal damage. Neuropsychologia 29: 1241–1249.
3. FULTON, J. F. 1951. Frontal Lobotomy and Affective Behavior. Norton. New York.
4. DAMASIO, A. R. & G. W. VAN HOESEN. 1983. Emotional disturbance associated with focal lesions of the limbic frontal lobe. *In* Neuropsychology of Human Emotion. K. M. Heilman & P. Satz, Eds.: 85–110. Guilford Press. New York.
5. LURIA, A. R. 1970. Traumatic Aphasia. Mouton. The Hague.
6. MILNER, B. 1964. Some effects of frontal lobectomy in man. *In* The Frontal Granular

Cortex and Behaviour. J. M. Warren & K. Akert, Eds.: 313–334. McGraw-Hill. New York.

7. HECAEN, H. & M. L. ALBERT. 1978. Human Neuropsychology. John Wiley and Sons. New York.

8. STUSS, D. T., E. F. KAPLAN, D. F. BENSON, W. S. WEIR, S. CHIULLI & F. F. SARAZIN. 1982. Evidence for the involvement of the orbito-frontal cortex in memory functions: An interference effect. J. Comp. Physiol. Psychol. **96:** 913–925.

9. MILNER, B., M. PETRIDES & M. L. SMITH. 1985. Frontal lobes and temporal organisation of memory. Hum. Neurobiol. **4:** 137–142.

10. SHALLICE, T. 1982. Specific impairments in planning. Philos. Trans. R. Soc. Lond. B. Biol. Sci. **298:** 199–209.

11. STUSS, D. T. & D. F. BENSON. 1986. Memory. *In* The Frontal Lobes. Raven Press. New York.

12. GOLDMAN-RAKIC, P. S. 1987. Circuitry of primate prefrontal cortex and regulation of behaviour by representational memory. *In* Handbook of Physiology. F. Plum & V. Mountcastle, Eds. Vol. 5: 373–17. The American Physiological Society. Washington, D.C.

13. FUSTER, J. M. 1989. The Prefrontal Cortex. 2nd edit. Raven Press. New York.

14. JACOBSEN, C. F. 1936. Studies of cerebral function in primates. Comp. Psychol. Monogr. **13:** 1–68.

15. BUTTERS, N. & D. PANDYA. 1969. Retention of delayed-alternation: Effect of selective lesion of sulcus principalis. Science **165:** 1271–1273.

16. STAMM, J. S. & S. C. ROSEN. 1969. Electrical stimulation and steady potential shifts in prefrontal cortex during delayed response performance by monkeys. Acta Biol. Exp. **29:** 385–399.

17. GOLDMAN, P. S., H. E. ROSVOLD, B. VEST & T. W. GALKIN. 1971. Analysis of the delayed-alternation deficit produced by dorsolateral prefrontal lesions in the rhesus monkey. J. Comp. Physiol. Psychol. **77:** 212–220.

18. KUBOTA, K. & H. NIKKI. 1971. Prefrontal cortical unit activity and delayed cortical unit activity and delayed alternation performance in monkeys. J. Neurophysiol. **34:** 337–347.

19. FUSTER, J. M. 1973. Unit activity in prefrontal cortex during delayed-response performance: Neuronal correlates of transient memory. J. Neurophysiol. **36:** 61–78.

20. FUSTER, J. M. & R. H. BAUER. 1974. Visual short-term memory deficit from hypothermia of frontal cortex. Brain Res. **81:** 393–400.

21. KOJIMA, S. & P. S. GOLDMAN-RAKIC. 1982. Delay-related activity of prefrontal neurons in rhesus monkeys performing delayed response. Brain Res. **248:** 43–49.

22. FUNAHASHI, S., C. J. BRUCE & P. S. GOLDMAN-RAKIC. 1993. Dorsolateral prefrontal lesions and oculomotor delayed response performance: Evidence for mnemonic "scotomas." J. Neurosci. **13:** 1479–1497.

23. JONIDES, J., E. E. SMITH, R. A. KOEPPE, E. AWH, S. MINOSHIMA & M. A. MINTUN. 1993. Spatial working memory in humans as revealed by PET. Nature **363:** 623–625.

24. PETRIDES, M., B. ALIVISATOS, A. EVANS & E. MEYER. 1993. Dissociation of human mid-dorsolateral from posterior dorsolateral frontal cortex in memory processing. Proc. Natl. Acad. Sci. USA **90:** 873–877.

25. MCCARTHY, G., A. M. BLAMIRE, A. PUCE, A. C. NOBRE, G. BLOCH, F. HYDER, P. S. GOLDMAN-RAKIC & R. G. SHULMAN. 1994. Functional magnetic resonance imaging of human prefrontal cortex activation during a spatial working memory task. Proc. Natl. Acad. Sci. USA **91:** 8690–8694.

26. SWARTZ, B. E., E. HALGREN, J. M. FUSTER & M. MANDELKERN. 1994. An [18]FDG-PET study of cortical activation during a short-term visual memory task in humans. Neuroreport **5:** 925–928.

27. MISHKIN, M. 1957. Effects of small frontal lesions on delayed alternation in monkeys. J. Neurophysiol. **20:** 615–622.

28. PASSINGHAM, R. 1975. Delayed matching after selective prefrontal cortex lesions in monkeys (*Macaca mulatta*). Brain Res. **92:** 89–102.

29. MISHKIN, M. & F. J. MANNING. 1978. Non-spatial memory after selective prefrontal lesions in monkeys. Brain Res. **143**: 313–323.
30. BACHEVALIER, J. & M. MISHKIN. 1986. Visual recognition impairment follows ventromedial but not dorsolateral prefrontal lesions in monkeys. Behav. Brain Res. **20**: 249–261.
31. FUNAHASHI, S., C. J. BRUCE & P. S. GOLDMAN-RAKIC. 1986. Perimetry of spatial representation in primate prefrontal cortex: Evidence for a mnemonic hemianopia. Soc. Neurosci. Abstr. **12**: 554.
32. WILSON, F. A. W., S. P. O'SCALHAIDE & P. S. GOLDMAN-RAKIC. 1993. Dissociation of object and spatial processing domains in primate prefrontal cortex. Science **260**: 1955–1958.
33. PANDYA, D. N. & D. L. BARNES. 1987. Architecture and connections of the frontal lobe. *In* The Frontal Lobes Revisited. E. Perecman, Ed.: 41–72. IBRN Press. New York.
34. DESIMONE, R. & L. G. UNGERLEIDER. 1989. Neural mechanisms of visual processing in monkeys. *In* Handbook of Neuropsychology. F. Boller & J. Grafman, Eds. Vol. 7: 267–299. Elsevier Science Publishers. Amsterdam.
35. NIKKI, H. & M. WATANABE. 1976. Prefrontal unit activity and delayed response: Relation to cue location versus direction of response. Brain Res. **105**: 79–88.
36. FUSTER, J. M., R. H. BAUER & J. P. JERVEY. 1982. Cellular discharge in the dorsolateral prefrontal cortex during a discrimination task with delay. Exp. Neurol. **77**: 679–694.
37. QUINTANA, J., J. M. FUSTER & J. YAJEYA. 1989. Effects of cooling parietal cortex on prefrontal units in delay tasks. Brain Res. **503**: 100–110.
38. PETRIDES, M. 1988. Performance on a nonspatial self-ordered task after selective lesions of the primate frontal cortex. Soc. Neurosci. Abstr. **14**: 2.
39. PETRIDES, M. 1995. Impairments on nonspatial self-ordered and externally ordered working memory tasks after lesions of the mid-dorsal part of the lateral frontal cortex in the monkey. J. Neurosci. **15**: 359–375.
40. BAUER, R. H. & J. M. FUSTER. 1976. Delayed-matching and delayed-response deficit from cooling dorsolateral prefrontal cortex in monkeys. J. Comp. Physiol. Psychol. **90**: 293–302.
41. QUINTANA, J. & J. M. FUSTER. 1993. Spatial and temporal factors in the role of prefrontal and parietal cortex in visuomotor integration. Cereb. Cortex **3**: 122–132.
42. CHOROVER, S. L. & M. COLE. 1966. Delayed alternation performance in patients with cerebral lesions. Neuropsychologia **4**: 1–7.
43. FREEDMAN, M. & M. OSCAR-BERMAN. 1986. Bilateral frontal lobe disease and selective delayed-response deficits in humans. Behav. Neurosci. **100**: 337–342.
44. VÉRIN, M., A. PARTIOT, B. PILLON, C. MALAPANI, Y. AGID & B. DUBOIS. 1993. Delayed response tasks and prefrontal lesions in man—Evidence for self-generated patterns of behaviour with poor environmental modulation. Neuropsychologia **31**: 1379–1396.
45. TEIXEIRA, C., M. VÉRIN, R. LEVY, B. PILLON, Y. AGID & B. DUBOIS. Effects of prefrontal lesions and fronto-striatal dysfunction on temporo-spatial working memory tasks in man. In preparation.
46. SQUIRE, L. R. 1989. Prefrontal cortex. *In* Memory and Brain. Oxford University Press. Oxford, UK.
47. PETRIDES, M. & B. MILNER. 1982. Deficits of subject-ordered tasks after frontal- and temporal-lobe lesions in man. Neuropsychologia **20**: 249–262.
48. SKINNER, J. E. & C. D. YINGLING. 1977. Central gating mechanisms that regulate event-related potentials and behavior. *In* Progress in Clinical Neurophysiology. J. E. Desmet, Ed. Vol. 1: 30–69. S. Karger. Basel.
49. KNIGHT, R. T., D. SCABINI & D. L. WOODS. 1989. Prefrontal cortex gating of auditory transmission in human. Brain Res. **504**: 338–342.
50. KNIGHT, R. T. 1994. Attention regulation and human prefrontal cortex. *In* Motor and Cognitive Functions of the Prefrontal Cortex. A. M. Thierry, P. S. Goldman-Rakic & Y. Christen, Eds. Springer-Verlag. Heidelberg.
51. CAVADA, C. & P. S. GOLDMAN-RAKIC. 1989. Posterior parietal cortex in rhesus monkey.

II. Evidence for segregated cortico-cortical networks linking sensory and limbic areas with the frontal lobe. J. Comp. Neurol. **287**: 422–445.

52. POSNER, M. I. & S. DEHAENE. 1994. Attentional networks. Trends Neurosci. **17**: 75–79.
53. INCISA DELLA ROCHETTA, A. & B. MILNER. 1993. Strategic search and retrieval inhibition: The role of the frontal lobes. Neuropsychologia **31**: 503–524.
54. PILLON, B., B. DEWEER, A. MICHON, C. MALAPANI, Y. AGID & B. DUBOIS. 1994. Are explicit memory disorders of progressive supranuclear palsy related to damage to striato-frontal circuits? Comparison with Alzheimer's and Huntington's disease. Neurology **44**: 1264–1270.
55. BADDELEY, A. 1986. Working memory. Clarendon Press. Oxford, UK.
56. MILNER, B. 1982. Some cognitive effects of frontal lobe lesions in man. Philos. Trans. R. Soc. Lond. Biol. Sci. **298**: 211–226.
57. PETRIDES, M. 1986. The effect of periarcuate lesions in the monkey on the performance of symmetrically and asymmetrically reinforced visual and auditory go, no-go tasks. J. Neurosci. **6**: 2054–2063.
58. MCANDREWS, M. P. & B. MILNER. 1991. The frontal cortex and memory for temporal order. Neuropsychologia **29**: 849–859.
59. LURIA, A. R. 1973. The frontal lobes and the regulation of behaviour. *In* Psychophysiology of the Frontal Lobes. K. H. Pibram & A. R. Luria, Eds.: 3–26. Academic Press. New York.
60. LURIA, A. R. & E. D. HOMSKAYA. 1964. Disturbances in the regulative role of speech with frontal lobe lesion. *In* The Frontal Granular Cortex and Behavior. J. M. Warren & K. Akert, Eds.: 353–371. McGraw-Hill. New York.
61. ROLLS, E. T. 1990. A theory of emotion, and its application to understanding the neuronal basis of emotion. Cognition & Emotion **4**: 161–190.
62. ROLLS, E. T., J. HORNAK, D. WADE & J. MCGRATH. 1994. Emotion-related learning in patients with social and emotional changes associated with frontal lobe damage. J. Neurol. Neurosurg. Psychiatry **57**: 1518–1524.
63. PARTIOT, A., M. VERIN, B. PILLON, C. TEIXEIRA, Y. AGID & B. DUBOIS. Delayed response tasks and basal ganglia lesions in man. Neuropsychologia In press.
64. ROSVOLD, H. E. & M. K. SWARCBART. 1964. Neural structures involved in delayed-response performance. *In* Frontal Granular Cortex and Behavior. J. M. Warren & K. Akert, Eds. McGraw-Hill. New York.
65. OLTON, D. S., J. J. BECKER & G. E. HEDELMANN. 1979. Hippocampus, space and memory. Behav. Brain Sci. **2**: 313–365.

Procedural Learning and Prefrontal Cortex

ALVARO PASCUAL-LEONE,[a,b] JORDAN GRAFMAN,[c]
AND MARK HALLETT[d]

[a]Instituto Ramón y Cajal
Consejo Superior de Investigaciones Científicas
and
Department of Physiology
University of Valencia
Valencia, Spain
[c]Cognitive Neuroscience Section
[d]Human Motor Control Section
National Institute of Neurological Disorders and Stroke
National Institutes of Health
Bethesda, Maryland 20892

Knowledge can be developed or expressed in various ways. Several pairings of concepts, for example, procedural versus declarative or implicit versus explicit, have been coined which are not mutually exclusive and require some clarification. *Procedural* knowledge is generally used to refer to a form of knowledge which can be measured by tasks in which memory is expressed by changes in performance as a result of prior experience. Procedural knowledge has been applied particularly to the acquisition of actions, habits, and skills. *Declarative* knowledge refers to the acquisition of facts and the deliberate recollection of information that is bound to a specific time and context. *Explicit* and *implicit* knowledge refer to whether or not the subject has a conscious awareness of the exposure to a task or information that eventually results in an improved performance. Therefore, procedural and declarative learning can be explicit or implicit. For example, on repeated testing, a subject may demonstrate improved performance on a task without consciously recalling being exposed to that task before. This would be a case of procedural-implicit knowledge. On the other hand, a subject may deliberately aim at improving performance in a task by repeated exposure to it, a case of procedural-explicit knowledge. Therefore, *procedural learning* may be used to refer to the process by which repeated exposure to a task, regardless of whether the subject does or does not form a conscious memory of this exposure, eventually results in improved performance on that task.

SERIAL REACTION TIME TEST

The serial reaction time test (SRTT)[1,2] is a task that allows the study of procedural-implicit and procedural-explicit learning. The subject sits in front of a com-

[b] Address correspondence to Prof. Dr. Alvaro Pascual-Leone, Departamento de Fisiología, Universidad de Valencia, Avda. Blasco Ibañez, 17, Valencia, 46010 Spain.

puter screen at eye level behind a response pad with four buttons numbered 1 to 4. The subject is instructed to push each button with a different finger of the right or left hand (index finger for button 1, middle finger for button 2, ring finger for button 3, and little finger for button 4). The "go" signal consists, for example, of an asterisk displayed on the screen aligned with the correct response button. Alternatively, the go signal may consist of a number (1, 2, 3, or 4) displayed in the middle of the screen corresponding to the numbered response buttons. In any case, upon appearance of the go signal, the subject has to push the appropriate response button as fast as possible with the appropriate finger. Response time (RT) is then measured from the go signal until the button press. When the correct response button is pushed, the go signal disappears and the next go signal appears 500 ms later. If an incorrect button is pushed, the go signal remains on until the subject makes the correct response.

The SRTT is performed in blocks of trials. In each block, the go signals might be presented in a random order (practice or control blocks of trials) or they might represent a sequence of cues whose order is repeated 10 times in each block of trials. However, in the latter case (repeating sequence), the subjects are not told about this repeating sequence. We have typically used blocks of 100 or 120 trials and repeating sequences of 10 or 12 cues, respectively.

Initially, during the SRTT, the subject exposed to blocks with a repeating sequence is unaware of the presence of such an order to the trials. Therefore, the learning that might take place is implicit. Eventually, after a variable number of blocks, the subject becomes aware of the repeating sequence although he or she does not know the exact structure of the sequence. At this point, we might assume that both implicit and explicit learning strategies are used. Finally, the subject achieves complete knowledge of the sequence, is able to reproduce it, and thus the learning becomes explicit. Thereafter, the subject's performance continues to improve, but the subject's strategy changes and he or she no longer reacts to the visual cues but rather anticipates them.

We have used this task to study the role of different neural structures in the acquisition of procedural knowledge and the correlates of the transition of implicit to explicit learning.

MODULATION OF CORTICAL MOTOR OUTPUTS DURING PROCEDURAL LEARNING

Acquisition of a new motor skill requires the adaptation of executive neural structures to the demands of the task. Cortical motor outputs to the muscles involved in the performance of the skill might need to be modulated to accommodate the new ability. The development of noninvasive neurophysiological techniques allows the study of these plastic phenomena in intact humans. We used serial cortical mapping with transcranial magnetic stimulation (TMS) to study the changes in cortical motor outputs associated with learning.[3] For example, we have shown that learning to perform a five-finger exercise on the piano is associated with a decrease in motor threshold and an increase in the area of cortical motor output to the finger flexors and extensors of the trained hand.[4] The same technique of TMS mapping might be used to explore the effects on cortical motor outputs of the development of implicit knowledge and of the transition of implicit to explicit knowledge in the SRTT.

At the beginning of the experiment,[5] we used focal TMS to map the cortical outputs to different muscles involved in the task. Keeping the stimulation intensity and the scalp positions constant, we repeated TMS mapping after every two blocks of SRTT. Therefore, we were able to compare performance of the task with the modulation of the cortical outputs to the muscles involved in the task. During the SRTT, the subjects exposed to blocks of trials with a repeating sequence of cues showed progressively shorter RTs and progressively larger maps of cortical outputs to the muscles involved in the task. This enlargement of the cortical output maps continued up to the time at which subjects achieved complete explicit knowledge of the repeating sequence. Thereafter, the maps rapidly went back to their baseline topography despite continued shortening of the RTs. Thus, a progressive improvement in RT during implicit learning is correlated with an enlargement in the maps of cortical motor outputs to the muscles involved in the task. On the other hand, the development of explicit knowledge and the resulting change in the subject's strategy (anticipation of the cue instead of reaction to it) is associated with a new modulation of the cortical motor outputs and possibly a shift in neural structures that assume the more active role in the execution of the task (FIG. 1).[5,6]

In another experiment,[7] we studied the intermanual transfer of implicit knowledge of sequential finger movements using a variation of the SRTT. In the first four blocks of trials, subjects had to press the appropriate response key to single visual cues using only one hand while not knowing that the cues appeared in a repeating sequence. Implicit learning was indicated by the shortening of RT in the absence of conscious awareness of the repeating sequence of visual cues. In blocks 5–8 all subjects had to use the other hand, and the order of the cues was changed into a random presentation (group 1), a completely new sequence (group 2), the parallel image (group 3), or the mirror image of the original sequence (group 4). In groups 1, 2, and 3, the hand switch resulted in increased RT during block 5 comparable to those observed in block 1. This result indicated a lack of intermanual transfer of knowledge. In group 4, the hand switch produced only a transient "plateau" in RT which then continued to shorten. Thus, intermanual transfer of implicit knowledge for sequential finger movements takes place only if the sequence practiced by the second hand is a mirror image of the sequence practiced by the first hand. These findings have significant implications in regard to the mode in which new procedural implicit knowledge is stored and thus is amenable to intermanual transfer.

Theoretically, sequences of finger movements can be stored primarily as *spatial coordinates of movements* or as *motor output patterns*. The information stored might reflect primarily the sequence of movements to be performed according to the sequence of targets in space and the sequence of changes in direction—that is, independent of which body parts perform each individual movement. Alternatively, the primary form of information stored might represent the sequence of body parts involved in the performance of a movement sequence without particular information about spatial location of targets or sequence of changes in movement direction. The fact that intermanual transfer of implicit knowledge is limited to the mirror version of the original sequence suggests that the knowledge was

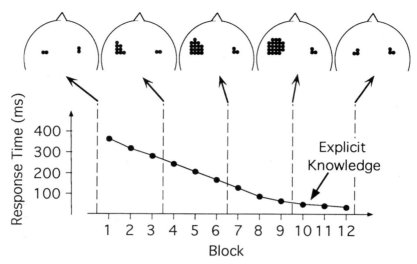

FIGURE 1. Modulation of motor cortical outputs in the course of procedural learning in the serial reaction time test (SRTT) when performing with the right hand. The graph shows the median response time in each block of the SRTT in a representative subject. The schematic representations of the head plot in form of a bubble diagram the number of scalp positions which, when stimulated with focal transcranial magnetic stimulation (TMS; single pulse, 110% of subject's baseline motor threshold intensity), evoke motor potentials in the contralateral forearm finger flexors of ≥60% of the subject's maximal baseline amplitude. Several TMS maps are shown for different time points during the SRTT. Note the increasing size of the cortical motor output maps to the forearm finger flexor muscle of the hand used in the task during the first several blocks of the SRTT and the rapid return to baseline following development of complete explicit knowledge of the sequence. For details see refs. 5 and 6.

coded in this latter fashion—that is, by motor output patterns. Therefore, when the homologous fingers have to be activated in the same order, the subject is at an advantage (mirror version). This advantage is lost when the fingers to be activated are different even though the spatial characteristics of the movements to be performed are held constant (parallel version). In this setting it is probably critical that the knowledge of the original sequence remained implicit. The transition of implicit to explicit knowledge is associated with a change in the strategy used by the subjects to complete the task and with a change in the pattern of motor cortical activation. It is likely that as complete explicit knowledge of the sequence is achieved brain structures other than the motor cortex assume more active roles in the execution of the task. We could hypothesize that, during the procedural acquisition of implicit knowledge, the new skill is principally *motor-output coded* and is stored in the form of plastic changes in the sensorimotor cortex. As the knowledge becomes explicit, other brain structures become involved in the learning process which may then become primarily *perceptually coded*.

In any case, our results show the important role of the modulation of cortical outputs during procedural learning, but they also raise a number of questions. The level of activation and thus the functional organization of motor cortical outputs are influenced by their rich connections to other neural structures—for example, basal ganglia, cerebellum, and prefrontal cortex. We might ask how these structures contribute to procedural learning and the associated modulation of cortical motor outputs.

ROLE OF THE BASAL GANGLIA IN PROCEDURAL LEARNING

Several studies have shown impairment of procedural learning in the presence of preserved declarative learning in patients with Huntington's disease,[8] patients with progressive supranuclear palsy,[9] and patients with Parkinson's disease (PD).[10–12] Using the SRTT, we have shown that patients with PD achieved procedural knowledge and used declarative knowledge of the task to improve performance, but required a larger number of repetitions of the task to develop explicit knowledge of the repeating sequence than normal subjects (Fig. 2).[13] This abnormality is only partially reverted with L-dopa treatment.

It might be argued that the necessary "energizing" influence of the basal ganglia on the prefrontal cortex is deficient in PD, thus accounting for abnormally slow access of information to and from "working memory" buffers. This would explain the greater difficulties of PD patients in procedural learning of longer repeating sequences and the need for a greater number of repetitions than normal to achieve explicit knowledge through motor performance.

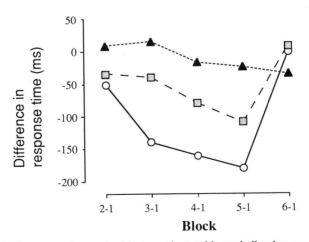

FIGURE 2. Performance of normal subjects, patients with cerebellar degeneration, and patients with Parkinson's disease in the serial reaction time test. Results represent the mean of 10 subjects in each group. Performance is expressed as difference between median response time in block 1 (random) and the rest of the blocks of trials in order to normalize for baseline motor performance impairments in the patient groups. For details see ref. 13. *Triangles*, cerebellar degeneration; *squares*, Parkinson's disease; *open circles*, normal.

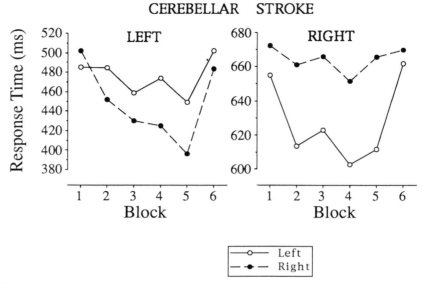

FIGURE 3. Representative results of the performance in the serial reaction time test (SRTT) of two patients with focal, hemispheric ischemic lesions of one cerebellar hemisphere. Results are given for performance with the right and left hand. The SRTT consists of 6 blocks of 100 trials. Blocks 1 and 6 are random, whereas blocks 2 to 5 consist of a repeating sequence of 10 trials. Note the differential impairment of performance with left versus right hand depending of the side of the cerebellar lesion. These results were obtained in collaboration with Dr. A. Sirigu and are presented here with her permission.

ROLE OF THE CEREBELLUM IN PROCEDURAL LEARNING

Selective impairment of procedural learning has also been reported in patients with cerebellar dysfunction.[14] In patients with cerebellar cortical degeneration, the SRTT reveals a profound alteration in procedural learning.[13] These patients do not show any significant performance improvement over the course of five blocks of trials (FIG. 2), fail to achieve explicit knowledge of the repeating sequence, and show only limited use of declarative knowledge of the task to improve their performance.

This deficient performance improvement (procedural knowledge) is linked to the absence of the normal modulation of motor cortical outputs to the muscles involved in the task.[15] Although the interpretation of these findings is difficult, it might be argued that an intact cerebello-cortical interaction is required to induce the plastic changes normally associated with procedural learning in the SRTT (FIG. 1).

Recently, we have had the opportunity to study several patients with focal, lateralized lesions of the cerebellar hemisphere (in collaboration with Dr. Angela Sirigu, INSERM, Paris). Preliminary results suggest that lesions in the right cerebellar hemisphere lead to impaired procedural learning in the SRTT only with the right hand, whereas lesions in the left cerebellar hemisphere impair selectively the performance improvement with the left hand (FIG. 3).

In the SRTT, the cerebellum may be required to provide a time index to the events and be therefore essential for the development of procedural knowledge. It appears that the role of the cerebellum is lateralized and selective for procedural learning with the hand ipsilateral to each cerebellar hemisphere. This raises the possibility that crossed connections between cerebellum and prefrontal cortex are critical in the role of the cerebellum in this form of learning.

ROLE OF THE PREFRONTAL CORTEX IN PROCEDURAL LEARNING

As we have briefly reviewed, procedural learning requires the normal function of cerebellar and basal ganglia structures[13] which are richly connected with the dorsolateral prefrontal cortex.[16–18] This suggests the hypothesis that the dorsolateral prefrontal cortex might be an essential component of the neural network responsible for procedural learning. We might argue that the integration of basal ganglia and cerebellar contributions takes place in prefrontal structures that provide the critical aspect of sequencing events in time, bridging temporal contingencies between individual trials, and thus provides the subject with the basis for recognizing the sequential nature of the task.

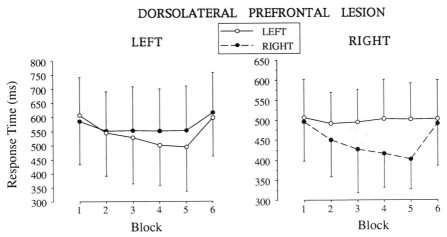

FIGURE 4. Representative results of the performance in the serial reaction time test (SRTT) of two patients with post-traumatic lesions of the dorsolateral prefrontal cortex. The two subjects had strictly unilateral, right- or left-sided lesions centered around area 46. Results are given for performance with the right and left hand. The SRTT consists of 6 blocks of 100 trials. Blocks 1 and 6 are random, whereas blocks 2 to 5 consist of a repeating sequence of 10 trials. Note the differential impairment of performance with left versus right hand depending of the side of the prefrontal cortical lesion.

Patients with post-traumatic brain lesions in the dorsolateral prefrontal cortex show abnormal performance in the SRTT. Patients with left-sided lesions do not show the expected performance improvement in the SRTT when using the right hand for the task. Conversely, right-sided prefrontal lesions result in deficient procedural learning when performing the SRTT with the left hand (FIG. 4). These lateralized effects of prefrontal lesions on procedural learning with the contralateral hand are consistent with the notion of the critical role of crossed cerebellar-prefrontal connections for the development of procedural knowledge in the SRTT.

The role of the prefrontal cortex in procedural learning can be further studied in normal volunteers using noninvasive neurophysiological techniques. Repetitive TMS, at frequencies of up to 30 Hz, allows the transient disruption of the function of a cortical area and thus produces an "experimental transient lesion."[3,19] In our experimental design, subjects performed five blocks of the SRTT (four with a repeating sequence of cues and the fifth with a random presentation of cues) in the absence of repetitive TMS and while TMS was being applied focally to the right or left dorsolateral prefrontal cortex. The stimulation coil was centered on the lateral convexity, 5 cm rostral to the optimal scalp position for the abductor pollicis brevis muscle. Stimulation was applied in trains of 5 Hz and 115% of the subject's motor threshold intensity. The stimulation trains started at the beginning of each block of trials and continued for a maximum of 60 s according to current safety guidelines.[20] In all cases, this was sufficient to assure stimulation from the beginning until completion of the block.

Repetitive TMS had profound lateralized effects on performance improvement.

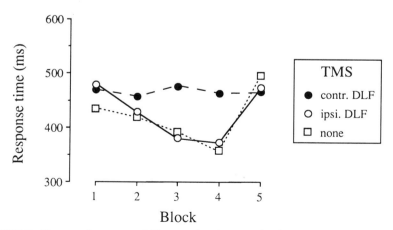

FIGURE 5. Mean performance of 10 normal volunteers in the serial reaction time test (SRTT) depending on whether or not repetitive transcranial magnetic stimulation (TMS) was being applied to the dorsolateral prefrontal cortex (DLF). The SRTT consisted of 5 blocks of 100 trials. Blocks 1 to 4 presented 10 repetitions of a 10-item sequence, whereas block 5 presented randomly appearing visual cues. Note the lack of performance improvement during contralateral dorsolateral prefrontal cortex stimulation. See text for details.

Stimulation of the dorsolateral prefrontal cortex led to an apparent block of procedural learning when performing with the contralateral hand (FIG. 5). Subjects tended to feel that performance was more difficult during stimulation to the contralateral dorsolateral frontal cortex. However, despite this subjective impression, we found no significant differences in RT and error rate in the last block of each set in which visual cues were randomly ordered. Therefore, it seems that TMS had no objective effect on response execution despite clearly disrupting procedural learning.

CONCLUSIONS

We reviewed findings that suggest that procedural learning is associated with a plastic modulation of the motor cortical outputs to the muscles involved in the task, and is dependent on a neural network that receives critical contributions from cerebellum, basal ganglia, and prefrontal cortex. Throughout this review we have presented several hypotheses, which we hope will lead to further experiments and discussions.

In the SRTT, procedural learning requires the implicit acquisition of the repeating sequence of events in time. Procedural learning in the SRTT cannot take place in the absence of the ability to compare a given visual cue with previous cues. The number of cues that have to be "stored" and compared with each new cue depends on the length of the sequence. This comparison has to be made on-line, while the subject is preparing to respond, and has to result in the modulation of the motor output system to allow progressively faster RTs. We suggest that the dorsolateral prefrontal cortex plays a critical role in the integration of contributions from cerebellum and basal ganglia to the learning task and in the induction of the appropriate plastic changes in motor cortical output.

REFERENCES

1. NISSEN, M. J. & P. BULLEMER. 1987. Attentional requirements of learning: Evidence from performance measures. Cogn. Psychol. **19:** 1–32.
2. WILLINGHAM, D. B., M. J. NISSEN & P. BULLEMER. 1989. On the development of procedural knowledge. J. Exp. Psychol. Learn. Mem. Cogn. **15:** 1047–1060.
3. PASCUAL-LEONE, A., J. GRAFMAN, L. G. COHEN, B. J. ROTH & M. HALLETT. 1995. Transcranial magnetic stimulation. A new tool for the study of higher cognitive functions in humans. *In* Handbook of Neurophysychology, Vol. 10. J. Grafman & F. Boller, Eds. Elsevier Science Publishers. Amsterdam.
4. PASCUAL-LEONE, A., L. G. COHEN, N. DANG, J. P. BRASIL-NETO, A. CAMMAROTA & M. HALLETT. Modulation of human cortical motor outputs during the acquisition of new fine motor skills. J. Neurophysiol. In press.
5. PASCUAL-LEONE, A., J. GRAFMAN & M. HALLETT. 1994. Modulation of cortical motor output maps during the development of implicit and explicit knowledge. Science **263:** 1287–1289.
6. PASCUAL-LEONE, A., J. GRAFMAN & M. HALLETT. 1994. Explicit and implicit learning and maps of cortical motor output. Science **265:** 1600–1601.
7. WACHS, K., A. PASCUAL-LEONE, J. GRAFMAN & M. HALLETT. 1994. Intermanual transfer of implicit knowledge of sequential finger movements. Neurology **44(Suppl. 2):** A329 (Abstr.).

8. KNOPMAN, D. & M. J. NISSEN. 1991. Procedural learning is impaired in Huntington's disease: From the serial reaction time task. Neuropsychologia 29: 245–254.
9. GRAFMAN, J., H. WEINGARTNER, P. A. NEWHOUSE, K. THOMPSON, F. LALONDE, I. LITVAN, S. MOLCHAN & T. SUNDERLAND. 1990. Implicit learning in patients with Alzheimer's disease. Pharmacopsychiatry 23: 94–101.
10. PHILLIPS, A. G. & G. D. CARR. 1987. Cognition and the basal ganglia: A possible substrate for procedural knowledge. Can. J. Neurol. Sci. 14: 381–385.
11. SAINT-CYR, J., A. E. TAYLOR & A. E. LANG. 1988. Procedural learning and neostriatal dysfunction in man. Brain 111: 941–959.
12. HARRINGTON, D. L., K. Y. HAALAND, R. A. YEO & E. MARDER. 1990. Procedural memory in Parkinson's disease: Impaired motor but preserved visuoperceptual learning. J. Clin. Exp. Neuropsychol. 12: 323–339.
13. PASCUAL-LEONE, A., J. GRAFMAN, K. CLARK, M. STEWART, S. MASSAQUOI, J.-S. LOU & M. HALLETT. 1993. Procedural learning in Parkinson's disease and cerebellar degeneration. Ann. Neurol. 34: 594–602.
14. SCHMAHMANN, J. D. 1991. An emerging concept. The cerebellar contribution to higher function. Arch. Neurol. 48: 1178–1187.
15. PASCUAL-LEONE, A., J. GRAFMAN & M. HALLETT. 1993. Modulación de los mapas de proyección cortical motora durante el aprendizaje implícito en enfermos con degeneración cerebelosa. Neurologia 8: 370 (Abstr.).
16. GOLDMAN-RAKIC, P. S. 1987. Circuitry of primate prefrontal cortex and regulation of behavior by representational memory. In Handbook of Physiology; Nervous System, Vol. 5. Higher Functions of the Brain, Part 1. F. Plum, Ed. American Physiological Society. Bethesda, MD.
17. FUSTER, J. M. 1989. The Prefrontal Cortex. Anatomy, Physiology, and Neuropsychology of the Frontal Lobe. 2nd edit. Raven Press. New York.
18. MIDDLETON, F. A. & P. L. STRICK. 1994. Anatomical evidence for cerebellar and basal ganglia involvement in higher cognitive function. Science 266: 458–461.
19. PASCUAL-LEONE, A., J. GRAFMAN & M. HALLETT. 1994. Transcranial magnetic stimulation in the study of human cognitive function. In New Horizons in Neuropsychology. M. Sugishita, Ed. 93–100. Elsevier Science Publishers. Amsterdam.
20. PASCUAL-LEONE, A., C. M. HOUSER, K. REESE, L. I. SHOTLAND, J. GRAFMAN, S. SATO, J. VALLS-SOLÉ, J. P. BRASIL-NETO, E. M. WASSERMANN, L. G. COHEN & M. HALLETT. 1993. Safety of rapid-rate transcranial magnetic stimulation in normal volunteers. Electroencephalogr. Clin. Neurophysiol. 89: 120–130.

Architecture of the Prefrontal Cortex
and the Central Executive

PATRICIA S. GOLDMAN-RAKIC

Department of Neurobiology
Yale University
New Haven, Connecticut 06510

INTRODUCTION

As this workshop signifies, the mind/brain discussion is now the subject of cross-disciplinary research with the result that mental phenomena are becoming recognized by brain researchers and the structure of the nervous system is being increasingly acknowledged by behaviorists and theorists. Nevertheless, scholars and scientists on both sides of the issue remain skeptical of one another's approach, and doubts prevail concerning whether neurobiology, based largely on the study of nonhuman experimental models and tissues, can add insight to cognition and mental processing, and, conversely, whether cognitive sciences can enrich an understanding of brain function. In this paper I hope to illustrate from recent research on nonhuman primates that (1) a genuine neurobiology of mental representation is possible, and (2) significant contributions concerning the organization of the human thought process can be derived from neurobiology. The work I will describe relies on behavioral analysis equally as much as on neurobiology.

THE SUPERVISORY ATTENTIONAL SYSTEM, CENTRAL EXECUTIVE, AND DOMAIN-SPECIFIC SLAVE SYSTEMS

One of the most powerful and influential ideas in cognitive psychology is Baddeley's working memory model.[1] This tripartite model of cognitive architecture invokes a supervisory controlling system called the Central Executive and two slave systems, the Articulatory Loop and the Visuospatial Scratch Pad or Sketch Pad, specialized for language and spatial material, respectively. The model, reproduced in FIGURE 1, recognizes the separation of informational domains for lower-level tasks handled by the "slave" systems, but retains the traditional notion of a general purpose, panmodal processor, the central executive, that manages control and selection processes, similar to the supervisory attentional system of Shallice.[2] It is interesting that Baddeley acknowledged that a single central controller was not essential to his model. "If the control functions could be carried out by the interaction of the various cognitive subsystems, as suggested by Barnard,[3] we would be happy to accept this" (ref. 1, p. 71). In what follows, I present evidence from experimental studies in nonhuman primates that decomposes the central executive into segregated information processing modules each with its own sensory, mnemonic, and motor control features. This multiple domain model reduces

71

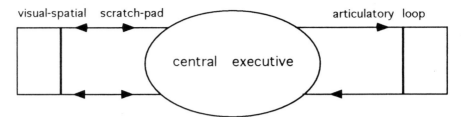

FIGURE 1. Diagrammatic representation of central executive according to Baddeley. Reproduced, with permission, from Baddeley.[1]

but does not necessarily eliminate "the residual area of ignorance" called the central executive. Our evidence is based mainly on the study of visuospatial working memory in nonhuman primates, and our premise is that understanding this information processing system will serve to explicate general principles applicable to other informational processing domains.

LOCALIZATION OF THE CENTRAL EXECUTIVE AND THE VISUOSPATIAL SKETCH PAD

The localization of the components of the working memory model has puzzled and challenged cognitive psychologists. Baddeley was himself very skeptical that neuroanatomical localization could be helpful to functional analysis and went so far as to comment with reference to the localization of long-term memory systems that "I would . . . argue that those aspects of the long-term memory deficit that have proved most amenable to interpretation through localization have shown the least theoretical development" (ref. 1, p. 237). Almost 10 years have passed since that statement and perhaps it is now possible to look more favorably on the contributions of cognitive neuroscience. The proposition we will support in this article is that the central executive is associated with a compartmentalized prefrontal architecture and a compartmental organization can explain a number of aspects of cognitive function. I review the findings from studies in monkeys that support the following tenets: (1) that working memory—the basic ability to keep track of and update information at the moment—is the cardinal specialization of the granular prefrontal cortex; (2) that the central executive is composed of multiple segregated special purpose processing domains rather than one central processor served by convergent slave systems; and (3) that each specialized domain consists of local and extrinsic networks with sensory, mnemonic, motor, and motivational control elements.[4] This process-oriented view explains the disorientation, perseveration, and distractibility of patients with frontal lobe lesions or dysexecutive syndromes as a default in the working memory system and accounts for dissociations in memory problems. According to this view, the prefrontal cortex has a specialized function that is replicated in many, if not all, of its various cortical subdivisions, and the interactions of these working memory centers with other areas in domain-specified cortical networks constitute the brain's machinery for higher-level cognition. This view is supported by a large experimental, clinical, and neurobiological data base (summarized in Goldman-Rakic[4]).

THE VISUOSPATIAL SKETCHPAD

We previously described a cortical area in the rhesus monkey with many if not all characteristics that could qualify as a visuospatial sketch pad. The region in question is area 46, which surrounds and lines the principal sulcus in the prefrontal cortex of the nonhuman primate brain (FIG. 2). Lesions restricted to this region have been shown repeatedly to impair performance on spatial delayed-response

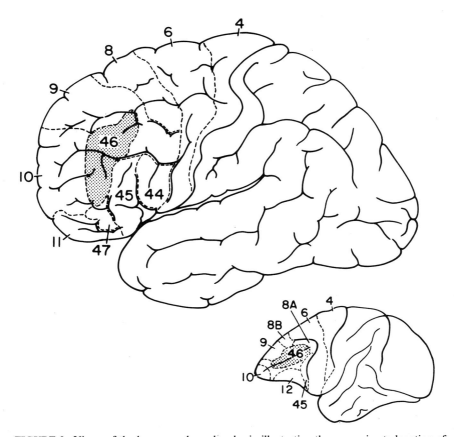

FIGURE 2. Views of the human and monkey brain illustrating the approximate location of area 46. Arabic numerals indicate the location of other cortical areas in the frontal lobe. The diagonal line that runs through area 46 on the monkey brain is the principal sulcus. This is the area associated with spatial working memory.

tasks that tax an animal's ability to hold information "in mind" for a short period of time and to update information from moment to moment. It is important to note that the same lesions do not impair performance which relies on associative memory or sensory-guided responses.[4,5] In general, the consistent rules of a task or its sensorimotor requirements do not cause a problem for the prefrontally lesioned animal. The monkey's difficulty lies in recalling information and using it to guide a correct response. Thus, on the basis of neuropsychological evidence, I have suggested that the brain obeys the distinction between working and associative memory, and that prefrontal cortex is preeminently involved in the former, whereas other areas—for example, the hippocampal formation and posterior sensory association regions—are critical for associative memory.[4]

Animal models are valuable because the phenomenon of working memory can be pursued at a number of different levels in order to fully comprehend the relevant neural circuit and cellular mechanisms and equally the cell biology of this unique process. Single-neuron recording in nonhuman primates has especially been used extensively to dissect the neuronal elements involved in working memory processes. In the oculomotor delayed-response (ODR) paradigm developed for this purpose, briefly presented visuospatial stimuli are remembered in order to provide guidance *from memory* for subsequent saccadic eye movements. The essential feature of this task is that the item to be recalled (in this case, the location of an object) has to be updated on every trial as in the moment-to-moment process of human mentation. The prefrontal cortex contains classes of neurons engaged respectively in registering the sensory cue, in holding it "on line," and in releasing the motor responses in the course of task performance.[6] These cells with diverse subspecializations are organized in modular or columnar units[7,8] and are thought to have common spatial selectivities.[9] In aggregate, dorsolateral prefrontal cortex contains a local circuit that encompasses the entire range of subfunctions necessary to carry out an integrated response: sensory input, retention in short-term memory, and motor signaling.

A particular focus in our laboratory are the prefrontal neurons that express "memory fields"; that is, the removal of a particular target from view is the trigger for an individual prefrontal neuron to increase its firing maximally and to remain activated until the end of the delay when the response is made (usually a period of 3–5,000 ms). The concept "memory field" is based on the finding that the same neuron appears to always code the same location and different neurons code different locations. In instances where the memory field of a neuron is not maintained throughout the delay and the activity falters, the animal is highly likely to make an error.[10] Thus, a default in the neuronal firing mechanism provides a neural basis for the oft-quoted phrase: "out of sight" is "out of mind." The finding that content-specific neuronal firing is directly associated with accurate recall provides an important example of how a compartmentalized and constrained architecture for memory processing can mirror the anatomical organization of the underlying neural circuitry. These and other results provide strong evidence at a cellular level for the theorized role of prefrontal neurons in working memory, that is, maintenance of representational information in the *absence* of the stimulus that was initially present. Accordingly, it is no wonder that monkeys and humans with prefrontal lesions have little difficulty in moving their eyes to a visible target or reaching for a desired object; their problem is directing these same motor responses to *remembered* targets and objects. At the same time, damage to the prefrontal cortex can and does spare knowledge about the outside world but destroys the ability to bring this knowledge to mind in order to guide behavior.

WORKING MEMORY: STORAGE AND PROCESS

It has been emphasized by cognitive theorists that working memory has at least two components—a storage component and a processing component.[1,11] The question can be raised as to whether working memory is sufficiently developed in nonhuman species and whether it can be studied in them. This question seems easily answered in the affirmative because monkeys are capable of remembering briefly presented information over short temporal delays and repeatedly updating that information as demonstrated by performance on the classical spatial delayed-response tasks (for review see refs. 4 and 12) as well as in the more demanding eight-item oculomotor version of that task,[10] in various match-to-sample paradigms,[13,14] and in "self-ordering" tasks.[15] It is less easily shown that monkeys can *process* information, that is, transform it mentally. A recent study in my laboratory addressed this issue in part by training monkeys on an anti-saccade task similar to that used by Guitton *et al.*[16] to study the effects of unilateral frontal cortical damage in humans. The anti-saccade paradigm required the monkeys to suppress the automatic or prepotent tendency to respond in the direction of a remembered cue and instead respond in the opposite direction, a transformation that is not particularly easy for human subjects. The anti-saccade task could be viewed as a member of a class of tasks such as the extremely valuable Stroop test that pit strong response tendencies against opponent responses. As is well known, the Stroop test requires the subject to overcome the prepotent tendency to read a printed word and instead name the discordant color of the ink in which it is printed.

We have recorded from the prefrontal cortex in our trained monkeys to isolate and characterize neuronal activity in the principal sulcus and surrounding cortex in a compound delayed-response paradigm in which, on standard trials, the monkey learned to make deferred eye movements to the same direction signaled by a brief visual cue (standard ODR task); on other trials, it learned to suppress that response and direct its gaze to the opposite direction. The type of trial was cued by a change in the color or size of the fixation point. The monkeys succeeded in learning this difficult task at high (85% and above) levels of accuracy. In itself, their acceptable learning performance indicates that monkeys are capable of holding "in mind" two sequentially presented items of information—the color of the fixation point and the location of a spatial cue—and of transforming the direction of response from left to right (or the reverse) based on a mental synthesis of that information. If "if-then" mental manipulations can be equated with propositional thought, the anti-saccade task may be a way of assaying the thought process in nonhuman species. Further, the task provides an elegant way of dissociating the direction of the cue from the direction of the response to allow us to determine the coding strategy of prefrontal neurons.

A. ODR task

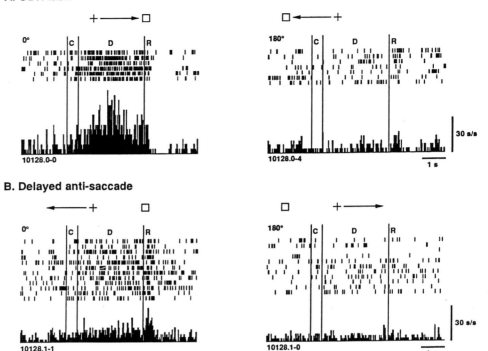

B. Delayed anti-saccade

FIGURE 3. The neuron shown in the figure was tested during concurrent administration of standard ocular delayed-response (ODR) and anti-saccade ODR trials. (**A**) On ODR trials, the cell's activity was significantly higher during the delay when the target to be recalled was to the right compared to the left. (**B**) This neuron was also activated in the delay period on the anti-saccade trials, even though the target on the right now signaled the animal to respond to the left. Thus, the neuron's activity was not dictated by the direction of responding, but by the direction of the remembered cue. This pattern of activity also indicates that the same neuron is engaged whether the monkey activates or inhibits a motor intention. (Modified from Funahashi et al.[37])

A major finding from these studies is that the great majority (approximately 60%) of prefrontal neurons was selectively activated during a silent 3-s period intervening between a particular antecedent stimulus and the prospective response, *regardless* of whether the intended movement was toward or away from the designated target. FIGURE 3 illustrates a neuron that exhibited enhanced activity in the delay-period of the ODR task whenever the visual cue to be remembered was presented on the right (FIG. 3A, left). For targets presented on the left, by contrast, delay-period activity was not above baseline (FIG. 3A, right). On the anti-saccade ODR trials, the neuron was again activated preferentially in the delay period when the visual cue was presented in the right, in spite of the fact that the monkey's response was now directed to the left at the end of the delay. The absence of motor planning activity in this neuron is further demonstrated by the absence of enhanced activity before saccades to the right in the anti-saccade task condition (FIG. 3B, right), demonstrating that it was not the rightward saccade in the ODR condition that was driving the unit. This result thus establishes that the same neuron involved in commanding an oculomotor response is also engaged when this response is suppressed and/or redirected. Such findings argue for at least a rudimentary form of propositional thinking on the part of nonhuman primates as well as point toward a cellular basis for mental processing in the nonhuman primate prefrontal cortex.

MULTIPLE WORKING MEMORY DOMAINS

According to the working memory analysis of prefrontal function, a working memory function should be demonstrable in more than one area of the prefrontal cortex and in more than one knowledge domain. Thus, different areas within prefrontal cortex will share in a common process—working memory; however, each will process different types of information. Thus, informational domain, not process, will be mapped across prefrontal cortex. Evidence on this point has recently been obtained in our laboratory from studies of nonspatial memory systems in prefrontal cortex.[17,18] In particular, we explored the hypothesis that the inferior convexity of the prefrontal cortex may contain specialized circuits for recalling the attributes of stimuli and holding them in short-term memory—thus processing nonspatial information in a manner analogous to the mechanism by which the principal sulcus mediates memory of visuospatial information. The inferior convexity cortex lying below and adjacent to the principal sulcus is a likely candidate for processing nonspatial—color and form—information. Lesions of this area produce deficits on tasks requiring memory for the color or patterns of stimuli (e.g., refs. 13 and 14), and the receptive fields of the neurons in the posterior portion of this area, unlike those in the dorsolateral cortex above, represent the fovea, the region of the retina specialized for the analysis of fine detail and color—stimulus attributes important for the recognition of objects.[19,20]

We recorded from the inferior convexity region in monkeys trained to perform delayed-response tasks in which spatial or feature *memoranda* had to be recalled on independent, randomly interwoven trials. For the spatial delayed-response (SDR) trials, stimuli were presented 13° to the left or right of fixation while the monkeys gazed at a fixation point on a video monitor. After a delay of 2500 ms, the fixation point disappeared, instructing the animal to direct its gaze to the location where the stimulus appeared before the delay. For the pattern delayed-response (PDR) trials, various patterns were presented in the center of the screen; one stimulus indicated that a left-directed and the other a right-directed response would be rewarded at the end of the delay. Thus, both spatial and feature trials required exactly the same eye movements at the end of the delay, but differed in the nature of the mnemonic representation that guided those responses.

We found that neurons were responsive to events in both delayed-response tasks. However, a given neuron was generally responsive to the spatial aspects or the feature aspects, but not both. Thus, a large majority of the neurons examined in both tasks were active in the delay period when the monkey was recalling a stimulus pattern that required a 13° response to the right *or* left. The same neurons did not respond above baseline during the delay preceding an identical rightward or leftward response on the PDR trials. Neurons exhibiting selective neuronal activity for patterned memoranda were almost exclusively found in or around area 12 on the inferior convexity of the prefrontal cortex, beneath the principal sulcus whereas neurons that responded selectively in the SDR were rarely observed in this region. Spatially responsive neurons appear instead in the dorsolateral cortical regions where spatial processing has been localized in our previous studies. In addition, we discovered that the neurons in the inferior convexity were highly responsive to complex stimuli, such as pictures of faces or specific objects. We subsequently used face stimuli as memoranda in a working memory task and demonstrated that such stimuli could indeed serve as memoranda in memory tasks. FIGURE 4 shows a neuron that encoded a face stimulus in the delay period of our working memory paradigm (FIG. 4A). The same cell was unresponsive on trials when the monkey had to remember a different face (FIG. 4B) as well as when patterns were used as memoranda (FIG. 4C and D). It should be noted that even though the same response is required on trials shown in FIGURE 4A and C, the neuron responds in the delay only in FIGURE 4A. These results provide strong

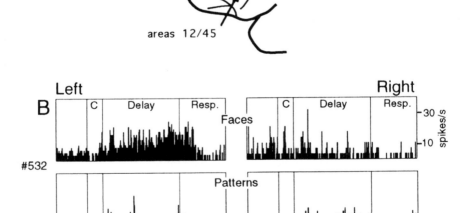

FIGURE 4. (**A**) Brain view of areas 12 and 45 from which neurons were recorded. PS, principal sulcus; AS, arcuate sulcus. (**B**) The neuron illustrated was activated in the delay when the stimulus to be recalled was a particular face (*left panel*), but not for another face (*right panel*). The same neuron was not differentially activated by the recall of patterned cues (*lower panels*). This result illustrates that prefrontal neurons can code selective features of or complex images in working memory. (Modified from Wilson *et al.*[18])

evidence that the neuron in question is encoding information about the identifying features of a stimulus and not about the direction of an impending response. Furthermore, different neurons encode different features. Altogether, our results establish that nonspatial aspects of an object or stimulus may be processed separately from those dedicated to the analysis of its spatial location and vice versa. Thus, feature and spatial memory—what and where an object is—are dissociable at both the area level and the single-neuron level. These findings support the prediction that different prefrontal subdivisions represent different informational domains rather than different processes and that more than one working memory domain exists in prefrontal cortex.

IMPLICATION FOR HUMAN COGNITION: ACTIVATION STUDIES USING POSITRON EMISSION TOMOGRAPHY

Numerous PET and several fMRI studies of the human brain support the role of the dorsolateral prefrontal cortex as a key site of activation during performance of working memory tasks.[21–28] The application of PET and other promising methods like fast scan magnetic resonance spectroscopy for the study of cognitive activation in human subjects offers an unprecedented opportunity to test hypotheses about cortical organization derived from studies of experimental animals and from human neuropsychology. The prefrontal cortex, in particular, is activated by working memory tasks, and several recent studies have pinpointed areas 9 and 46 as functional sites in the normal performance of spatial working memory processes. McCarthy et al.,[26,27] Smith et al.,[29] and Sweeney et al.[28] have all examined spatial working memory paradigms that were similar to those that have been employed in studies of spatial working memory in nonhuman primates. Petrides et al.[22] found similar areal activation in a spatial self-ordering task. In all of these studies of spatial cognition in humans, the functional organization of the cortex bears a remarkable correspondence to that observed in nonhuman primates.

With respect to nonspatial working memory, the results are less clear. Petrides et al. have recently provided evidence that area 46 was activated in a verbal[23] working memory task. Likewise, Frith et al.[30] have reported that area 46 was activated during tasks calling for the open-ended generation of words or finger movements. As with spatial working memory tasks, these nonspatial tasks had a working memory component in that the information needed to guide correct responses was not present in the immediate environment and had to be recalled and/or generated de novo at the time of response. The differentiation between spatial and object memory thus remains an issue.

The clearest dissociations that can so far be discerned in imaging studies appear to be between tasks that involve explicit verbal processing, on the one hand, and explicit spatial or location processing, on the other. Less clear differences have been observed between location versus object memory, as would be expected from the monkey lesion and neurophysiological literature. At present, the variety of findings with respect to regional localization of spatial and nonspatial working memory tasks raise several possibilities that need to be considered in future research. It is possible that in the human prefrontal cortex, functions that are distributed within a hemisphere of the nonhuman primate have been allocated to different hemispheres in line with the increased hemispheric specialization that appears to be a hallmark of human cortical organization. Many studies report a predominant right hemisphere activation for spatial tasks, and a left hemisphere predominance for verbal paradigms. A second consideration is the strong potential for interactions with verbal mediation in human studies. In spite of efforts to prevent verbal mediation in many studies, spatial as well as nonspatial tasks could have engaged verbal encoding, and, conversely, nonspatial tasks could have engaged spatial processes, depending on how the stimuli are presented. "Functional cross-overs" might explain to some degree the overlap in regional localization that is commonly observed when comparing spatial versus nonspatial processing in prefrontal cortex. Perhaps the most nagging problem in the PET and to a considerable extent the fMRI studies is that of spatial resolution. If an object or feature processing and visuospatial modules were close to one another as they are in the rhesus monkey, and further if they were coactivated during task performance because of problems inherent in task design, it would be difficult to tease them apart.

WHERE THEN IS THE CENTRAL EXECUTIVE?

Studies in nonhuman primates are beginning to model the basic processes that are central to cognitive operations. The modular parallel organization of memory circuits in the macaque cerebral cortex suggests a neural basis for similarly modular and segregated cognitive processing systems demonstrable in humans behaviorally, and by neuropsychological deficits following relatively circumscribed injuries, and by noninvasive imaging of the brain during cognitive processing.

It is important to underscore that although the domains of information processing are modular and parallel, the process carried out within these systems is complex, integrative, and temporally regulated. An outstanding feature of the memory cells of the prefrontal cortex is that a different groups of cells respond at different time points as the process unfolds within a trial. Assuming conservatism in evolution of cortical structure and function, experimental studies in experimental animals may help to decide controversial issues in cognitive psychology and may also shed light on the phylogenetic origins and neural basis of intelligence. Currently, the comparative analysis of working memory functions across monkeys and humans favors the idea of multiple working memory domains—that is, multiple special purpose systems organized in parallel rather than the concept of a central panmodal executive processor to account for the diversity and complexity of the human thought process. As suggested in FIGURE 5, these working memory domains have the complexity of neural machinery necessary to accommodate both passive storage functions for specified information and the processing of that very same information. Presumably, the more demand placed on the system, the more neurons within a domain would be recruited to meet that demand within the limits of the particular system. The activation of prefrontal loci would require a sufficient load to be resolved by PET or fMRI. If a task is insufficiently demanding, too few neurons might be activated to be resolved by present imaging modalities. Negative findings in PET and fMRI studies or in neuropsychological investigation

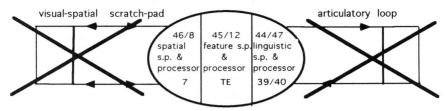

central executive

FIGURE 5. Provisional neurologically based model of the central executive proposed in this paper: Domain-specific working memory modules can register information, hold it "on line," *and* process it by interacting with the relevant sensory and motor areas with which each is connected. The number of neurons engaged by any given task will depend upon the level or depth of processing.

should therefore be interpreted cautiously when drawing inferences about localization of function. On the other hand, positive findings must also be regarded with caution if behavioral analysis is insufficient to confirm the strategy employed by versatile human subjects. The same cautions apply to nonhuman primate research where monkeys can and do at times outwit investigators with respect to behavioral strategies.

It may be argued that the organization of the human brain differs in architecture from the nonhuman primate brain by virtue of its greater cognitive and linguistic capacity, and, accordingly, the human brain may have a cortical center or network that is truly a central processor oblivious to informational domain. If so, imaging studies could in the future reveal the location of this area but thus far they have not. What area would we expect it to be? The architecture of cognitive processing in human and nonhuman primates is a topic of great challenge and one which can only be enriched by collaborative efforts among researchers from neurobiology and psychology and allied fields.

REFERENCES

1. BADDELEY, A. 1986. Working Memory: 1–289. Oxford University Press. London.
2. SHALLICE, T. 1982. Specific impairments in planning. Phil. Trans. R. Soc. Lond. B. **298:** 199–209.
3. BARNARD, P. 1985. Interacting cognitive subsystems: A psycholinguistic approach to short-term memory. *In* Progress in the Psychology of Language. Vol. 2. A. Ellis, Ed.: 197–258. Lawrence Erlbaum. London.
4. GOLDMAN-RAKIC, P. S. 1987. Circuitry of primate prefrontal cortex and regulation of behavior by representational memory. *In* Handbook of Physiology, The Nervous System, Higher Functions of the Brain. F. Plum, Ed.: 373–417. American Physiological Society. Bethesda, MD.
5. GOLDMAN, P. S. & H. E. ROSVOLD. 1970. Localization of function within the dorsolateral prefrontal cortex of the rhesus monkey. Exp. Neurol. **27:** 291–304.
6. GOLDMAN-RAKIC, P. S., S. FUNAHASHI & C. J. BRUCE. 1990. Neocortical memory circuits. Q. J. Quant. Biol. **55:** 1025–1038.
7. GOLDMAN-RAKIC, P. S. 1984. Modular organization of prefrontal cortex. Trends Neurosci. **7:** 419–424.

8. KRITZER, M. & P. S. GOLDMAN-RAKIC. 1995. Intrinsic circuit organization of the major layers and sublayers of the dorsolateral prefrontal cortex in the rhesus monkey. J. Comp. Neurol. **359:** 131–143.
9. GOLDMAN-RAKIC, P. S. 1995. Cellular basis of working memory. Neuron **14:** 477–485.
10. FUNAHASHI, S., C. J. BRUCE & P. S. GOLDMAN-RAKIC. 1989. Mnemonic coding of visual space in the monkey's dorsolateral prefrontal cortex. J. Neurophysiol. **61:** 331–349.
11. JUST, M. A. & P. A. CARPENTER. 1985. Cognitive coordinate systems: Accounts of mental rotation and individual differences in spatial ability. Psychol. Rev. **92:** 137–172.
12. FUSTER, J. M. 1989. The Prefrontal Cortex, 2nd edit.: 1–255. Raven Press. New York.
13. PASSINGHAM, R. E. 1975. Delayed matching after selective prefrontal lesions in monkeys (*Macaca mulatta*). Brain Res. **92:** 89–102.
14. MISHKIN, M. & F. J. MANNING. 1978. Non-spatial memory after selective prefrontal lesions in monkeys. Brain Res. **143:** 313–323.
15. PETRIDES, M. 1991. Functional specialization within the dorsolateral frontal cortex for serial order memory. Proc. R. Soc. Lond. B **246:** 293–298.
16. GUITTON, D., H. A. BUCHTEL & R. M. DOUGLAS. 1985. Frontal lobe lesions in man cause difficulties in suppressing reflexive glances and in generating goal-directed saccades. Exp. Brain Res. **58:** 455–472.
17. O SCALAIDHE, S. P., F. A. W. WILSON & P. S. GOLDMAN-RAKIC. 1992. Neurons in the prefrontal cortex of the macaque selective for faces. Soc. Neurosci. Abstr. **18:** 705.
18. WILSON, F. A. W., S. P. O SCALAIDHE & P. S. GOLDMAN-RAKIC. 1993. Dissociation of object and spatial processing domains in primate prefrontal cortex. Science **260:** 1955–1958.
19. MIKAMI, A., S. ITO & K. KUBOTA. 1982. Visual response properties of dorsolateral prefrontal neurons during a visual fixation task. J. Neurophysiol. **47:** 593–605.
20. SUZUKI, H. & M. AZUMA. 1983. Topographic studies on visual neurons in the dorsolateral prefrontal cortex of the monkey. Exp. Brain Res. **53:** 47–58.
21. JONIDES, J., E. E. SMITH, R. A. KOEPPE, E. AWH, S. MINOSHIMA & M. A. MINTUN. 1993. Spatial working memory in humans as revealed by PET. Nature **363:** 623–625.
22. PETRIDES, M., B. ALIVISATOS, A. C. EVANS & E. MEYER. 1993a. Dissociation of human mid-dorsolateral from posterior dorsolateral frontal cortex in memory processing. Proc. Natl. Acad. Sci. USA **90:** 873–877.
23. PETRIDES, M., B. ALIVISATOS, E. MEYER & A. C. EVANS. 1993b. Functional activation of the human frontal cortex during the performance of verbal working memory tasks. Proc. Natl. Acad. Sci. USA **90:** 878–882.
24. COHEN, J. D., S. D. FORMAN, T. S. BRAVER, B. J. CASEY, D. SERVAN-SCHREIBER & D. C. NOLL. 1994. Activation of prefrontal cortex in a non-spatial working memory task with functional MRI. Hum. Brain Map **1:** 293–304.
25. SWARTZ, B. E., E. HALGREN, J. FUSTER, F. SIMPKINS, M. GEE & M. MANDELKERN. 1995. Cortical metabolic activation in humans during a visual memory task. Cereb. Cortex **3:** 205–214.
26. MCCARTHY, G., A. M. BLAMIRE, A. PUCE, A. C. NOBRE, G. BLOCH, F. HYDER, P. S. GOLDMAN-RAKIC & R. SHULMAN. 1994. Functional magnetic resonance imagining of human prefrontal cortex activation during a spatial working memory task. Proc. Natl. Acad. Sci. USA **91:** 8690–8694.
27. MCCARTHY, G., A. PUCE, R. T. CONSTABLE, J. H. KRYSTAL, J. GORE & P. S. GOLDMAN-RAKIC. 1996. Activation of human prefrontal cortex during spatial and object working memory tasks measured by functional MRI. Cereb. Cortex. In press.
28. SWEENEY, J. A., M. A. MINTUN, B. S. KWEE, M. B. WISEMAN, D. L. BROWN, D. R. ROSENBERG & J. R. CARL. A positron emission tomography study of voluntary saccadic eye movements and spatial working memory. J. Neurophysiol. In press.
29. SMITH, E. E., J. JONIDES & R. A. KOEPPE. 1996. Dissociating verbal and spatial working memory using PET. Cereb. Cortex. In press.

30. FRITH, C. D., K. FRISTON, P. F. LIDDLE & R. S. J. FRACKOWIAK. 1991. Willed action and the prefrontal cortex in man. Proc. R. Soc. Lond. B **244:** 241–246.
31. RAJKOWSKA, G. & P. S. GOLDMAN-RAKIC. 1995. Cytoarchitectonic definition of prefrontal areas in the normal human cortex: II. Variability in locations of areas 9 and 46 and relationship to the Talairach Coordinate System. Cereb. Cortex **5:** 323–337.
32. STUSS, D. T. & D. F. BENSON. 1986. The Frontal Lobes.: 1–303. Raven Press. New York.
33. PAULESCU, E., C. D. FRITH & F. S. J. FRACKOWIAK. 1993. Localization of a human system for sustained attention by positron emission tomography. Nature **362:** 342–345.
34. ZATORRE, R. J., A. C. EVANS, E. MEYER & A. GJEDDE. 1992. Lateralization of phonetic and pitch discrimination in speech processing. Science **256:** 846–849.
35. PETERSEN, S. E., P. T. FOX, M. I. POSNER, M. MINTUN & M. E. RAICHLE. 1988. Positron emission tomographic studies of the cortical anatomy of single-word processing. Nature **331:** 585–589.
36. MCCARTHY, G., A. M. BLAMIRE, D. L. ROTHMAN, R. GRUETTER & R. G. SHULMAN. 1993. Echo-planar magnetic resonance imaging studies of frontal cortex activation during word generation in humans. Proc. Natl. Acad. Sci. USA **90:** 4952–4956.
37. FUNAHASHI, S., M. V. CHAFEE & P. S. GOLDMAN-RAKIC. 1993. Nature **365:** 753–756.

Functional Organization of the Human Frontal Cortex for Mnemonic Processing

Evidence from Neuroimaging Studies

MICHAEL PETRIDES

Montreal Neurological Institute
McGill University
3801 University Street
Montreal, Quebec, Canada H3A 2B4

Damage to the human lateral frontal cortex does not result in a general mnemonic impairment.[1] For instance, patients with lesions of the lateral frontal cortex perform well on standard tests of recognition memory and on various tests of short-term memory, such as story recall or the digit span.[1] Performance on such tasks can be normal even when the lesions are bilateral, as several studies of patients who had undergone frontal lobotomies have shown.[1-3] Frontal cortical damage, however, results in severe impairments on certain specific aspects of mnemonic performance that depend on the expression of a number of executive processes.[1] The frontal cortex is not a homogeneous region of the brain; it comprises several architectonic areas that differ markedly in terms of their connections with other cortical and subcortical areas.[4] Elucidating the contribution of the frontal cortex to mnemonic processing, as well as other cognitive processing, will ultimately depend on understanding the nature of the specific functional interactions between the different frontal cortical areas and the other brain areas with which they are connected. A recent theoretical model has postulated distinct contributions of different frontal cortical areas to mnemonic processing, based on an analysis of the mnemonic impairments of patients and monkeys with lesions restricted to various parts of the frontal cortex.[5] The present article describes this model briefly and focuses on a description of recent attempts in our laboratory to test it by means of functional neuroimaging studies with positron emission tomography (PET). A detailed description of the model and the work on which it is based has been published elsewhere.[5]

A TWO-LEVEL HYPOTHESIS OF THE INVOLVEMENT OF THE MID-LATERAL FRONTAL CORTEX IN MEMORY

As several physiological and neurobehavioral studies have shown, specialized cortical systems, originating in the primary sensory cortical areas, underlie the processing of exteroceptive sensory input (e.g., visual, auditory, somatic). The information is processed in a series of sensory-specific areas, and it is finally interpreted in modality-specific and multimodal areas of the posterior association cortex, where a coded representation of it is achieved (FIG. 1). The interpretation of incoming information is largely the result of relating this new information with older stored representations. In the present model, the transient storage of information (i.e., working memory) while it is being integrated with new and recalled information is assumed, to a large extent, to result from processing within these modality-specific and multimodal posterior cortical association areas. Thus, a considerable amount of information processing that in the cognitive psychological literature is subsumed by the concept of working memory is carried out in these posterior cortical regions (see ref. 5 for details).

What then is the specific contribution of the lateral frontal cortical areas to mnemonic processing? The posterior cortical association areas, where recently processed information is temporarily held while it is being integrated with incoming and recalled information, are connected with the ventrolateral frontal cortical region. In the monkey, this region lies below the sulcus principalis, occupying the inferior frontal convexity, and comprises architectonic areas 47/12, 45, and the ventralmost part of area 46 that lies below the sulcus principalis[6] (FIG. 2). In the human brain, the ventrolateral frontal cortical region largely occupies the inferior frontal gyrus (FIG. 2). According to the present model,[5] functional interaction between this ventrolateral frontal region and the posterior association cortex is critical for the expression within memory of various executive processes, such as active selection, comparison, and judgment of stimuli held in short-term and long-term memory. This type of interaction is necessary for active (explicit) encoding and retrieval of information, that is, processes initiated under conscious effort by the subject and guided by the subject's plans and intentions. It is important to distinguish here between these *active forms of encoding and retrieval,* which depend on the lateral frontal cortex, from the *more passive forms of encoding and retrieval,* which result when incoming or recalled stimuli automatically trigger stored representations (e.g., on the basis of strong preexisting associations or matching to stored representations). These latter aspects of mnemonic processing do not critically depend on the lateral frontal cortex, and, according to the present model, this accounts for the normal performance of patients and monkeys with lateral frontal lesions on several mnemonic tasks.

Furthermore, the model postulates that a fundamental distinction exists between the middle portions of the dorsolateral and the ventrolateral frontal cortical regions. The mid-dorsolateral frontal cortex, which includes most of areas 46 and 9, is a specialized region where information held on-line can be monitored and manipulated. The essential nature of this type of mnemonic processing is captured in the self-ordered working memory tasks that were first developed for work with patients in the late 1970s.[7] Patients with lateral frontal excisions are severely impaired on the self-ordered tasks, despite the fact that they have no primary memory impairment, performing very well on recognition memory tests and on other short-term memory tasks.[1,7] Work in the monkey has shown that lesions limited to the mid-dorsal part of the lateral frontal cortex (i.e., dorsal area 46 and area 9) impair performance on these and other similar tasks, such as the externally ordered tasks that require monitoring of the occurrence of stimuli from an expected set.[8]

In the self-ordered task, the subjects are presented with different arrangements

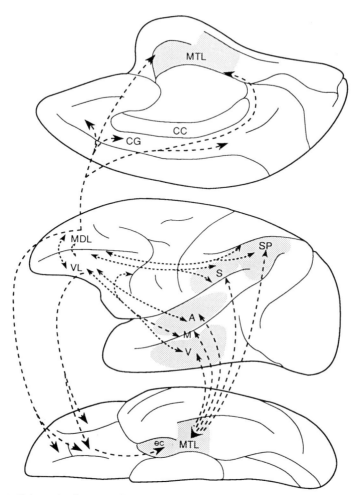

FIGURE 1. Schematic diagram of the brain of the macaque monkey to illustrate some of the functional interactions postulated to underlie mnemonic processing (see text and ref. 5 for details). The final stage of information processing, which originates in the primary sensory areas, occurs in unimodal and multimodal areas of the posterior association cortex. (S, somatic; SP, spatial; A, auditory; V, visual; and M, multimodal information processing areas in the posterior association cortex). In the human brain, linguistic information is processed, primarily in the left hemisphere in the region of the parietotemporal junction, that is, supramarginal gyrus in parietal cortex and middle and posterior temporal cortex. Processing in these posterior association cortical areas is assumed to underlie not only perception and long-term storage, but also transient maintenance of information for further processing. These areas interact with ventrolateral (VL) frontal cortical areas when executive processing, such as decision making, comparison, reproduction of information held in memory, is involved. The mid-dorsolateral (MDL) part of the frontal cortex, which is connected with the ventrolateral frontal cortex and the memory system of the medial temporal lobe (MTL), both directly and indirectly, exercises a higher-order control of mnemonic processing when monitoring and manipulation of information in working memory are required. CC, corpus callosum; CG, cingulate gyrus; ec, entorhinal cortex.

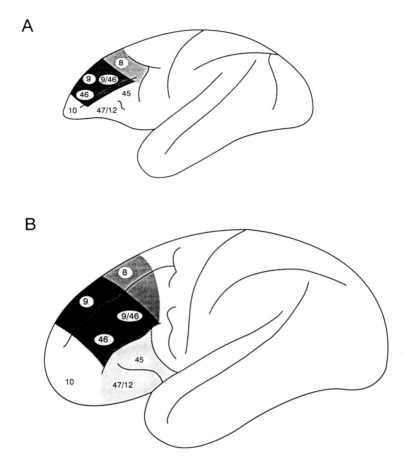

FIGURE 2. Schematic diagrams of the lateral surface of the macaque monkey (**A**) and the human (**B**) frontal cortex to illustrate the location of the mid-dorsolateral frontal region (areas 46, 9, and 9/46) and the ventrolateral frontal region (areas 45 and 47/12) discussed in the text. The term mid-dorsolateral frontal cortex is used to distinguish, in the rostrocaudal direction, this region of the middle and superior frontal gyri from the frontopolar cortex (i.e., area 10) and the posterior dorsolateral frontal cortex (i.e., area 8 and rostralmost area 6). In the human brain, ventrolateral frontal cortical areas 45 and 47 occupy the pars triangularis and pars orbitalis of the inferior frontal gyrus, respectively. In a recent comparative architectonic study,[6] we found that area 47 of the human ventrolateral frontal cortex corresponds to a large part of area 12 in the ventrolateral frontal cortex of the macaque monkey. These areas are thus labeled as area 47/12 in both the human and the monkey brain to acknowledge this architectonic correspondence.

of the same set of stimuli and have to select a different stimulus, on each trial, until all the stimuli are selected. Thus, from the moment they start responding, the subjects must constantly compare the responses that they have already made with those still remaining to be carried out. In other words, each selection must be marked in the subject's mind and simultaneously considered in relation to the others that still remain to be selected. This is what we termed monitoring of events within working memory.[5,7,8] It is the simultaneous consideration of each stimulus to be selected with the other possible selections. Monitoring within working memory is to be distinguished from simple attention to a stimulus held in memory. There are many mnemonic situations in which a stimulus in memory is attended to and the other stimuli exist as a background—that is, they are not in the center of current awareness. These situations do not challenge monitoring within working memory in the sense used here. Monitoring within working memory, as this term is used to describe the function of mid-dorsolateral frontal cortex, implies attention to the stimulus that is currently under consideration together with active consideration (i.e., attention) of several other stimuli whose current status is essential for the decision to be made.

The analysis of the impairment of monkeys with mid-dorsolateral frontal lesions on the self-ordered and externally ordered tasks is consistent with the above analysis.[8] Monkeys with such lesions can remember stimuli as demonstrated by normal performance on recognition memory tests and on other short-term memory tasks (e.g., object alternation where the emphasis is on switching between two recurring stimuli).[8] The fundamental problem of these animals on the self-ordered and on the externally ordered working memory tasks has been shown to stem from the monitoring requirements of these tasks, that is, the number of stimuli that must be kept in mind and considered as responses are being made.[8] The mid-dorsolateral part of the frontal cortex therefore appears to be a specialized area of the cerebral cortex in which information can be held on-line for monitoring (in the sense described above) and manipulation of stimuli. Note that the manipulation of stimuli implies simultaneous consideration of several stimuli together and thus monitoring. It is precisely for this reason that, in the early 1980s, we introduced the concept of an impairment in active working memory to describe the essential characteristic of the deficit of patients with frontal lesions on the self-ordered task.[7]

Thus, according to the two-level hypothesis of the involvement of the lateral frontal cortex in mnemonic performance, processing within the ventrolateral frontal cortex (areas 45 and 47/12) constitutes one level of executive interaction with information held in posterior cortical association areas. The ventrolateral frontal cortex is critical for the active (i.e., strategic) encoding and retrieval of specific information held in posterior cortical regions and thus in selecting, comparing, or deciding on information held in short-term and long-term memory. The mid-dorsolateral frontal cortex (areas 9 and 46), on the other hand, constitutes another level of interaction and is involved when several pieces of information in working memory need to be monitored and manipulated on the basis of the requirements of the task or the subject's current plans.[5] The fundamental distinction between these two regions of the frontal lobe is therefore in terms of the nature of the executive processing that is being carried out, although within the dorsolateral and ventrolateral frontal regions there may be further specialization according to the sensory modality of the information processed. Finally, it must be emphasized that the two levels of mnemonic executive processing posited above are likely to be involved in several tasks and often simultaneously. The successful demonstration of the specific contribution of the different areas will therefore depend on selective lesion studies (e.g., in nonhuman primates) in which impaired performance on certain mnemonic tasks is contrasted with normal performance on other similar tasks and on neuroimaging studies with normal human subjects in which experimental tasks are differentially loaded with requirements thought to involve one or the other area.

FUNCTIONAL ACTIVATION OF THE HUMAN MID-DORSOLATERAL FRONTAL CORTEX

In our recent studies with PET, it has been possible to extend to the human brain the demonstration from the animal work[8] that the mid-dorsolateral frontal cortex constitutes a specialized region for the monitoring, within working memory, of self-ordered and externally ordered responses.[9,10] In these studies, we measured with PET the distribution of cerebral blood flow (CBF) (i.e., a marker of local neuronal activity) in normal volunteer subjects as they performed various mnemonic tasks. By comparing the distribution of CBF between the experimental conditions of interest and appropriate control conditions, CBF changes specific to the particular cognitive requirements of the experimental tasks could be isolated.

In one of our first studies with PET, we measured CBF during the performance of a nonspatial visual self-ordered task, a visual matching control task, and a visual conditional task.[9] The same eight visual stimuli (abstract designs) were used in all three tasks, and these stimuli were presented in a different random arrangement on each trial. The subjects were required to indicate their response by pointing to particular stimuli. Thus, the only difference between the three tasks lay in their cognitive requirements. In the self-ordered task, which was directly analogous to those we had previously used with patients[7] and monkeys,[8] the subjects were required to select a different stimulus on each trial until all had been selected. The subjects were therefore required to consider actively (i.e., monitor) their earlier selections as they were preparing their next response. In the matching control task, the subjects had to search and find the same stimulus on each trial. This task therefore involved the same visual stimuli and searching behavior as the self-ordered task, but did not require that the subjects consider their earlier responses in relation to the current one. In the conditional task, the subjects had learned, prior to scanning, associations between the stimuli and particular color cues. During scanning, they were required to select the stimulus that was appropriate for the color cue presented. Thus, the searching among the stimuli was the same as in the self-ordered task, but since the stimulus to be selected, on each trial, was completely determined by the color cue presented, no monitoring within working memory of prior selections was required. Performance of the self-ordered task, in comparison with either the matching control or the conditional task, resulted in significantly greater activity within the mid-dorsolateral frontal cortex (areas 46 and 9), particularly within the right hemisphere. There was no activation in this region when CBF in the conditional task was compared with that of the control task, although there was now significant activity within the posterior dorsolateral frontal cortex in area 8, a region that is known to be critical for visual conditional learning.[11] The contrast in the activation patterns between the self-ordered and the conditional tasks emphasizes the specificity of activation within the mid-dorsolateral frontal cortex in relation to the monitoring requirements of the self-ordered task.[9]

Another study examined activation patterns in relation to the performance of a verbal self-ordered task and a verbal externally ordered task.[10] In the self-ordered task, the subjects had to generate randomly numbers from the set 1 to 10, avoiding repetition of any number until all the numbers from the set had been generated. In the externally ordered task, the subjects had to monitor random presentations from the same set of numbers in order to identify the number that was left out on each trial. The control task, which required counting forwards from 1 to 10, involved the same cognitive processes for generating and pronouncing numbers as the two experimental tasks, but without their special mnemonic requirements. When CBF in the control task was subtracted from either one of the two experimental tasks, there was significant bilateral activity in the mid-dorsolateral frontal cortex.[10] These findings are in complete accord with predictions from the animal work[5,8] which demonstrated the critical role of the mid-dorsolateral frontal cortex in the active monitoring of information within working memory.

ACTIVATION OF THE VENTROLATERAL AND THE ORBITAL FRONTAL CORTEX

The above PET studies were designed to reveal specific activation within the mid-dorsolateral frontal cortex so that the contribution of this region of the lateral frontal cortex in mnemonic processing could be better understood. In another series of experiments, we attempted to activate specifically the ventrolateral or the orbital frontal cortex. In the latter experiments, we tried to equalize the tasks in terms of the memory requirements thought to involve the mid-dorsolateral frontal cortex (see above) and to load the tasks differentially in terms of mnemonic processes hypothesized to involve the ventrolateral or the orbital frontal cortex, respectively.

The orbitofrontal cortex maintains strong connections with the medial temporal limbic region[4,12] which is critically involved in mnemonic processing, as shown both by work with patients[13] and experimental animals.[14,15] Furthermore, there is evidence from work in the monkey that large lesions of the orbital and medial (cingulate and subcallosal) frontal cortex yield a severe recognition memory disorder, suggesting that these structures are an integral part of the limbo-thalamic system underlying recognition memory.[16] Related to this is the observation that monkeys with orbital frontal lesions fail to habituate to the repeated presentation of stimuli.[17] These findings suggested to us that the orbital frontal cortex may be preferentially involved in the early reactions to novel stimuli and may therefore participate in their automatic encoding. On the other hand, it has been argued that the ventrolateral frontal cortex is involved when explicit judgments about events in memory are required (see above and ref. 5).

On the basis of the above considerations, we designed a PET study to test the hypothesis that the ventrolateral frontal cortex may be specifically active when explicit judgments on information held in memory must be made, whereas activity within the orbital frontal cortex may be differentially sensitive to the relative familiarity of stimuli (Petrides *et al.*, unpublished experiment). The subjects were scanned under the following conditions: (1) observing familiar stimuli, (2) observing novel stimuli, and (3) making explicit recognition judgments between novel and familiar stimuli. In the novelty condition, the subjects saw pairs of novel stimuli appearing on the screen and were simply required to look at these stimuli and to touch the screen to advance to the next pair. In the familiarity condition, the subjects saw pairs of familiar stimuli, and, as in the novelty condition, they had to touch the screen to advance to the next pair. In the recognition condition, the subjects again saw pairs of abstract designs, but now one of the stimuli was familiar and the other was novel. The subjects were required to make an explicit judgment about which of the two stimuli was the novel one and to touch it in order that the next pair be presented. In all conditions, the stimuli were colored abstract designs appearing, in pairs, on a touch-sensitive screen, and the subjects responded by touching the screen. Thus, the nature of the stimuli, the mode of stimulus presentation, and the way the subjects indicated their response were identical in the three scanning conditions; the only difference between these conditions lay in their cognitive requirements.

We subtracted CBF measured in the familiarity condition from that in the novelty condition to test the hypothesis that significant activation would be found within the human orbitofrontal cortex as a result of the inspection of a series of novel stimuli and therefore their automatic encoding. This subtraction revealed greater activity in the orbitofrontal cortex and the adjacent limbic cingulate region in the novelty condition as compared with the familiarity condition. The activation in the orbitofrontal cortex was bilateral. Note that no area of lateral frontal cortex exhibited changes in CBF as a result of the mere inspection of novel stimuli and therefore their encoding. The fact that the novel stimuli were encoded during the scanning period was verified in a post-scanning recognition test.

The second hypothesis investigated in this experiment was that the mid-ventrolateral frontal cortex would be differentially involved in various executive processes such as those that underlie the capacity to make decisions (e.g., explicit judgments) on information held in memory.[5] Note that in the novelty or familiarity conditions the only mnemonic experience is the automatic awareness that stimuli are novel or familiar. In the recognition condition, however, an explicit judgment is required as to which stimulus is familiar and which one is novel. Significant activation of the ventrolateral frontal cortex was present in the recognition condition in comparison with either the novelty or the familiarity condition. It is noteworthy that the peak of this activation was located between the horizontal ramus and the lateral orbital sulcus, namely, within area 47/12. In the monkey, this part of the ventrolateral frontal cortex has been shown to be strongly connected with the inferotemporal cortex, which is the final stage in the analysis of visual pattern information.[4,18] Thus, the present findings with PET provided strong confirmation of the hypothesis that the mid-ventrolateral frontal cortex plays a major role when explicit judgments concerning mnemonic information are being made.

It is important to note the absence of differential activation within the mid-dorsolateral frontal cortex in any of these subtractions. This lack of activation is consistent with work in nonhuman primates demonstrating that the dorsolateral frontal cortex is not critically involved in the performance of recognition memory tasks.[8,16] The visual stimuli used in the present investigation were similar to those used in our earlier working memory study that revealed strong activation in human mid-dorsolateral frontal cortex (i.e., areas 46 and 9).[9] In the earlier work, activation due to the explicit judgments made in the experimental self-ordered task was controlled (i.e., subtracted out), because it was also present to the same extent in the matching control task. Thus, the differential activation between the self-ordered and the control tasks was due to the additional monitoring requirements of the self-ordered task.

DIFFERENTIAL INVOLVEMENT OF THE MID-DORSOLATERAL AND THE VENTROLATERAL FRONTAL CORTEX IN MEMORY

The above findings demonstrated differential activation of the mid-dorsolateral and the ventrolateral frontal cortex during the performance of nonspatial visual mnemonic tasks. It was shown that the relative activation in these frontal cortical regions is dependent on the nature of the required executive processing. In other related work, we observed similar results with visuospatial[19] and auditory[20] stimuli. We found that when the monitoring requirements of the task were extensive, there was differential activation within the mid-dorsolateral frontal cortex. On the other hand, when the task emphasized explicit judgments on stimuli held in short-term memory or the simple repetition of a sequence in which the stimuli were displayed, the ventrolateral frontal cortex was differentially activated. Strategic retrieval of information from long-term memory also activates the ventrolateral frontal cortex.[21,22]

The arguments made above are also consistent with the results of studies of patients who had undergone excisions of frontal or temporal cortex for the treatment of epilepsy. In one experiment, the patients were tested on a self-ordered task in which they had to generate digits randomly from a given set and on a digit span test in which they had to reproduce a series of digits presented by the experimenter (Petrides, unpublished experiments). The results were strikingly different for the two verbal short-term memory tasks. The patients with lesions invading the dorsolateral frontal cortex were severely impaired on the verbal self-ordered task, but performed normally on the digit span task. A related observation in the monkey is relevant here. Monkeys with mid-dorsolateral frontal lesions are severely impaired on the self-ordered and externally ordered tasks, but perform normally on a fixed sequence task in which they have to learn to select from a set of stimuli according to a fixed order.[8]

How can we explain the above observation of normal performance on the digit span task coupled with severely impaired performance on the self-ordered digit task by patients with lesions invading the dorsolateral frontal cortex? According to the model presented earlier, in the digit span task, the sequence of the presented numbers is analyzed and held in short-term mnemonic form in posterior association cortex. If the subject has to repeat this sequence, the executive processes being tapped are primarily those of the ventrolateral frontal cortex, namely, the retrieval (i.e., selection) of specific information from working memory. Once the first number has been retrieved, the process is repeated with the next number in line, and so on, until all the numbers have been reproduced. In attentional terms, we could say that the subject needs to attend to the first stimulus in the series held in working memory, and, having repeated (i.e., acted on) that digit, the subject can now attend to the next one in the series, and so on, until all have been repeated. Thus, although six or seven numbers may be held in short-term memory in posterior association cortex, from the executive point of view—that is, repetition of the digits—attention is directed to the numbers seriatim. This is in sharp contrast to the self-ordered task in which the subject, having randomly selected one or more numbers from the set, must now constantly consider (i.e., attend to) the selected numbers *in relation to* the nonselected ones, as each move is being planned. In other words, the monitoring demands of the self-ordered task, in the sense in which this term has been used to describe mid-dorsolateral frontal function,[5] are significantly greater than those of the digit span task.

The above analysis is consistent not only with the results of lesion studies but also with current neuroimaging studies. As mentioned above, we found strong activation within the mid-dorsolateral frontal cortex in a verbal working memory task in which the subjects had to monitor either their self-generated choices from a set of digits or the external generation of digits from the set.[10] In our study, the executive requirements (i.e., monitoring) of the working memory tasks were designed to be greater than those of the control task. In another study of verbal working memory with PET,[23] however, in which the monitoring requirements of the experimental and control tasks did not differ, only posterior association cortex was activated and, in addition, the ventrolateral frontal cortex when articulatory rehearsal was required.

Functional activation studies of spatial working memory have yielded what appear to be inconsistent results. Jonides *et al.*[24] reported activation in ventrolateral frontal cortex (area 47/12), whereas McCarthy *et al.*[25] reported activation in mid-dorsolateral frontal cortical area 46. These conflicting findings can be reconciled when the requirements of the two spatial working memory tasks are carefully considered. In the study by Jonides *et al.*, the subjects were presented with three locations and, after a delay, a probe appeared and they had to decide whether the probed location was one of the three previously shown. In other words, the subjects had to match a given probe with information stored in spatial working memory—that is, they had to retrieve a specific piece of information from short-term memory. This is exactly the type of executive process that, in the model presented above, is assumed to depend on the ventrolateral frontal cortex. By contrast, the task used by McCarthy *et al.*[25] required extensive monitoring within working memory because the subjects had to judge whether each stimulus, in a long series, was located in a position that had been occupied earlier in the series.

This task taxed the type of monitoring process subserved by the mid-dorsolateral frontal cortex. Similar results were obtained on spatial working memory tasks studied in our laboratory.[19] We have observed activation of the mid-dorsolateral or the ventrolateral frontal cortex or both, depending on whether the monitoring or the retrieval of specific information from spatial working memory was taxed.

In conclusion, activation of the mid-dorsolateral frontal cortex and the ventrolateral frontal cortex has been reported with a variety of stimuli (e.g., visual nonspatial, visuospatial, auditory and visual verbal, and auditory nonverbal) in a number of neuroimaging studies. The present article has argued that the nature of the required executive processing, rather than the nature of the stimulus material, is the critical factor determining whether the mid-dorsolateral and the ventrolateral frontal cortex are differentially active. This is not to deny that, *within* the mid-dorsolateral and the ventrolateral frontal cortex, some differentiation according to the modality of the stimulus material may exist.

REFERENCES

1. PETRIDES, M. 1989. Frontal lobes and memory. *In* Handbook of Neuropsychology. F. Boller & J. Grafman, Eds. Vol. 3: 75–90. Elsevier. Amsterdam.
2. JUS, A., K. JUS, A. VILLENEUVE, A. PIRES, R. LACHANCE, J. FORTIER & R. VILLENEUVE. 1973. Studies on dream recall in chronic schizophrenic patients after prefrontal lobotomy. Biol. Psychiatry **6:** 275–293.
3. STUSS, D. T., E. F. KAPLAN, D. F. BENSON, W. S. WEIR, S. CHIULLI & F. F. SARAZIN. 1982. Evidence for the involvement of orbitofrontal cortex in memory functions: An interference effect. J. Comp. Physiol. Psychol. **96:** 913–925.
4. PANDYA, D. N. & C. L. BARNES. 1987. Architecture and connections of the frontal lobe. *In* The Frontal Lobes Revisited. E. Perecman, Ed. The IRBN Press. New York.
5. PETRIDES, M. 1994. Frontal lobes and working memory: Evidence from investigations of the effects of cortical excisions in nonhuman primates. *In* Handbook of Neuropsychology. F. Boller & J. Grafman, Eds. Vol. 9: 59–82. Elsevier. Amsterdam.
6. PETRIDES, M. & D. N. PANDYA. 1994. Comparative architectonic analysis of the human and the macaque frontal cortex. *In* Handbook of Neuropsychology. F. Boller & J. Grafman, Eds. Vol. 9: 17–58. Elsevier. Amsterdam.
7. PETRIDES, M. & B. MILNER. 1982. Deficits on subject-ordered tasks after frontal- and temporal-lobe lesions in man. Neuropsychologia **20:** 249–262.
8. PETRIDES, M. 1995. Impairments on nonspatial self-ordered and externally ordered working memory tasks after lesions of the mid-dorsal part of the lateral frontal cortex in the monkey. J. Neurosci. **15:** 359–375.
9. PETRIDES, M., B. ALIVISATOS, A. C. EVANS & E. MEYER. 1993. Dissociation of human mid-dorsolateral frontal cortex in memory processing. Proc. Natl. Acad. Sci. USA **90:** 873–877.
10. PETRIDES, M., B. ALIVISATOS, E. MEYER & A. C. EVANS. 1993. Functional activation of the human frontal cortex during the performance of verbal working memory tasks. Proc. Natl. Acad. Sci. USA **90:** 878–882.
11. PETRIDES, M. 1987. Conditional learning and the primate frontal cortex. *In* The Frontal Lobes Revisited. E. Perecman, Ed. The IRBN Press. New York.
12. BARBAS, H. 1988. Anatomic organization of basoventral and mediodorsal visual recipient prefrontal regions in the rhesus monkey. J. Comp. Neurol. **276:** 313–342.
13. MILNER, B. 1972. Disorders of learning and memory after temporal lobe lesions in man. Clin. Neurosurg. **19:** 421–446.
14. MISHKIN, M. 1982. A memory system in the monkey. Philos. Trans. R. Soc. Lond. B **298:** 85–95.

15. SQUIRE, L. R. & S. ZOLA-MORGAN. 1991. The medial temporal lobe memory system. Science **253:** 1380–1386.
16. BACHEVALIER, J. & M. MISHKIN. 1986. Visual recognition impairment follows ventromedial but not dorsolateral prefrontal lesions in monkeys. Behav. Brain Res. **20:** 249–261.
17. BUTTER, C. M. 1964. Habituation of responses to novel stimuli in monkeys with selective frontal lesions. Science **144:** 313–315.
18. UNGERLEIDER, L. G., D. GAFFAN & V. S. PELAK. 1989. Projections from inferior temporal cortex to prefrontal cortex via the uncinate fascicle in rhesus monkeys. Exp. Brain Res. **76:** 473–484.
19. OWEN, A. M., A. C. EVANS & M. PETRIDES. Evidence for a two-stage model of spatial working memory processing within the lateral frontal cortex: A positron emission tomography study. Cereb. Cortex. In press.
20. PERRY, D. W., M. PETRIDES, B. ALIVISATOS, R. J. ZATORRE, A. C. EVANS & E. MEYER. 1994. Functional activation of human frontal cortex during tonal working memory tasks. Soc. Neurosci. Abstr. **20:** 435.
21. PETRIDES, M., B. ALIVISATOS & A. C. EVANS. 1995. Functional activation of the human ventrolateral frontal cortex during mnemonic retrieval of verbal information. Proc. Natl. Acad. Sci. USA **92:** 5803–5807.
22. BUCKNER, R. L., S. E. PETERSEN, J. G. OJEMANN, F. M. MIEZIN, L. R. SQUIRE & M. E. RAICHLE. 1995. Functional anatomical studies of explicit and implicit memory retrieval tasks. J. Neurosci. **15:** 12–29.
23. PAULESU, E., C. D. FRITH & R. S. J. FRACKOWIAK. 1993. The neural correlates of the verbal component of working memory. Nature **362:** 342–344.
24. JONIDES, J., E. E. SMITH, R. A. KOEPPE, E. AWH, S. MINOSHIMA & M. A. MINTUN. 1993. Spatial working memory in humans as revealed by PET. Nature **363:** 623–625.
25. MCCARTHY, G., A. M. BLAMIRE, A. PUCE, A. C. NOBRE, G. BLOCH, F. HYDER, P. GOLDMAN-RAKIC & R. G. SHULMAN. 1994. Functional magnetic resonance imaging of human prefrontal cortex activation during a spatial working memory task. Proc. Natl. Acad. Sci. USA **91:** 8690–8694.

Human Rehearsal Processes and the Frontal Lobes: PET Evidence

EDWARD AWH,[a] EDWARD E. SMITH, AND JOHN JONIDES

Department of Psychology
University of Michigan
Ann Arbor, Michigan 48109

INTRODUCTION

Our research is focused on *working memory*. This is a storage system that holds a limited amount of information for a brief time, with that information rapidly accessible and changeable from moment to moment. Such a system is essential for dealing with problems that require one to record features of a constantly changing environment, and to keep these features "on line" as they are used to guide behavior.

Extensive research supports two basic claims about the neural implementation of working memory in both human and nonhuman primates: (1) Working memory is implemented in the brain by heightened neural activity in particular regions, which notably include prefrontal and parietal cortex;[1,2] and (2) different kinds of working memories correspond to different kinds of information. This is indicated by findings in nonhuman primates that neurons in different regions of the prefrontal cortex are active when monkeys have to store spatial information versus object information,[3] and by the PET findings with humans that different networks of cortical regions are active depending on whether people have to remember spatial, object, or verbal information.[4] In this paper, we emphasize human data, and try to go beyond the above two generalizations by decomposing each working memory into two basic constituents. We advance the following hypotheses:

1. Each working memory itself consists of a passive *storage* buffer and an active maintenance or *rehearsal* process. (The storage process may consist of either a separate structure or merely continued activation of perceptual processes; the rehearsal process consists of any operations that intentionally lengthen the duration of a representation.)
2. The storage and rehearsal processes may be implemented by different brain regions. In verbal working memory, rehearsal seems to be mediated by frontal regions, whereas storage may be mediated by posterior regions.

First we consider *verbal* working memory, and present evidence that it conforms to hypotheses 1 and 2. Then we consider *spatial* working memory and provide preliminary evidence characterizing the storage and rehearsal of information about location.

---

[a] Address correspondence to Edward Awh, 525 E. University Avenue, Ann Arbor, MI 48109-1109.

STORAGE AND REHEARSAL IN VERBAL WORKING MEMORY

Background

The idea that verbal working memory includes both storage and rehearsal components is a cornerstone of behavioral research on working (or short-term) memory.[5,6] One of the best pieces of evidence for the distinction is the *word length effect*. When a subject is presented a short list of words and asked to recall the words in order, accuracy is greater for words that take less time to pronounce.[7] The simplest account of this finding is that subjects are rehearsing the words to themselves between presentation and recall, and the faster they can do so, the less likely that any particular word in store will decay before it is produced. A second piece of evidence for the storage-rehearsal distinction is the *articulatory suppression effect*. If subjects in a verbal working memory task are also required to articulate a familiar item concurrently (e.g., "the"), memory accuracy declines, and this decline cannot be attributed to simple distraction.[6] The explanation of this result is that the concurrent articulation task disrupts or suppresses the subjects' implicit rehearsal, which in turn leads to decay of some of the items in store, and a decline in recall.

To follow up on this behavioral evidence, we conducted two PET experiments that investigate the storage-rehearsal distinction in verbal working memory.[8]

Item Recognition Experiment

Rationale and Method

In any verbal working memory task with a retention interval of a second or more, we would expect subjects to rehearse the material during the interval (as well as during the response period).[9] Such rehearsal seems to consist of covert speech. Accordingly, it might involve the same neural mechanisms as does overt speech, which include Broca's area and other left-hemisphere frontal regions that appear to mediate the planning of speech. Thus, activation in these regions was expected in our task.

The first verbal working memory task that we studied was a variant of the widely used *item recognition* task developed by Sternberg.[10] It is schematized at the top of FIGURE 1. Each trial consisted of four events: (1) a fixation cross presented for 500 ms; (2) four targets, each one an uppercase letter, exposed for a total of 200 ms; (3) a return to the fixation cross for a retention interval of 3000 ms; and (4) a probe, available for 1500 ms, that consisted of a single lowercase letter. The subjects' task was to decide whether or not the probe had the same name as any of the targets, and to indicate their decision by pressing a response button once for matches and twice for nonmatches. Because the targets and probe were in different cases, subjects were induced to represent the targets with a verbal code (phonological or articulatory). Successful performance on this task requires processes in addition to remembering verbal information, for example, attending to the inputs and selecting and executing a response. To remove the effects of these nonmemory processes from the PET images, a control condition

Item Recognition Task

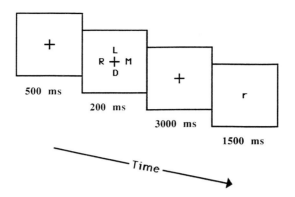

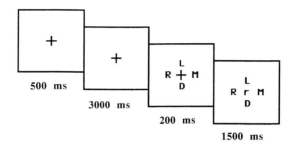

Item Recognition Control

FIGURE 1. Schematic drawing of the events on each trial of the Item Recognition (*top*) and Item Recognition Control (*bottom*) tasks.

was devised that included these processes but not memory (this follows the subtraction methodology developed by Posner *et al.*[11]). In the *item recognition control* task (FIG. 1 bottom), the sequence of trial events consisted of (1) a fixation cross; (2) continuation of the fixation cross for another 3000 ms; (3) four uppercase target letters presented for a total of 200 ms; and (4) a lowercase probe letter presented along with the four uppercase target letters. Again the subjects' task was to indicate whether or not the probe was identical in name to any of the targets, but in this case the decision could be made without any stored information. In both tasks, the probe matched one of the targets about half the time.

With regard to the PET procedure, subjects were first familiarized with the PET apparatus. Then each subject had an intravenous catheter inserted into his or her right arm for administration of the radioactive tracer. The subject was positioned in the scanner with a band across the forehead attached to a head holder to constrain head movement. Eleven subjects were tested. They had three scans each of the item recognition task and the control condition, in which each scan consisted of 20 trials in sequence. The sequence began just prior to the injection of the radionuclide, at which time a bolus injection of 66 mCi of [^{15}O]-labeled water was given. PET acquisition (using a Siemens/CTI-931/08-12) began 5 s after the count rate was observed to increase above the background level and continued for 60 s thereafter, during which time the sequence of items continued to be presented. The trials continued until after the PET scan was completed. Scans were performed at intervals of 14 min, allowing time for the oxygen-15 to decay.

The PET images for each subject were first transformed to a stereotactic coordinate system,[12,13] and then linearly scaled to the dimensions of a standard atlas brain.[14] After normalizing pixel values for global flow-rate differences among scans,[15] the data were averaged across subjects, thereby obtaining means and variances for the two conditions of interest. The difference image was created by subtracting activation in the control task from that in memory task; this image was then analyzed by performing post-hoc t tests on a voxel-by-voxel basis and correcting the outcomes for multiple comparisons.[16,17]

Results and Discussion

The analysis resulted in a map of cerebral areas that showed significant increases in regional cerebral blood flow. FIGURE 2 presents four brain images showing the significant areas of activation in the item-recognition task. The number below each image gives its z-coordinate (an indication of how inferior or superior the relevant brain region is with respect to anterior-posterior commissure line). The areas of activation have been superimposed on a composite magnetic resonance image so as to provide some anatomical localization. The coordinates defining each area of activation are given in TABLE 1.

Note first that most of the significant areas of activation are in the left hemisphere. These regions include: Area 7 ("area" is shorthand for "Brodmann area") and area 40 in parietal cortex (see FIG. 2, top right image), along with three regions in frontal cortex, corresponding to area 44 (Broca's area), the inferior aspect of area 6 (the premotor area), and the superior aspect of area 6 (the supplementary motor area, or SMA). Broca's area is evident in the bottom left image, whereas the premotor area and SMA are visible in the top left image. The three left-hemisphere frontal regions are known to play a role in explicit speech,[18] and hence are likely to mediate implicit speech, or rehearsal, as well. The two parietal regions may be involved in mediating the passive storage function. Indeed, area 40 in left parietal cortex is the most frequent site of damage in patients who have impaired verbal working memory.[19,20]

Other regions were activated as well. Two of these have surfaced in other PET studies of cognition: a right-hemisphere cerebellar site and a midline structure, the anterior cingulate. The cerebellar site has been argued to mediate aspects of the planning and execution of speech,[21] so it too may play a role in implicit speech

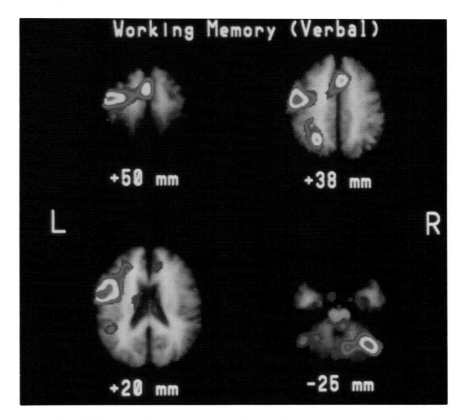

FIGURE 2. PET images of the statistically significant activation sites in the item Recognition minus Item Recognition Control subtraction analyses [Working Memory (Verbal)]. Each image is superimposed on an MRI image of a composite brain in order to illustrate anatomical localization of the activation foci. Stereotaxic coordinates of the significant foci of activation are given in TABLE 1.

or rehearsal (the right cerebellum receives projections from the *left* cerebral hemisphere). The anterior cingulate has been found active in other studies of cognitive tasks,[22] and has typically been interpreted as reflecting attentional processes. The remaining two areas of activation in the verbal task were the left-hemisphere thalamus and insular cortex (these are not shown in FIG. 2); we have no ready explanation for their involvement in the verbal task, nor are they typically found in other PET studies of working memory.

In sum, the known functionality of the activated areas supports the claim that different neuroanatomical regions mediate rehearsal and storage. In particular, whereas parietal regions may implement storage, frontal regions very likely implement rehearsal. Two of the frontal regions involved, the premotor area and SMA,

TABLE 1. Significant Activation Foci for Memory Minus Control (Item Recognition Task)

Stereotaxic Coordinates				
x	y	z	Z-Score	Brain Area
				Left hemisphere
24	−55	43	5.3	Posterior parietal (areas 40 and 7)
55	3	20	5.7	Broca's area (area 44)
44	12	22	5.0	Broca's area (area 44)
1	5	52	4.4	SMA (area 6)
48	−6	40	5.8	Premotor cortex (area 6)
28	14	4	5.3	Insular cortex
17	−4	9	4.3	Thalamus
				Right hemisphere
−33	−60	−25	5.4	Cerebellum
				Midline
−6	19	38	4.6	Anterior cingulate (area 32)

SMA, supplementary motor area.

are known to be involved in the high-level preparation and planning of movement in general for nonhuman primates as well as humans.[23] It is no surprise, then, that these two areas also play a role in the planning of human speech.[18] The other frontal region involved, Broca's area, is, of course, known to play a crucial role in overt speech; prior imaging work indicates it is also activated during internal speech,[24] a result consistent with the present findings. Presumably, Broca's area mediates a more downstream function than that accomplished by the premotor area and SMA; for example, Broca's area may be responsible for specifying the articulatory features of the utterance to be internally generated.

Continuous Memory Experiment

Rationale and Method

One purpose of this study was simply to replicate the critical parietal (storage) and frontal (rehearsal) activations in a different kind of verbal working memory task. A second goal of this study was to provide more direct evidence that the frontal regions involved—Broca's, premotor, and SMA—mediate rehearsal. Our logic was similar to that used by Paulesu et al.[21] These authors obtained PET measures during various tasks, which included an item recognition task similar to the one we used in the experiment just described and a rhyming task in which subjects had to decide whether or not each of a series of test letters rhymed with a target syllable. The item recognition task produced activations like those we obtained, including posterior parietal areas as well as frontal speech and motor sites. Assuming (as we do) that the item recognition task involved both rehearsal and storage, and assuming further that the rhyming task involved rehearsal but not storage, Paulesu et al. subtracted the activations in the rhyming task from those in the item recognition task. They found a reduction in the activation in the frontal regions but not in the parietal ones, and argued that this result supports the claim that the frontal regions mediate rehearsal. A problem with this logic, however, is that it is not clear that the rhyming task requires much by way of rehearsal—only one syllable needed to be maintained in the entire task. In lieu of this, we used as one of our conditions a task in which subjects were explicitly instructed to continuously rehearse letters. Presumably, this task reflects a purer measure of rehearsal, and subtracting its activation pattern from that obtained in our memory condition should come closer to "subtracting out rehearsal."

The verbal working memory task we used is referred to as "2-back" and is presented schematically at the top of FIGURE 3. Subjects were presented a continuous stream of single letters, each for 500 ms with a 2500-ms interval between successive letters; each letter appeared at the center of the screen. The subjects' task was to decide whether or not each letter matched the one presented two back (not the previous letter, but the one prior to that). One-third of the letters provided matches that required positive responses (there were also three matches 1-back and 3-back so that subjects could not use mere familiarity as the basis of their responses).

There were two control conditions. One was a *search* task that presumably includes the nonmemory components of the 2-back task (e.g., encoding the letters, selecting and executing a motor response). This search condition is presented in the middle of FIGURE 3. The same sequence of letters as in the 2-back task was presented, but now subjects had only to decide whether or not each letter matched a target letter given at the beginning of the block. Subtracting the activation in this condition from that in the 2-back condition should reveal the neural bases of rehearsal and storage, which should match the results obtained in the previous study. The second control was a simple *rehearsal* task, and it is presented at the bottom of FIGURE 3. Again the same sequence of letters as in the 2-back task was presented, but now subjects had to push a button when each letter appeared, continuously say the name of the letter to themselves until the next one appeared, and so on. Subtracting the activation in this condition from that in the 2-back condition should remove some of the neural underpinnings of rehearsal, but leave the neural basis of storage unaffected.

The PET procedure was the same as that in the previous experiment, except that now nine subjects were tested, and every subject had three scans of each of the three conditions. The analysis of the PET images paralleled that in the first experiment.

Results and Discussion

We are again interested in difference images, but now two subtractions are of particular interest: 2-back minus search and 2-back minus rehearsal. FIGURE 4 presents the difference images for 2-back minus search; the coordinates defining each significant area of activation are given in the top of TABLE 2.

The most important result is that all areas that were significantly activated in the first study are again significant here, with the exception of the two regions for which interpretation was unclear: thalamus and insular cortex. Again, there is

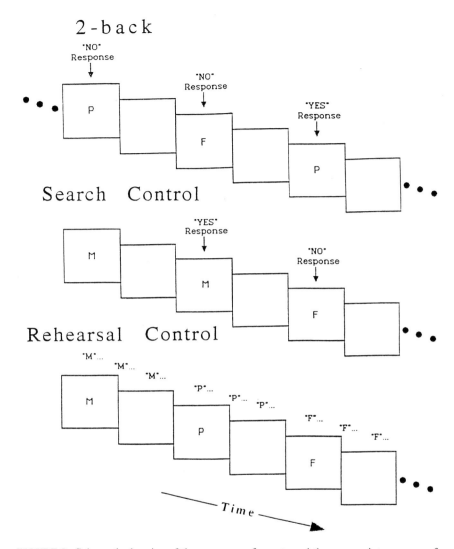

FIGURE 3. Schematic drawing of the sequence of events and the appropriate response for each item in a sample series from the 2-Back (*top*), Search (*middle*), and Rehearsal (*bottom*) conditions.

TABLE 2. Significant Activation Foci for 2-Back Minus Search

Stereotaxic Coordinates				
x	y	z	Z-Score	Brain Area
				Left hemisphere
33	− 46	38	5.4	Posterior parietal (area 40)
17	− 60	45	5.7	Superior parietal (area 7)
42	17	22	4.4	Broca's area (area 44)
28	1	52	6.0	SMA, premotor (area 6)
26	− 67	− 50	5.1	Cerebellum
6	3	54	5.2	SMA
				Right hemisphere
− 12	− 64	47	5.3	Superior parietal (area 7)
− 26	− 55	50	4.6	Superior parietal (area 7)
− 24	3	52	5.5	SMA, premotor (area 6)
− 1	− 64	− 25	4.8	Cerebellar vermis
− 33	− 60	− 25	5.4	Cerebellum
				Midline
3	12	40	5.0	Anterior cingulate (area 32)

SMA, supplementary motor area.

activation in the three frontal regions that presumably mediate rehearsal—Broca's area, premotor area, and SMA—as well as in the posterior parietal regions that presumably implement storage. Furthermore, the areas common to our two studies have also been found in studies of other investigators of verbal working memory.[21,25] This convergence of results strengthens our belief that we are indeed seeing evidence of the neural basis of verbal working memory.

In addition to these common areas of activation, three additional areas proved significant in the 2-back minus search subtraction. All three are right-hemisphere regions homologous to those activated in the left hemisphere, and include Area 7 in the superior parietal cortex, along with the premotor area and SMA in frontal cortex. The degree of activation in these right-hemisphere areas is consistently less than that in the left-hemisphere homologues. These findings suggest that the right-hemisphere activations under discussion may reflect the functional recruitment of right-hemisphere mechanisms to assist in an unusually demanding version of what is normally a left-hemisphere task.[26]

Consider now the 2-back minus rehearsal subtraction, which should reveal activations in brain areas that mediate storage with areas related to rehearsal subtracted out. FIGURE 5 presents the difference images; the coordinates defining each significant area are given in TABLE 3. As expected, this subtraction reveals a loss of significant activation in Broca's area and premotor area, both of which presumably mediate rehearsal. Furthermore, the activation in left posterior parietal cortex remains significant, supporting the hypothesis that this area participates in storage. However, there is still activation in SMA and right cerebellar cortex after subtraction, despite the fact that these areas have also been associated with rehearsal. One possibility is that our rehearsal control was not sufficiently demanding to engage a full complement of rehearsal processes. Alternatively, these areas may mediate processes unrelated to rehearsal.

The 2-back minus rehearsal subtraction also reveals activation in the thalamus,

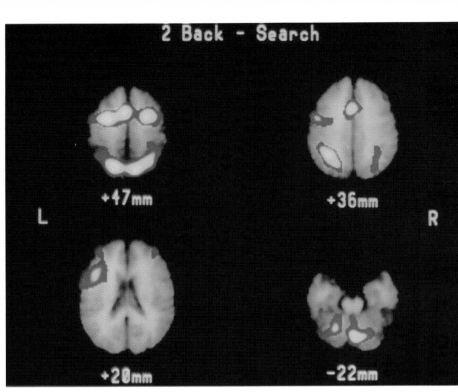

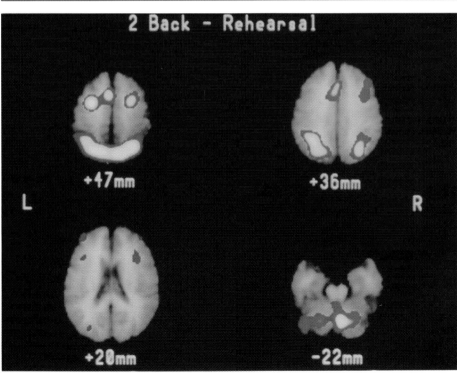

TABLE 3. Significant Activation Foci for 2-Back Minus Rehearsal

Stereotaxic Coordinates				
x	y	z	Z-Score	Brain Area
				Left hemisphere
17	−60	43	5.8	Posterior and superior parietal (areas 40 and 7)
28	1	50	5.5	SMA
3	14	43	4.8	SMA
				Right hemisphere
−26	−58	45	5.3	Superior parietal (area 7)
−12	−64	47	5.7	Superior parietal (area 7)
−26	3	50	4.5	SMA (area 6)
−3	−17	2	4.7	Thalamus
−3	−62	−25	4.8	Cerebellar vermis
−28	−60	−38	4.6	Cerebellum

SMA, supplementary motor area.

for which we have no interpretation. Finally, the activation in anterior cingulate cortex that appeared in the 2-back minus search subtraction drops out in this subtraction. The lack of anterior-cingulate activation casts doubt on interpretations that center on an attentional role for this brain region because the attentional difference between 2-back and rehearsal seem similar to that between 2-back and the search control.

In sum, these results provide two sources of evidence for the claim that verbal rehearsal is mediated by regions in frontal cortex. First, using a very different working memory task than that employed in the first study, we again found significant activation in Broca's area, premotor area, and SMA—regions whose known functionality involves the planning of speech. Second, we also provided "subtraction" evidence for the claim of interest. We selected two tasks—2-back and rehearsal—which at the *cognitive level* seem to require implicit rehearsal, and then showed at the *neural level* that the active regions they have in common tend to be those that mediate implicit rehearsal.

A weak link in the above argument is the assumption that, at the cognitive level, both the 2-back and rehearsal tasks require rehearsal. Such an assumption calls for behavioral evidence. Accordingly, we performed a follow-up behavioral experiment in which we sought to establish an articulatory suppression effect, which is a behavioral indicator of rehearsal (see our earlier discussion). Subjects

←———————————————————————————————

FIGURE 4 (Top). PET images of the statistically significant activation sites in the 2-Back minus Search subtraction analyses. Each image is superimposed on an MRI image of a composite brain. Stereotaxic coordinates of the significant foci of activation are given in TABLE 2.

FIGURE 5 (Bottom). PET images of the statistically significant activation sites in the 2-Back minus Rehearsal subtraction analyses. Each image is superimposed on an MRI image of a composite brain. Stereotaxic coordinates of the significant foci of activation are given in TABLE 3. Note the loss of significant activation in anterior regions associated with rehearsal (i.e., Broca's area and premotor area), whereas left posterior parietal activations remain significant.

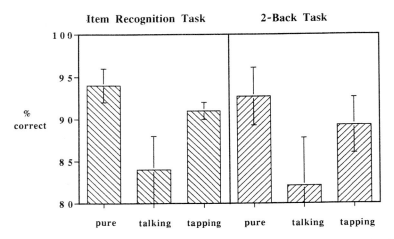

FIGURE 6. Graphs depicting Item Recognition (*left*) and 2-Back (*right*) accuracies during pure task performance, articulatory suppression, and tapping. In both tasks, only articulatory suppression caused significant decrements in performance. Because two-thirds of the 2-back trials required negative responses, there could have been an overall bias to say "no"; hence, only the data from match trials are presented (this pattern of accuracies is also statistically significant across all trials).

performed the 2-back task or the item recognition task from the first study, either alone or concurrently with another task. One concurrent task required subjects to continuously say aloud the names of the digits 1–4, whereas the other secondary task required subjects to continuously tap with the fingers of the left hand at a prescribed rate; only the "say aloud" or articulation task should interfere with implicit rehearsal, and hence this task should be more detrimental to memory performance than the tapping task. Exactly this difference was found in both the 2-back and the item recognition tasks (see FIG. 6). Thus the behavioral results converge with the PET findings in indicating that rehearsal is involved in the memory tasks that we studied.

Summary

Our PET results are broadly consistent with the generalization that part of the neural network mediating working memory is in the frontal cortex.[1] However, in our studies the frontal cortex contribution to working memory involves rehearsal not sheer storage. Of course, the results discussed thus far concern only verbal materials; whether our notion of rehearsal processes applies to nonverbal working memory is a topic which we next address.

REHEARSAL IN SPATIAL WORKING MEMORY

Previous Hypotheses

Research on spatial working memory has focused mainly on its independence from other working memory systems. There have been few hypotheses regarding the specific subcomponents of this system. Baddeley[6] has suggested that implicit eye movements (i.e., operation of an eye-movement control system without overt eye movements) to target positions may serve as a rehearsal mechanism for spatial positions. He reports that a secondary task requiring overt eye movements disrupts the performance of a spatial memory span task. Smyth and Scholey[27] hypothesize that spatial working memory depends on shifts of spatial attention. They demonstrated that spatial span (assessed by a version of the Corsi Blocks task) is reduced by concurrent tasks that require shifts of spatial attention. It is still unclear, however, exactly how spatial attention might mediate the rehearsal of location information. In the following sections, we provide a hypothesis that makes explicit the role of spatial selective attention.

A Specific Hypothesis

Research on spatial selective attention emphasizes improvements in processing efficiency at attended locations in space.[28] Thus, although it is well known that stimuli falling in the center of the visual field enjoy faster and more sensitive perceptual processing (the retinal acuity effect), visual processing advantages independent of this factor can be demonstrated when attention is oriented to a particular region of space without shifts of gaze. Current research suggests that spatial selective attention may operate by enhancing the processing of early perceptual systems in a location-specific manner.[29] Thus, visual processing may be improved in the particular cortical regions that process the attended region of space. (Recall that visual cortex is topographically organized—that is, independent locations in cortex can be mapped onto independent locations in the environment.)

We propose a model of spatial rehearsal in which an interaction of attentional and perceptual mechanisms mediates the "on line" maintenance of spatial information. By this account, the rehearsal of spatial information *corresponds* to spatial selective attention, creating a location-specific change in visual processing mechanisms. Two forms of support for this view are offered: First, a review of evidence suggests a strong correspondence between the neuroanatomical regions mediating spatial selective attention and those that we have found to mediate spatial working memory. Second, a preliminary behavioral study provides evidence of interaction between the psychological mechanisms of spatial selective attention and spatial working memory.

Brain Circuitry Involved in Spatial Selective Attention

Evidence for Enhancement of Early Visual Processing

A recent study by Heinze *et al.*[29] supports the idea that visual processing in extrastriate cortex is modulated by spatial selective attention. Subjects in these experiments were instructed to attend to either the left or right side of bilateral stimulus arrays to perform a visual target detection task. Combined PET and ERP measures showed increased activation in extrastriate cortex (contralateral to the attended side) that began as early as 80–130 ms after stimulus onset. Thus, both the timing and localization of these neuronal responses suggest that spatial selective attention causes location-specific changes in early visual processing.

Parietal Cortex

The neural network mediating spatial selective attention has also been shown to include regions of parietal cortex.[30] When attention was tonically maintained to a specific spatial location, increased activation occurred in parietal-occipital cortex (once again, contralateral to the attended side of space). In addition, similar contralateral increases were observed in the inferior occipital association cortex. The interpretation of these results was that the visual responses in these areas were enhanced by orienting of selective attention. Furthermore, in a task where subjects continuously shifted attention to various peripheral locations, enhanced responses were observed in superior parietal cortex.

Frontal Cortex

In a detection task, the activity of neurons in the monkey prefrontal cortex was recorded.[31] Visual stimuli were presented extrafoveally while the monkey gazed at a fixation point. In one condition, the monkey was attending the peripheral visual stimulus (because the behavioral response depended on the offset of this stimulus). In another condition, the peripheral stimulus did not have behavioral significance. When neurons in the prearcuate and periprincipalis areas (putatively homologous to dorsolateral prefrontal cortex in humans[32]) were compared in these two conditions, significantly higher neuronal responses were found to *attended* visual stimuli. These results provide support for a role of prefrontal cortex in the selection of visual stimuli.

It should be noted that frontal lobe regions were also activated in the studies by Heinze *et al.*[29] and Petersen *et al.*[30] In particular, both studies showed that area 6 (including premotor and supplementary motor areas) is activated by orienting of spatial attention. Further evidence comes from a recent review of the effects of frontal lobe damage in humans.[33] The authors concluded that regions of frontal cortex are critical to the proper functioning of spatial selective attention. For example, a study of patients who had undergone unilateral frontal or temporal lobe excisions[34] revealed that frontal lobe patients were less able to take advantage of a cue that indicated the location of an impending visual target. From this and other studies, Foster *et al.* concluded that the *right* frontal lobe is particularly important for visuospatial orienting.

Summary of Spatial Selective Attention Circuitry

The following cortical regions have been implicated in spatial selective attention: (1) visual processing areas, including extrastriate and parietal-occipital regions; (2) superior parietal cortex; and (3) frontal cortex, including dorsolateral prefrontal cortex and area 6 (supplementary motor and premotor). Next, we consider the overlap between these regions and those that mediate spatial working memory.

Spatial Working Memory Experiment

Method

The spatial working memory task we used is referred to as "spatial 3-back" and is illustrated in FIGURE 7. This task is very similar to the continuous verbal memory experiment described previously. Subjects fixed their gaze on a centrally located cross while a sequence of 42 consonants was presented, each for 500 ms, with a 2500-ms interval between successive letters. The letters appeared at randomly chosen locations around an imaginary circle (whose radius was 6.6° of visual angle). Their task was to decide whether the spatial position of each letter matched the position of the letter presented three back. This spatial memory experiment was part of a larger study that also tested verbal working memory; however, only the spatial working-memory results will be discussed here.

The control condition was a *spatial search* task designed to include the perceptual and motor components of the spatial 3-back task. The stimulus display for the search task was identical to the one used in the spatial 3-back task, but the subjects' task here was simply to search for the occurrence of one of three previously memorized spatial positions. Subtracting the activation in this spatial search task from that in the spatial 3-back task should reveal the brain regions that mediate storage and rehearsal of spatial information.

Again, the PET procedure was identical to that used in the continuous verbal memory study, except that eight subjects were tested; each subject had two scans of the spatial 3-back condition, and two scans of the search condition. The analysis

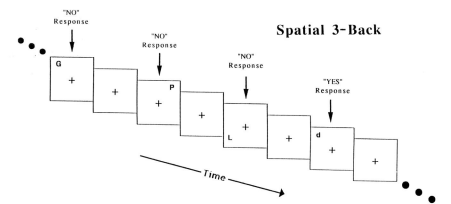

FIGURE 7. Schematic drawing of the sequence of events and the appropriate response for each item in a sample series from the Spatial 3-Back condition.

techniques on the difference images are consistent with the other PET experiments
in this report.

Results and Discussion

The difference images for spatial 3-back minus spatial search are presented in
FIGURE 8. The coordinates and z-score for each activation focus are shown in
TABLE 4.

The most striking feature of these results is the strong overlap with the neural
circuitry associated with spatial selective attention. Specifically, the subtraction
analyses reveal a bilateral pattern of activation in superior and inferior parietal
cortex (areas 7 and 40), dorsolateral prefrontal cortex (areas 9, 10, and 46), and
supplementary motor cortex (area 6). *All* of these sites have been implicated in
the neural circuitry underlying spatial selective attention. Moreover, the frontal
and posterior parietal activations show a clear right-hemisphere dominance (as
indicated by the z-scores for the right- and left-hemisphere sites), consistent with
neuropsychological evidence on spatial attention.[33]

The extrastriate region is the only cortical area implicated in the selective
attention studies that was not found in the present analysis. However, there is
reason to believe that the particular control task we used may have caused this
anomaly. Recall that subjects were searching for the occurrence of any of three

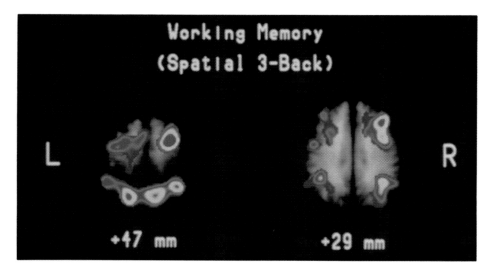

FIGURE 8. PET images of the statistically significant activation sites in the Spatial 3-Back
minus Search subtraction analyses. Each image is superimposed on an MRI image of a
composite brain. Stereotaxic coordinates of the significant foci of activation are given in
TABLE 4. Note the relative dominance of right-hemisphere activation in this task.

TABLE 4. Significant Activation Foci for Spatial 3-Back Minus Spatial Search

Stereotaxic Coordinates				
x	y	z	Z-Score	Brain Area
				Left hemisphere
44	−46	43	5.5	Posterior parietal (area 40)
19	−67	50	5.0	Superior parietal (area 7)
26	−53	40	4.8	Posterior and superior parietal (areas 40 and 7)
33	44	20	4.7	Dorsolateral prefrontal (areas 46 and 10)
12	−1	58	4.7	SMA (area 6)
				Right hemisphere
−42	−49	40	7.4	Posterior parietal (area 40)
−30	3	47	6.9	SMA (area 6)
−35	28	29	5.5	Dorsolateral prefrontal (areas 46 and 9)
−12	−64	50	4.6	Superior parietal (area 7)

SMA, supplementary motor area.

previously memorized spatial positions during the search task. Post-experimental questionnaires revealed that the predominant strategy for monitoring these locations involved *imagery* of the three positions, a process known to activate occipital cortex.[35] Thus, we may have subtracted out occipital activations in this study. In line with this reasoning, we did find occipital activations in a previous spatial memory study that utilized a simpler control condition.[2]

In summary, our study of spatial working memory shows a striking overlap in the brain regions that mediate spatial selective attention and spatial working memory. This provides support for the hypothesis that the brain regions subserving spatial attention may also mediate spatial memory.

Dual-Task Memory Experiment

A Prediction

In addition to predicting correspondence in the neural circuitry of spatial memory and attention, the proposed model of spatial working memory makes a behavioral prediction. If spatial rehearsal involves selective orienting to memorized locations, then the typical effect of orienting spatial selective attention—improved processing efficiency at attended locations—should be observable at memorized locations.

Method

To test this prediction, a dual-task spatial memory experiment was designed (illustrated in FIG. 9). Each trial consisted of the following sequence of events: (1) The appearance of a central fixation cross marked the beginning of each trial

Dual Task Memory Experiment

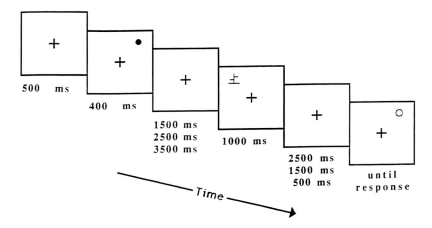

FIGURE 9. Schematic drawing of the sequence of events in each trial of the Dual-Task Spatial Memory experiment. A 50-ms warning tone occurred at the onset of the fixation cross. Choice stimuli (*middle panel*) occurred at intervals varying randomly from 1500, 2500, and 3500 ms after the offset of the dot. The retention interval totaled 5000 ms.

(a warning tone also occurred during the first 50 ms of this period). (2) The memory stimulus (a simple dot) was presented for 400 ms (the potential locations of the dot included 36 positions on each of three concentric circles, at 4, 5.5, and 7° of visual angle; the dot fell on each circle and position with equal likelihood). (3) A 5000-ms retention interval ensued, during which a choice reaction time stimulus appeared for 1000 ms (potential locations were from the same set as the memorized locations). The choice stimulus occurred at an interval varying randomly between 1500, 2500, and 3500 ms after the offset of the memory stimulus; (4) 5000 ms after the offset of the dot, a probe circle appeared on the screen and remained visible until the subject indicated with a key press whether or not it encircled the original dot.

The probe matched the memorized location with probability .5 (hit trials). When the probe did not fall in the memorized location (miss trials), the distance between the probe and the dot was varied systematically between .7, 2, 2.7, and 3.7° of visual angle. With probability .25, the choice stimulus appeared in the same location as the one held in memory (constituting a "choice match"). In order to control for retinal acuity effects, choice matches and choice mismatches were equally distributed on the three circles.

Eight university students served as subjects. Subjects were instructed to regard the memory task as primary, and not to let the choice task interfere with memory accuracy. Subjects were instructed to maintain fixation throughout each trial, and they were monitored with a video camera in order to ensure compliance. Trials in which eye movements were detected were excluded.

Results

Results on the memory task were orderly. Mean accuracy on hit trials was .87. Accuracy on the miss trials increased monotonically as the distance of the probe from the memorized location increased. This distance effect shows that subjects were probably using a spatial coding strategy to perform the primary memory task.

The critical variable in this experiment is reaction time to the choice matches compared to choice mismatches. If subjects are selectively attending the memorized locations, there should be a corresponding decrease in reaction time to the choice matches. The results confirmed this prediction. Subjects were significantly faster to respond to choice matches than to choice mismatches (598 vs. 615 ms), $[f(1,7) = 10.6, p < .025]$. Although accuracy on this task was virtually at ceiling, subjects were also reliably more accurate on choice match trials than choice mismatch trials (99.3 vs. 97.9%), $[t(7) = 2.1, p < .05$, one-tailed], eliminating the possibility of a speed/accuracy trade-off.

Although these results support the hypothesis that spatial rehearsal is mediated by orienting of spatial selective attention, they should be interpreted with caution. Further control experiments are needed to assess potential alternative explanations of these data. For instance, it is possible that the dot marking the memorized location caused automatic orienting of spatial attention to the memorized location (regardless of whether this orienting might subserve rehearsal). Although the interval between the memory stimulus and the choice stimulus (minimum 1500 ms) exceeds previously demonstrated durations of exogenous orienting,[36] this possibility should be considered. Also, it is possible that subjects adopted a voluntary orienting strategy (not in service of, but in addition to, the memory task). Although the memory dot matched the choice location only with probability .25, it is still possible that subjects adopted the (nonoptimal) strategy of attending to the memorized location in order to facilitate performance on the choice task.

Conclusions

Preliminary behavioral evidence shows that when subjects hold a location in working memory, visual processing benefits attributable to spatial selective attention can be observed at that location. Electrophysiological, neuroimaging, and clinical evidence suggests a strong correspondence between the neurological substrates of spatial selective attention and spatial working memory. Thus, behavioral and brain evidence converge to suggest a role for spatial selective attention in the maintenance of information in spatial working memory.

The dissociation of storage and rehearsal processes is less clear in spatial working memory than it is in verbal working memory; however, the distinction between the *source* and the *site* of attentional effects[37] may provide a useful perspective. That is, if the visual processing areas are regarded as the site of attentional effects, whereas frontal and superior parietal regions serve as the source of these effects, a pleasing analogy can be drawn between the site/source distinction, and the storage/rehearsal distinction. By this view, the location-specific change in visual processing regions could constitute storage in spatial working memory, whereas the active maintenance of these changes by frontal and parietal cortices could constitute rehearsal.

GENERAL CONCLUSIONS

Consistent with our initial hypotheses, neuroanatomical and behavioral evidence shows that verbal working memory involves dissociable storage and rehearsal processes. Verbal storage recruits mechanisms in posterior brain regions, whereas anterior regions mediate articulatory rehearsal. In addition, we advanced a hypothesis in which spatial selective attention mediates the active maintenance of information in spatial working memory. This model is supported by both neuroanatomical and behavioral evidence. Here again, frontal brain regions may play an important role in rehearsal (along with other attentional mechanisms in parietal cortex), whereas posterior (visual processing) brain regions may be viewed as a passive buffer for location information.

REFERENCES

1. GOLDMAN-RAKIC, P. S. 1987. *In* Handbook of Physiology: The Nervous System. F. Plum, Ed. American Physiological Society. Bethesda, MD.
2. JONIDES, J., E. E. SMITH, R. A. KOEPPE, E. AWH, S. MINOSHIMA & M. MINTUN. 1993. Spatial working memory in humans as revealed by PET. Nature 363: 623–625.
3. WILSON, F. A. W., S. P. O'SCALAIDHE & P. S. GOLDMAN-RAKIC. 1993. Dissociation of object and spatial processing domains in primate prefrontal cortex. Science 260: 1955–1958.
4. SMITH, E. E., J. JONIDES, R. A. KOEPPE, E. AWH, E. H. SCHUMACHER & S. MINOSHIMA. Spatial vs. object working memory: PET investigations. J. Cognit. Neurosci. 7: 337–358.
5. SPERLING, G. 1967. Successive approximations to a model for short-term memory. Acta Psychologica 27: 285–292.
6. BADDELEY, A. D. 1986. Working Memory. Clarendon Press. Oxford, UK.
7. BADDELEY, A. D., N. THOMPSON & M. BUCHANAN. 1975. Word length and the structure of short-term memory. J. Verb. Learn. Verb. Behav. 14: 575–589.
8. AWH, E., J. JONIDES, E. E. SMITH, E. H. SCHUMACHER, R. A. KOEPPE & S. KATZ. Dissociation of storage and rehearsal in verbal working memory: Evidence from PET. Psychol. Sci. In press.
9. COWAN, N. 1994. Mechanisms of verbal short-term memory. Curr. Directions Psychol. Sci. 3(6): 185–189.
10. STERNBERG, S. 1966. High speed scanning in human memory. Science 153: 652–654.
11. POSNER, M. I., S. E. PETERSEN, P. T. FOX & M. E. RAICHLE. 1988. Localization of cognitive operations in the human brain. Science 240: 1627–1631.
12. MINOSHIMA, S., K. L. BERGER, K. S. LEE & M. A. MINTUN. 1992. An automated method for rotational correction and centering of three-dimensional functional brain images. J. Nucl. Med. 33: 1579–1585.
13. MINOSHIMA, S., R. A. KOEPPE, M. A. MINTUN, K. L. BERGER, S. F. TAYLOR, K. A. FREY & D. E. KUHL. 1993. Automated detection of the intercommissural line for stereotactic localization of functional brain images. J. Nucl. Med. 34: 322–329.
14. TALAIRACH, J. & P. TOURNOUX. 1988. A Co-Planar Stereotaxic Atlas of a Human Brain. Thieme. Stuttgart.
15. FOX, P. T., J. M. FOX, M. E. RAICHLE & R. M. BURDE. 1985. The role of cerebral

cortex in the generation of saccadic eye movements; a positron emission tomography study. J. Neurophysiol. **54:** 348–368.

16. FRISTON, K. J., C. D. FRITH, P. F. LIDDLE & R. S. J. FRACKOWIAK. 1991. Comparing functional (PET) images: The assessment of significant change. J. Cereb. Blood Flow Metab. **11:** 690–699.

17. WORSLEY, J. J., A. C. EVANS, S. MARRETT & P. NEELIN. 1992. A three-dimensional statistical analysis for CBF activation studies in the human brain. J. Cereb. Blood Flow Metab. **12:** 900–918.

18. PETERSEN, S. E., P. T. FOX, M. I. POSNER, M. MINTUN & M. E. RAICHLE. 1988. Positron emission tomographic studies of the cortical anatomy of single-word processing. Nature **331:** 585–589.

19. MCCARTHY, R. A. & E. K. WARRINGTON. 1990. *In* Cognitive Neuropsychology: A Clinical Introduction. Academic Press. San Diego, CA.

20. VALLAR, G. & T. SHALLICE. 1990. Neuropsychological Impairments of Short Term Memory. Cambridge University Press. Cambridge, UK.

21. PAULESU, E., C. D. FRITH & R. S. J. FRACKOWIAK. 1993. The neural correlates of the verbal component of working memory. Nature **362:** 342–343.

22. PARDO, J. V., P. J. PARDO, K. W. JANER & M. E. RAICHLE. 1990. The anterior cingulate cortex mediates processing selection in the Stroop attentional conflict paradigm. Proc. Natl. Acad. Sci. USA **87:** 256–259.

23. FUSTER, J. M. 1995. Memory in the Cerebral Cortex. MIT Press. Cambridge, MA.

24. ROLAND, P. E. & L. FRIBERG. 1985. Localization of cortical areas activated by thinking. J. Neurophysiol. **53:** 1219–1243.

25. PETRIDES, M., B. ALIVISATOS, E. MEYER & A. EVANS. 1993. Functional activation of the human frontal cortex during the performance of verbal working memory tasks. Proc. Natl. Acad. Sci. USA **90:** 878–882.

26. SMITH, E. E., J. JONIDES & R. A. KOEPPE. Dissociating verbal and spatial working memory using PET. Cereb. Cortex. In press.

27. SMYTH, M. M. & K. A. SCHOLEY. 1994. Interference in immediate spatial memory. Memory & Cognition **22(1):** 1–13.

28. POSNER, M. I. 1980. Orienting of attention. Q. J. Exp. Psychol. **32:** 3–25.

29. HEINZE, H. J., G. R. MANGUN, W. BURCHERT, H. HINRICHS, M. SCHOLZ, T. F. MUNTE, A. GOS, M. SCHERG, S. JOHANNES, H. HUNDESHAGEN, M. S. GAZZANIGA & S. A. HILLYARD. 1994. Combined spatial and temporal imaging of brain activity during visual selective attention in humans. Nature **372:** 543–546.

30. PETERSEN, S. E., M. CORBETTA, F. M. MIEZIN & G. L. SHULMAN. 1994. PET studies of parietal involvement in spatial attention: Comparison of different task types. Can. J. Exp. Psychol. **48(2):** 319–338.

31. KODAKA, Y., A. MIKAMI & K. KUBOTA. 1994. Attention to a visual stimulus enhances neuronal responses in monkey prefrontal cortex (poster). Presented at the Society of Neuroscience meeting. Washington, D.C.

32. PETRIDES, M. & D. N. PANDYA. 1994. Comparative architectonic analysis of the human and the macaque frontal cortex. *In* F. Boller & J. Grafman, Eds.: 17–57. Handbook of Neuropsychology, Vol. 9. Elsevier. Amsterdam.

33. FOSTER, J. K., G. A. ESKES & D. T. STUSS. 1994. The cognitive neuropsychology of attention: A frontal lobe perspective. Spec. Issue: The cognitive neuropsychology of attention. Cogn. Neuropsychol. **11(2):** 133–147.

34. ALIVISATOS, B. & B. MILNER. 1989. Effects of frontal or temporal lobectomy on the use of advance information in a choice reaction time task. Neuropsychologia **27:** 495–503.

35. KOSSLYN, S. M., N. M. ALPERT, W. L. THOMPSON, V. MALIJKOVIC, S. WEISE, C. F. CHABRIS, S. E. HAMILTON, S. L. RAUCH & F. S. BUONANNO. 1993. Visual mental imagery activates topographically organized visual cortex: PET investigations. J. Cognit. Neurosci. **5(3):** 263–287.

36. MUELLER, H. J. & P. M. RABBITT. 1989. Reflexive and voluntary orienting of visual attention: Time course of activation and resistance to interruption. J. Exp. Psychol. Hum. Percept. Perform. **15(2):** 315–330.

37. POSNER, M. I. & S. E. PETERSEN. 1990. The attention system of the human brain. Annu. Rev. Neurosci. **13:** 25–42.

Frontal Lobes, Memory, and Aging

MORRIS MOSCOVITCH[a,b] AND GORDON WINOCUR[b,c]

a Department of Psychology
University of Toronto
Erindale Campus
Mississauga, Ontario L5L 1C6, Canada
b Rotman Research Institute
Baycrest Centre for Geriatric Care
3560 Bathurst Street
Toronto, Ontario M6A 2E1, Canada
c Department of Psychology
Trent University
Peterborough, Ontario K9J 7B8, Canada

Research on the neuropsychology of aging and memory is concerned with changes in memory with age that are related to corresponding changes in the nervous system. Studies of neurological patients have identified a number of structures which, when damaged, lead to a variety of memory disorders. Principal among these structures is the hippocampus and associated cortex in the medial temporal lobes as well as anatomically related structures in the limbic system and diencephalon. Damage to any of these structures can lead to a deficit in encoding and retention of new information and, perhaps, in impairment of some aspects of retrieval.

There has also been a growing appreciation of the contribution of the frontal lobes and its related structures to memory. Unlike the hippocampus, the frontal lobes contribute to organizational aspects of memory at encoding and retrieval; the use to which memory is put rather than its mere storage and reactivation. Recent positron emission tomography (PET) activation studies suggest that involvement of the frontal lobes in memory may be more extensive than has been suspected on the basis of focal-lesion studies.[1]

Age-related changes in hippocampal and frontal systems are likely to be associated with failing memory in the elderly. However, memory is a complex function that consists of a number of separable components, each likely to be mediated by structures in addition to the hippocampal and frontal systems. Support for this idea is based on evidence from studies of normal and brain-damaged people that different memory functions are dissociable one from another.

With this evidence as a guide to an extensive review of the literature on memory and aging, we found that the patterns of impaired and preserved memory functions in the elderly corresponded closely to those observed in patients with lesions to the brain structures mentioned.[2] This paper, an update of our earlier review, will focus on the relation between frontal lobe function and memory in older adults. Although the bulk of the paper is concerned with humans, studies of nonhuman animals are also included both to provide corroborating evidence and, more importantly, to supply information when relevant data from studies on humans are not available.

TABLE 1. Tests Sensitive to Frontal-Lobe Damage on which Older Adults Were Impaired: A Representative Sample (*see text for more*)

Test	Frontal Patients	Older Adults
Wisconsin Card Sorting Task	Milner[5,14]	Benton et al.[30] Leach et al.[31]
Verbal fluency	Milner[5,14] Benton[15]	Benton et al.[30] Leach et al.[31]
Stroop	Golden[34] Perret[35]	Cohn et al.[37] Comalli et al.[38]
EXPLICIT MEMORY		
Recency judgments	Milner[39] Milner et al.[40] Butters et al.[43]	McCormack[52]
Temporal ordering	Shimamura et al.[41]	Kinsbourne[49] Naveh-Benjamin[50] Vriezen[51] LeFever & Kumkova[55] Parkin et al.[56]
Conditional associative learning	Petrides[69]	Vriezen[51]
Source amnesia	Schacter et al.[82] Janowsky et al.[85]	McIntyre & Craik[86] Dywan & Jacoby[87] Schacter et al.[89,90] Kausler & Puckett[91] Light et al.[92] Mitchell et al.[93] Rabinowicz[94] Hashtroudi et al.[95,98] Cohen & Faulkner[96] Guttentag & Hunt[97] Koriat et al.[99] Craik et al.[101] Spencer & Raz[102] Glisky et al.[105]
Frequency estimation (deficit for high, but not low, frequency of occurrence)	Smith & Milner[106]	*High (deficit)* McCormack[53] Freund & Witte[109] Kausler et al.[110] Kowler et al.[111] *Low (no deficit)* Kausler et al.[58] Attig & Hasher[112] Ellis et al.[113]
Release from proactive inhibition	Moscovitch[116] Freedman & Cermak[118]	Dobbs et al.[121] (review) Moscovitch & Winocur[122]
Feeling of knowing (deficit at long but not at short delays)	Janowsky et al.[117]	Butterfield et al.[126] *(short delay, no deficit)* Lachman et al.[127] *(short delay, no deficit)*
Free recall of organized material	Janowsky et al.[117] Mayes[137] Wheeler et al.[139] (review) Incisa della Rochetta[141] Incisa della Rochetta & Milner[142]	Parkin & Lawrence[125] Craik & Jennings[129] Craik[131]
Recognition (strategic/organized)	Wheeler et al.[139] (review) Stuss et al.[225]	Parkin & Walter[143]
Serial reaction time test	Doyon et al.[190]	Howard & Howard[160,186]

(Continued)

TABLE 1. (*Continued*)

Test	Frontal Patients	Older Adults
IMPLICIT MEMORY		
Stem completion	Shimamura et al.[226] (no deficit)	*Deficit* Davis et al.[173] Chiarello & Hoyer[182] Hulstch et al.[183] Winocur et al.[184]
		No deficit Light & Lavoie[162] (review) Light & Singh[169]
Associative stem completion priming	Mayes & Gooding[157]	Howard et al.[158]
Reading transformed script	Wilson & Baddeley[153] Martone et al.[156]	Moscovitch et al.[166] Hashtroudi et al.[179]

Serial reaction time test
  (hierarchical structure
  or temporal sequence)
	Pascual-Leone et al.[194]	Jackson & Jackson[187,195]

FRONTAL LOBES

The functions of the frontal lobes are diverse and elusive. Structurally, the frontal cortex is heterogeneous,[3] consisting of a number of anatomically distinct areas that have different phylogenetic and ontogenetic histories.[4] Whereas it has been known for some time that two large subdivisions of the prefrontal cortex, the orbitofrontal and dorsolateral regions, have different functions,[5-7] recent evidence suggests that even smaller regions within these subdivisions have specialized functions that can be distinguished from one another.[8,9] Given this apparent diversity, it is small wonder that there is little agreement about the functions of the frontal lobes. Although some constructive and commendable attempts have been made at presenting unifying theories of frontal lobe function,[7,8,10,11] none has been comprehensive enough to accommodate the range of findings in the literature. Two camps or points of view can be identified. One camp believes that there is a common underlying function that expresses itself in diverse ways determined by the anatomical connections in each region and their respective domains. Goldman-Rakic's[7] view that frontal lobes are involved in working memory falls into this camp. The other camp does not assume a functional link among the various regions but rather argues for greater functional independence among them.[8,12] Until one can formulate with greater clarity and precision what the functions of the prefrontal cortex are, it will remain difficult to adjudicate between these two general viewpoints.

The organization of this paper will reflect these two points of view. In the first part, we will catalogue the deficits associated with focal damage to the frontal cortex, specifying the affected subregions when we can. We will then examine the literature on aging to determine if comparable deficits are found in elderly people. A list of representative studies is provided in TABLE 1. In the second part, we will consider unifying frameworks that attempt to integrate the available evidence, and suggest directions for future research and theoretical development.

PSYCHOMETRIC TESTS OF FRONTAL FUNCTIONS

A number of psychometric test batteries contain tests purported to be sensitive to frontal lobe lesions. We will not review them in detail,[13] but instead simply escribe briefly those that are used most commonly. Among these are tests of verbal fluency and the Wisconsin Card Sorting Test (WCST), which is a test of hypothesis formation and set-shifting. Milner[5,14] showed that lesions of the dorsolateral prefrontal cortex, usually on the left side, lead to a difficulty in shifting sets (or hypotheses) that is marked by perseveration on previously correct, but currently incorrect, responses. Deficits in the fluency with which words can be generated from a given initial letter are associated with left orbitofrontal lesions.[15] Generating category names, however, is more likely to be affected by left temporal lobe lesion.[16] Tests of nonverbal fluency, in which subjects are required to generate meaningless designs, are affected more by right- than left-frontal lesions.[17,18]

Recently, a number of investigators have shown, however, that diffuse damage or focal lesions of other structures including the left- and right-temporal lobe can lead to deficits on verbal fluency[19-22] and on WCST.[23-25] It is difficult to adjudicate between these different claims. The procedures used for testing verbal fluency and WCST in the various studies were different as, in some cases, were the etiology of the patients' damage. Because performance on verbal fluency and WCST, like that on other psychometric tests, may be determined by multiple factors, changes in some aspects of the test may alter the critical components of the test so that the contribution of nonfrontal structures becomes more prominent. For example, Teuber et al.[26] modified the WCST by changing sets after every 10 trials, rather than after 10 errorless trials. Under these conditions, patients with frontal lesions were no more impaired than normal subjects. Similarly, warning the patient that a set change is about to occur,[27] using cards whose stimuli are symmetrically arranged[23] rather than asymmetrically,[14] or using different scoring procedures, may also eliminate the specific frontal lobe deficit. The conclusion to be drawn from these studies is not that the frontal lobes are not required for successful performance on the WCST; rather these studies suggest that frontal deficits most clearly emerge when strong response sets are developed and set-shifting is dependent on internal monitoring of outcomes. This conclusion is supported by the predominance of perseverative responses in patients with lesions to the prefrontal cortex as compared to patients with lesions in other areas.[5,23,24] More recently, Raz and his colleagues[28,29] have shown that the volume of the dorsolateral prefrontal cortex as measured by magnetic resonance imaging (MRI) is correlated significantly with the number of perseverative errors on WCST in normal young and old people. With regard to letter fluency, if patients with diffuse damage or epilepsy without surgical intervention are removed from the sample,[19] then the findings show that deficits are greatest in patients with left-frontal lesions, though patients with right-frontal lesions are also impaired.

Age-related deficits have been observed on both WCST and tests of verbal fluency but not consistently. Some agreement seems to exist that the likelihood of finding such deficits increases greatly as individuals enter their eighth decade. The performance of adults in their sixties and seventies may be more variable, which may account for reports of normal[30] and of impaired performance.[31]

Another test that has gained some popularity is the Stroop test,[32,33] which has recently been standardized for use with clinical populations.[34] In this test, subjects are shown a list of color patches and two lists of color names. One list is written in black, the other in a color that does not correspond to the name (e.g., the word red written in blue). The subject's task is to name the color patches, read the black list, and then name the color in which the word is written in the colored list. Successful performance with the colored list requires that the subject overcome the interfering effect of the word in order to name the color. Even in normal young adults, naming times are longer and errors are greater for the colored list than for the other two. This increase in errors and latency is known as the Stroop effect.

As might be expected, patients with frontal lesions show a larger Stroop effect than intact controls, presumably because frontal patients have greater difficulty in suppressing the interfering effects of the written color name (red).[34,35] Here, too, however, there is some concern that greater Stroop interference is not a hallmark of frontal-lobe damage and can also occur with lesions to other sites.[36] Nonetheless, it is the case that elderly people show greater Stroop interference than do young adults.[33,37,38]

EXPERIMENTAL TESTS

In addition to psychometric tests, a number of experimental tests have been developed that are sensitive to frontal-lobe lesions. Unfortunately, many of the tests also involve a memory component that may be affected by temporal-lobe lesions. Because frontal- and temporal-lobe lesions are presumed to affect different components of the test, the nature of the impairment should be different in the two cases. In evaluating the performance of patients with cortical lesions, it is important, where possible, to note the pattern of deficits in an attempt to distinguish between lesions to the frontal lobes and lesions to other cortical structures. For example, patients with frontal lesions are impaired at judging which of two stimuli appeared more recently in a list even though they remember having seen both stimuli earlier. Patients with temporal-lobe lesions, on the other hand, fail the recency judgments only when their memory of the stimuli themselves is impaired. When they recognize the stimuli as "old," they can determine as well as normal people which of the two occurred more recently.[39,40]

Temporal Order

In addition to judgments of recency, other tests of temporal order are affected by frontal- and temporal-lobe lesions. Shimamura *et al.*[41] have shown that both amnesic patients and patients with frontal lesions are impaired in reproducing the order both of a recently presented list of words and of world events that occurred during the last 30 years. What is important from our perspective is that the deficit in temporal ordering was not related to the severity of the amnesia. This is consistent with Milner's[39,40] finding regarding the contribution of frontal lobes and hippocampus to judgments of recency (see above). Interestingly, if the stimuli are manipulated instead of merely observed, recency judgment is intact following frontal lesions.[42]

Some tests of list differentiation (see next section) may also be considered as tests of temporal order. In these tests, two lists of items are presented with each list separated from the other by a large or small interval that is usually filled by some activity. Subjects are then tested for their ability to recall or recognize the items and to assign them to the correct list or temporal order. As expected, Butters *et al.*[43] showed that patients with frontal-lobe lesions were impaired at judging whether test items which consisted of representational line drawings belonged to the first or second list they had studied. They confirmed with frontal patients what had been suspected on the basis of studies of Korsakoff patients. Deficits on tests of list differentiation in Korsakoff patients may also be related to the frontal dysfunction that is associated with their amnesia. Huppert and Piercy[44] showed that even when Korsakoff patients recognized the words they studied, they were poor at reporting whether they had studied the words recently or 24 hours earlier, or whether the words were part of list 1 or list 2. In a later study, Squire[45] showed that Korsakoff patients' poor performance on a test of list differentiation was correlated with their performance on a battery of tests of frontal function.

Studies of Parkinsonian patients, whose profile of cognitive deficits includes frontal dysfunction, show they are similarly impaired on tests of temporal order[46] and of dating events.[47,48] Patients with Alzheimer's disease, on the other hand, who have a profound memory loss due to medial temporal-lobe degeneration, tend to be less impaired on similar tests if they can recognize the material.

Memory for temporal order is worse in old than in young adults. Old adults have greater difficulty than young adults in reconstructing the order of a list of words or pictures,[49–51] and in judging the relative recency of two items,[52] though on some studies the effect does not reach significance.[53,54] In tests of temporal order that are more akin to list differentiation, LeFever & Kumkova[55] and Parkin *et al.*[56] have reported age-related deficits. In the latter study, Parkin *et al.* found that the degree of impairment was correlated with performance on frontal-lobe tests measuring spontaneous flexibility, such as different types of fluency tests, but not with performance on tests measuring reactive flexibility, such as the WCST (see Eslinger and Grattan[57] on flexibility). Parkin *et al*'s finding suggests that age-related declines in memory for temporal order (or list differentiation) is associated with deterioration of some frontal functions but not of others, though the particular processes and mechanisms involved have yet to be determined.

It is not completely certain whether the temporal-order deficit in elderly people can be attributed solely to frontal dysfunction or whether there is also a temporal-lobe component to it.[51] The finding of age-related deficits in temporal ordering of performed activities[58] suggests that the deficit may also be related to hippocampal dysfunction (see section on list differentiation for other tests that have a temporal component).

Judgments of temporal order or recency may also figure in tests such as delayed response, spatial alternation, object reversal, and spatial reversal. In the alternation task, the correct response alternates from trial to trial. In reversal, the subject must first reach a criterion of correct responses with respect to one location or object, before reversal to another location or object occurs. In delayed response, subjects must match one of two items to a previously presented target. When the targets and test items are chosen from a small set of recurring items, successful performance involves the temporal segregation of the current target from targets presented on previous trials that are no longer relevant. On the alternation and reversal tasks, the subject must again focus on the immediately preceding trial to guide performance and ignore the responses of prior targets. Frontal lesions produce deficits on these tests in humans,[59] monkeys,[6,7,60,61] and rats[62] which are exacerbated when the subject must overcome a strong, prepotent response, as demonstrated in the reversal studies in which no deficits are found in establishing the initial pre-reversal response. Lesions of the medial temporal lobes will also lead to impaired performance on these tests. The temporal-lobe deficits, however, are linked more to the delay between the target and test items or to the delay between trials rather than to the size of the stimulus set or to the establishment of prepotent responses.[63,64]

Tasks with a spatial component, such as spatial alternation, are difficult for animals with hippocampal lesions even if no delay is involved. However, their error pattern is different from that of animals with frontal lesions. Whereas hippocampal animals either choose randomly[65] or develop a position preference, frontal animals tend to perseverate on the previously correct response.[66]

Aged rats and monkeys are impaired on a variety of alternation and reversal tasks that are sensitive to both hippocampal and frontal lesions. On the reversal tasks, aged monkeys, like monkeys with frontal lesions, perseverate on the previously correct response, but like monkeys with hippocampal lesions they also have difficulty in learning a new response once the perseverative tendency is overcome.[67] In most studies, therefore, it is difficult to know the cause of the poorer performance in aged rats. An exception is the study by Winocur[68] on delayed, go–no-go alternation with rats. In these tests, we see a decrement in performance of aged rats that is indicative of both frontal and hippocampal dysfunction. Their performance, impaired even at short delays as a result of frontal dysfunction, becomes worse at longer delays due to impaired hippocampal function.

Conditional Associative Learning

Conditional associative learning has also been used to investigate the effects of frontal and medial temporal-lobe lesions in animals and humans. In this paradigm, the subject must learn to associate by trial and error specific responses to different stimuli. In humans, damage to either the right or left frontal lobes produces impairment on verbal and nonverbal versions of this test.[69] In contrast, patients with unilateral temporal-lobe lesions with large hippocampal removals in the left hemisphere are impaired only on the verbal versions of the test, whereas those with removals on the right hemisphere are impaired on the pictorial, nonverbal version. These results confirm the hypothesis that hippocampal removals interfere with encoding of hemisphere-specific information into long-term memory and not with the conditional aspects of the task. In work with monkeys, Petrides[12] has identified Brodmann's areas 6 and 8 as the frontal regions that are critical for conditional associative learning. Recent work with PET scans has shown that homologous regions are involved in this test in humans.[70,71]

Impaired performance on the conditional associative learning test has also been found in normal elderly people, but it is difficult to determine with certainty whether the deficit is related to frontal or hippocampal dysfunction or to both (see Vriezen[51] for more details). Vriezen administered two versions of this test: a trial-and-error version similar to the one used by Petrides[69] and a correction version in which the correct answer was supplied if an error was made. The latter version may be more sensitive to hippocampal than to frontal dysfunction. The elderly people were equally impaired on both. Unfortunately, the study was not designed to assess predictions about the respective contributions of the two brain regions. Nonetheless, the pattern of correlation of each of the versions of the conditional associative learning test with another frontal test, temporal ordering, proved informative. Performance on the trial-and-error version correlated significantly with temporal ordering in the Parkinsonian patients but not in the normal, aged controls.[46]

The distinction between frontal-lobe and hippocampal involvement in conditional associative learning has also been demonstrated in rats.[72] Rats were taught to press a bar on the left or right depending on the side on which a light appeared. The amount of time between light onset and the opportunity to respond was varied. Rats with hippocampal lesions were not impaired in learning the basic conditional discrimination at short intervals, but their performance deteriorated as the interval between stimulus and response was increased. However, rats with frontal-lobe lesions were severely and equally impaired at all intervals. These results support the hypothesis that the hippocampus is critical for retention, whereas the frontal lobes are necessary for the conditional aspects of the task. Again, as predicted, old rats performed more poorly than did young rats on this test. The pattern of performance of the old rats was indicative of both frontal and hippocampal dysfunction. Some deficit was noted at short delays (frontal) which was exacerbated at long delays (hippocampal).

Self-Ordered Pointing and Radial Arm Mazes

In self-ordered pointing, patients are required to select an item from an array of items pictured on a page.[73] Having done so, the patient turns to the next page in which the same array appears, although the items are arranged differently. The task is to select a different item on every page. This procedure is repeated for as many pages as there are items. Patients with frontal-lobe damage, in the vicinity of areas 46 and 9, are impaired on this test with left and right frontal lesions producing the greatest impairment on a verbal and nonverbal version of this test, respectively. The same regions are shown to be active on PET scans that are conducted while normal people perform this task.[70,71] Comparisons between old and young people are not available for the self-ordered pointing task.

Analogues of this test have been developed for use with monkeys.[8,74] In these tests, animals are presented with several stimuli and are rewarded for responding to a different stimulus in each trial. Frontal lesions in areas homologous to those in humans produce deficits on these tests, but again no data are available on the performance of old monkeys.

The radial arm maze, used extensively with rats, can be considered to be a spatial analogue of the self-ordered pointing task. The rat is rewarded for selecting a new arm on each trial. Deficits are again observed following frontal lesions.[75] As expected, aged rats perform more poorly than young rats.[76,77]

It should be noted that in humans, monkeys, and rats, damage to the medial temporal lobes will also lead to impaired performance on the various versions of self-ordered tests. As yet, it is not always possible to distinguish between the effects of lesions to the two regions on the basis of performance measures.

Learning Other Complex Mazes

Aged rats are impaired at learning complex mazes, tasks which are also sensitive to frontal and hippocampal lesions.[78–80] Winocur and Moscovitch[79,80] have shown that hippocampal and frontal contribution to maze learning can be dissociated, with the former implicated in retaining maze-specific information and the latter in acquiring a general maze-learning skill. Aged rats are impaired on both components. Studies of maze learning in humans have shown that patients with right hippocampal lesions are impaired on this task because they fail to remember the path traced,[81] whereas patients with right frontal lesions perform poorly because they do not adhere to the rules. Although elderly people also have difficulty in learning complex mazes, no studies have been reported that dissociate frontal from hippocampal effects.

List Differentiation—Memory for Sources and Contexts

Event-monitoring, a component of self-ordered pointing and radial arm maze tasks, is also a component on tests that require the subject to identify the source of the information they remember. For example, subjects are taught a set of facts, some by one experimenter, and the remainder by another. Their task is to remember the facts as well as the source of the information. As expected, amnesic patients with various etiologies have difficulty remembering both facts and sources. When the amnesic patients' fact memory was equated with that of normal people by testing the amnesics at much shorter delays, the extent of their deficit on memory for sources varied according to the degree of frontal dysfunction as measured by WCST and verbal fluency,[82] and not according to the severity of their amnesia. Moreover, whereas normal people and nonfrontal amnesic patients often forgot which of the two experimenters taught them a particular fact (source attribution errors), they rarely, if ever, attributed their knowledge to an extraexperimental source. The term "source amnesia" was used to describe this more extreme form of the deficit, which was a much more common error for the frontal amnesics. The results were replicated by Shimamura and Squire[83] and Parkin et al.[84] As a direct test of the hypothesis that "source amnesia" is related to frontal lobe damage, Janowsky et al.[85] tested nonamnesic patients with focal frontal-lobe lesions. Their patients demonstrated the predicted source amnesia.

Elderly adults, like frontal patients, are deficient in identifying the source of the events they have experienced. In the extreme, they have difficulty distinguishing whether they learned a fact in the laboratory or elsewhere[86] or whether their knowledge about the fame of individuals was based on laboratory or real-world experience.[87,88] More common is their difficulty in source monitoring or context attribution within the experimental setting. Thus, elderly people are poor at remembering which of two experimenters presented a target,[86,89,90] or what the physical attributes of the target were—for example, whether it was heard in a male or female voice,[91] whether it was seen in capital or small letters,[91] whether it was seen or heard,[92] whether they saw it or generated it,[93,94] and even whether they or someone else said something[95] or they only imagined or intended to say something or perform an action.[94,96-100] In short, elderly people have severe attribution errors and occasionally even source amnesia.

Craik et al.[101] provide supportive evidence of a link between age-related deficits on these tests and frontal dysfunction. They showed that performance on the source or context attribution test in elderly people is correlated with the number of perseverative errors on the WCST, a test of frontal function. Their finding was replicated by Schacter et al.[89] and by Spencer and Raz[102] with respect to the ability of older adults to identify the context (room, set of cards, and color) in which the stimuli were presented.

In highlighting the elderly person's difficulties with source attribution, one should not lose sight of the fact that it is very likely that the same subjects will also have poorer memory than the young for the targets. Our point is that these are different deficits attributable to disruption of different mechanisms. Source memory failure results from a decline in frontal-lobe function, whereas target memory failure is related to medial temporal/hippocampal impairment. To underscore this point, amnesic patients without frontal damage, who are typically poor at remembering both types of information, can perform normally on the source attribution test if their target memory is equated with that of controls. However, elderly people (like patients with frontal damage) are not as good as the young in recollecting the context of an event even when their memory for the content of it is intact.[89,90,100,103,104]

Glisky et al.[105] provide the most compelling evidence from studies of normal aging that memory for targets (or facts) is dissociable from memory for source, and that the two are mediated by the medial-temporal and frontal lobes, respectively. They found a functional double dissociation between memory for items and for the voice in which the item was read, and performance on standard tests sensitive to medial-temporal and frontal lobe damage (see Moscovitch and Winocur,[2] for an extended discussion on the importance of such functional double-dissociation tests for studies on the neuropsychology of aging and memory).

Frequency Estimation

Another example of a deficit that may be related to monitoring is found in tests of frequency estimation. Here subjects are presented with a series of items some of which are repeated various numbers of times. The subject's task is to estimate the frequency with which an item was presented. Smith and Milner[106] found that at high frequencies, patients with left or right frontal lesions underestimated the number of presentations more than normal people and patients with temporal-lobe lesions. The evidence on age-related deficits in frequency estimation is contradictory.[107,108] Whereas many investigators report that elderly people are worse at estimating frequency than the young,[53,109-111] others found no age differences.[58,112,113] It should be noted that frontal patients were impaired most noticeably at high frequencies for which performance even among normal people was inaccurate. The deficits in the elderly are, therefore, also expected to occur primarily when the frequency estimation task is sufficiently difficult to challenge their frontal lobes. The contradictory findings in the literature on normal aging may be reconciled if this factor is taken into account. As Freund and Witte[109] elegantly demonstrated, age-related deficits in frequency estimation emerge only at high frequencies (above) when presentation rate is slow but at lower frequencies when presentation is increased.

Release from Proactive Inhibition

In release from proactive inhibition (PI), subjects are presented with lists of words from a single taxonomic category followed by a list from a different category. Recall, tested after each list, declines as PI builds up in the same category condition. When the category is shifted, recall improves which is indicative of release from PI. Korsakoff patients typically fail to release from PI,[114,115] a condition attributed to frontal dysfunction in many of these amnesics. As a direct test of this hypothesis, Moscovitch[116] found that patients with left unilateral frontal lobectomies also failed to show normal release from PI especially if they were impaired on the WCST. Using a different test, Janowsky et al.[117] found no differences between frontal-lobe patients and normal controls. Based on their findings that only those frontal patients who were also amnesic failed to show normal release from PI, Freedman and Cermak[118] suggested that PI release failure is likely to occur in frontal patients only if there is an accompanying memory disorder.

Failure of older adults to release from PI has been reported by some investigators but not by others.[119–121] Here, too, the neurological literature is instructive in helping to resolve the contradictory evidence. As noted, release from PI is typically normal in community-dwelling elderly but is consistently impaired in institutionalized, but nondemented, elderly people.[122] Deficits on both frontal and hippocampal tests are even more widespread, and certainly more severe, in institutionalized elderly people than among the community-dwelling elderly.[79,80,123,124] As in patients, failure to release from PI seems to occur most reliably in elderly people who have frontal dysfunction superimposed on a memory disorder.

The type of frontal dysfunction is also important. Parkin and Lawrence[125] found that release from PI is related to performance on frontal tests of spontaneous, but not of reactive, flexibility. Because the test of spontaneous flexibility involved category generation, it may be the case that temporal-lobe functions were also implicated. If so, these results lend further support for the idea that both memory and frontal-lobe functions are compromised in people with poor release from PI.

Metamemory

Metamemory refers to a self-monitoring process whereby individuals gain insight into the operation and capacity of their own memory. It is often reported that patients with frontal-lobe lesions lack insight into their memory (as well as in other domains), often even being unaware of severe amnesia or other cognitive, sensory, or motor impairment (anosagnosia). Few studies, however, have tested metamemory directly in patients with frontal-lobe lesions. An exception is the study by Janowsky et al.[117] on "feeling of knowing." In their test, subjects had to recall obscure facts in response to questions. For facts they failed to recall, they were asked to gauge their "feeling of knowing" the forgotten fact by estimating whether a cue might help them recall or recognize it. The patients were tested immediately or after a delay of 1–3 days. They were also tested for "feeling of knowing" of factual information that they had acquired premorbidly. Janowsky et al. report that patients with frontal lesions were impaired on the metamemory task only when tested 1–3 days later. In contrast, Korsakoff amnesic patients were impaired at all intervals. Non-Korsakoff amnesic patients performed normally on the metamemory task, suggesting that the Korsakoff deficit on this test was related to the frontal dysfunction that commonly accompanies their memory disorder. To obtain large "feeling of knowing" deficits both disorders must be present.

Many more studies on metamemory have been conducted in elderly people than in patients with frontal damage. A variety of paradigms and abilities have been subsumed under the label of metamemory. These include test of people's ability to choose appropriate mnemonic strategies, to reflect on their memory performance in everyday life, to predict their performance on memory tests, to evaluate how well they performed and to adjust study times according to the difficulty of the memory test. Not surprisingly, given the diversity of the techniques, the results have been mixed. Sometimes old people are not as good as the young, but in most cases there are no age differences. In a test of feeling of knowing, for which there are comparable data on patients with frontal-lobe lesions, Butterfield et al.[126] and Lachman et al.[127] found no age-related decline if metamemory was tested shortly after study, consistent with the finding that deficits are absent in immediate tests even with frontal patients.

Many metamemory tests may vary in their sensitivity to frontal damage.[117] Even for those that are sensitive, clear deficits may emerge only in subjects who have pronounced frontal dysfunction with a superimposed memory disorder. This may account for the relatively few studies that report age differences in metamemory in normal elderly people. What is needed are independent measures of medial-temporal function and of different types of frontal function in the elderly that can be correlated with their performance on metamemory tests. It would be desirable in this regard to compare community-dwelling elderly with healthy, institutionalized elderly because the latter group is known to have memory loss compounded by conspicuous signs of frontal dysfunction.

Free Recall, Cued Recall, and Recognition

In contrast to metamemory, age-related deficits in free recall are among the most robust and reliable findings in the psychological literature. Smaller but reliable age-related deficits in recognition have also been reported. Comparing the extent of age-related deficits on the two tasks is difficult because the baseline conditions, the difficulty, and the scales are usually dissimilar (but see Calev[128]).

Nonetheless, a number of investigators (see Craik and Jennings[129]) have argued that aging affects recall more than recognition. Because encoding and retention processes are presumably equivalent in recall and recognition, what distinguishes one from the other must be the processes involved at retrieval. Whereas recognition benefits from presentation of the target item which acts as a retrieval cue that can automatically reactivate the stored information, free recall is dependent on self-initiated retrieval processes that involve searching and generating the appropriate cue before the automatic retrieval process is triggered. According to Craik,[130,131] recognition receives much greater environmental support than does recall and, as a result, makes fewer demands on cognitive resources. Because Craik believes that cognitive resources are diminished with age, recall is likely to suffer more than recognition as one gets older.

From a neuropsychological perspective, the memory processes common to recognition and recall are those likely to be mediated by the hippocampal system, which is involved in consolidation, retention, and the automatic aspects of retrieval (ecphory[132]) that are triggered by the appropriate cue.[132–135] Patients with damage to the hippocampal system perform poorly on tests of both recall and of recognition. Whether amnesic patients have a disproportionate deficit in recall as compared to recognition is currently in dispute.[83,136,137]

To attribute the greater deficit on recall than on recognition in the elderly solely to deterioration of the hippocampal system would ignore the strategic, self-initiated retrieval component that is a hallmark of many tests of recall but not of most tests of recognition. We believe that this strategic retrieval component is mediated by the frontal lobes and its related structures.[133–135] The greater deficit in recall than in recognition in elderly people is therefore likely to be a function both of hippocampal and frontal system deterioration that occurs with age.

A recent PET activation study on recognition memory for faces in young and old adults is instructive. Grady et al.[138] found increased activation (in comparison to a baseline perceptual matching task) of right hippocampus, left prefrontal and temporal cortex during encoding in young, but not in old, adults. During testing for recognition, however, both groups showed increased activation of right prefrontal cortex, a region which has been implicated in retrieval in a number of PET activation studies.[1] The results are consistent with our view that the age-related impairment in recognition, when it occurs, is due to inadequate cortical and hippocampal activation during encoding. Our view predicts that if recall had been tested, age-related differences in activation of prefrontal structures associated with retrieval would have been found.

It is important to note that patients with lesions restricted to the lateral or orbital surface of the frontal lobes are often unimpaired on many tests of recall and recognition which measure learning and retention. Wheeler et al.'s[139] recent review and meta-analysis of the literature on the effects of frontal-lobe lesions on memory bear this out. They found a noticeable impairment on tests of free recall, some deficit on cued recall, and little or no impairment on recognition.[225] Although Wheeler et al. did not stress this, Moscovitch[2,118,133,140] observed that an impairment is noted when organizational abilities at encoding or retrieval are required for successful performance. Thus, impaired performance in frontal-lobe patients has been reported on recall of stories and of categorized lists of words.[117,137,141,142]

In both cases the material is structured and allows for self-generated organizational factors to come into play and aid recall. When encoding and retrieval strategies are supplied by the experimenter, the memory deficit associated with frontal lesions is reduced or eliminated.[142] Similarly, when strategic factors are minimized, free recall of unstructured word lists and learning of pairs of randomly associated words are relatively spared after frontal lesions, but impaired after hippocampal damage.

Two studies by Parkin and his colleagues speak directly to the issue of the relation between frontal-lobe deterioration and differential memory loss in recall and recognition in older adults. Using Calev's[128] test for matching recognition and recall, Parkin and Lawrence[125] found that the size of the discrepancy between performance on recall and recognition in older adults was correlated with performance on WCST, a frontal test of reactive flexibility, but not on verbal fluency, a frontal test of spontaneous flexibility. What is interesting in light of the foregoing discussion, is that Calev's recall test involves categorized lists of words which is just the type of test that is likely to be sensitive to frontal-lobe contribution at retrieval.

In another study, Parkin and Walter[143] examined the relation between frontal-lobe function and aging on two aspects of recognition: a recollective component that is assumed to involve contextual, reconstructive processes similar to those associated with recall, and a component which is based only on the item's familiarity without recollection of its context. As predicted, Parkin and Walter found that the extent of the older adults' recollective experience, but not their familiarity with the item, was significantly correlated with their performance on WCST.

Memory with and without Awareness

Memory with awareness involves conscious recollection of the past and is typically measured by explicit tests such as recognition and recall. Memory without awareness does not require conscious reflection on the past. Instead, retention of the past is inferred from performance on implicit tests which measure changes in behavior with experience or practice. For example, having read a word or seen a face, the subject is likely to identify either one more quickly on subsequent viewing, often without consciously remembering the initial presentation.

The distinction between implicit and explicit tests of memory is an old one, but it is only recently that the significance of the distinction for theories of memory has been appreciated. Concern with dissociations among different forms or tests of memory has fueled empirical and theoretical work which, in turn, has led to major advances in our understanding of normal memory and of memory disorders. Major reviews on the topic have appeared in recent years and the interested reader is referred to them (see Roediger and McDermott,[144] Moscovitch et al.[145,146] for recent reviews). Our purpose is not to adjudicate among the various theories or among some of the controversies in the empirical literature. Instead, we will review some of the basic, reliable findings in the literature on normal young adults and relate them to neuropsychological research on memory disorders in humans and animals. Taken together, the observed dissociation among different tests of memory suggest that different critical components, at both the functional and structural level, are involved in each of the tests. An examination of the neuro-psychological literature will help us identify some of these components. We will then discuss these findings in relation to the corresponding literature on normal aging.

The picture that emerges is that the cortical or subcortical region involved in processing a certain type of information also mediates performance on implicit tests of memory that pertain to that information. This suggests that these regions are modified by the information they have processed and have stored a representation of it. For many implicit tests, particularly those that are perceptual, reactivation of that representation or some aspects of it are both a necessary and sufficient condition for eliciting strong repetition priming effects.[133–135,140,147–150]

Some implicit tests, however, depend on an additional strategic or organizational component that may involve the frontal lobes. For example, improvement with practice at solving puzzles such as the Tower of Hanoi requires planning, organization of response sequences, and monitoring of responses in addition to mere repetition. Other tests may fall between these two poles. Shallice[151] and Saint-Cyr et al.[152] have shown that mastering the Tower of Hanoi depends, in part, on the integrity of the frontal lobes and related structures. Even improvement in learning simple jigsaw puzzles may be impaired in patients with frontal dysfunction.[153] There is suggestive evidence that the frontal lobes may contribute to performance on still other implicit tests of memory. Work on normal people has indicated that repetition effects on reading transformed script and word stem–completion are influenced by semantic or lexical search variables as well as perceptual ones.[144,154,155] It is significant that patients with considerable frontal dysfunction,[156] such as Huntington's disease patients or patients with severe closed head injury,[153] show little improvement in learning to read transformed script. Working with Korsakoff amnesic patients who also frequently have frontal-lobe deficits, Mayes and Gooding[157] found that on implicit paired-associate, stem-completion tests, performance correlated significantly with frontal-lobe impairment but not with severity of amnesia. Howard et al.[158] reported deficits on similar implicit, paired-associated tests in old people, but did not examine whether performance was correlated with frontal dysfunction.

In light of these observations, a hypothesis worth pursuing is that the frontal lobes contribute to those implicit tests that require organizational skills or have a strategic, lexical or semantic search component.

Implicit Tests of Memory in Aging

Experiments have been conducted in the elderly on a variety of implicit tests of memory (for reviews see Graf,[159] Howard and Howard,[160,161] Light and Lavoie[162]). Our working assumption is that age-related deficits will appear only on those tests that involve the hippocampus and frontal lobes. Performance on many implicit tests of memory should, therefore, be unaffected by age. In line with our hypothesis, no age differences in repetition effects were found on lexical decision tasks,[163] picture naming,[164,165] speeded reading,[166] category judgment tasks,[167] word-fragment completion,[168] perceptual identification of words[169] and pictures,[170] homophone spelling,[171-173] category exemplar generation,[174,175] preferences for novel patterns,[161,176] and skin conductance responses to studied versus new words.[177,178] Except for homophone spelling and exemplar generation, all these tests can be considered to be primarily perceptual repetition priming tests that do not involve the hippocampus. The absence of a significant, semantic search component precludes frontal-lobe involvement on these tests.

However, age-related changes have been reported on implicit tests of memory that are thought to have a substantial frontal contribution or basal ganglia contribution. Moscovitch et al.[166] reported that institutionalized elderly people, whose frontal dysfunction is prominent in comparison to community-dwelling elderly people,[79,80] have difficulty learning to read transformed script and show little repetition effects for that material. Even normal elderly people show an impaired ability to acquire this reading skill, a finding confirmed by Hashtroudi et al.[179] Age-related deficits were reported in a pursuit-rotor task and a mirror-tracing task,[180] both of which are known to be impaired in patients with basal ganglia pathology and frontal dysfunction.[181]

A similar "frontal" (or basal ganglia) explanation likely accounts for the discrepancies in the literature on age-related deficits on word-stem completion. Initial reports by Light and Singh[168,169] claimed that there was a slight, but statistically nonsignificant, age-related deficit on word-stem completion. Shimamura et al.'s[226] report of normal stem-completion in patients with frontal-lobe lesions was consistent with Light and Singh's finding. In subsequent research, Chiarello and Hoyer[182] and Hultsch et al.[183] found significant deficits on the same tests in the elderly. Indeed, all authors argue, and Hultsch et al. demonstrate, that the initial failure to find a significant deficit was related to the weak statistical power of the Light and Singh study. Moreover, stem completion was the only one among a number of perceptual repetition priming tests on which Hultsch et al. found an age-related decline.

To test directly the hypothesis that age differences on stem completion are related to frontal-lobe function, Winocur et al.[184] correlated performance on stem completion and fragment completion with performance on WCST and letter fluency, two standard tests of frontal-lobe function. Consistent with previous findings, they found that old people performed significantly worse than the young on stem completion but not on fragment completion. More interestingly, only performance on stem completion correlated with performance on WCST and verbal fluency in the older adults. Winocur et al. also found that older adults were impaired on explicit memory versions of both stem and fragment completion, that is, on stem and fragment cued recall. Unlike accuracy in the implicit versions, accuracy of cued recall on the explicit versions did not correlate with performance on the frontal tests, but instead correlated with performance on tests of verbal and nonverbal (Rey-Osterrieth figure) delayed recall, which are sensitive to medial temporal-lobe damage. These results provide evidence of a correlational or functional double dissociation between implicit stem-completion and stem cued recall. To explain these results, Winocur et al. proposed that the stem-completion test has a strategic, semantic generative component that involves the frontal lobes whereas fragment completion is a more purely perceptual test that depends primarily on posterior neocortical structures. Gabrieli et al. (submitted) provide a similar interpretation to account for the deleterious effects of dividing attention on tests of stem completion but not of perceptual identification. To explain the pattern of results on the explicit version of the tests, Winocur *et al.* proposed that the stems and fragments act as cues that directly elicit the correct response via the medial temporal/hippocampal system with minimal involvement of strategic, frontal operations.

It is interesting to note that implicit memory for a recurring serial pattern[185] is not impaired in old people although explicit memory for that pattern is.[161,186] One might have expected, given the sequential nature of the task, that the frontal lobes would be involved and that elderly people might therefore be impaired. One possibility worth investigating is the type of organization involved in acquiring and executing the task. In the typical test, an asterisk appears in one of four locations on a screen and the task is to push the button under the asterisk as soon as possible. The recurring sequence can be learned by acquiring simple associations that reflect the statistical transition probabilities between adjacent elements or by forming larger-scale units or hierarchies that reflect the complex serial order.[187,188] As Cohen *et al.*[189] recently demonstrated, it is only learning patterns among many elements of the sequential, hierarchical component of the implicit test that is disrupted by a concurrent, attention-demanding task. It is also this component that is most likely to require frontal involvement and be sensitive to the effects of aging. Consistent with this prediction, impaired learning on the serial reaction time test has been reported in patients with frontal-lobe lesions[190] and in patients with Parkinson's[191] and Huntington's disease[192,193] who have frontal dysfunction, as well as in normal people with experimentally induced frontal deactivation (see Pascual-Leone *et al.*[194]). Jackson and Jackson[195,196] have recently shown that it is also learning of the sequential, hierarchical component that is impaired in old age and in patients with Parkinson's disease.

In the literature on animals, no age-related deficit is associated with performance on analogues of implicit tests of memory that do not involve the frontal lobes. Thus, performance in aged rats is normal on discrimination learning,[197,198] operant conditioning tasks such as learning to press a lever on a continuous reinforcement schedule,[68,199] and one-way active avoidance learning. On the other hand, there is growing evidence that old rats, like old people, are impaired on "implicit tests" that do have a frontal component. Acquisition of a maze-learning skill and conditional rule-learning can be considered two such tests because rats with hippocampal lesions perform normally on them. Performance on both tests, however, is impaired by prefrontal lesions indicating a strong frontal contribution to them. Consistent with our hypothesis, old rats are deficient on these tests.[72,79,80]

SUMMARY

A remarkable consistency exists between the memory deficits seen in human patients and experimental animals with frontal lesions and those seen in normal aging. Indeed, not one instance of a significant discrepancy is found if the same test is administered to both frontal patients and older adults. Moreover, in a number of instances, performance on the frontal memory tests correlated significantly with performance on non-mnemonic tests of frontal function in the elderly but not with performance on other tests, thereby satisfying the criterion of at least functional, single dissociation. Evidence of functional and structural double dissociation is necessary to establish unequivocally that decline in performance with age on the various frontal memory tests is indeed related to the deterioration of the frontal cortex and not to a general deterioration associated with aging.[2]

PSYCHOSOCIAL INFLUENCES

This paper has focused on decline in learning and memory functions associated with the prefrontal cortex. It is important to emphasize that cognitive function does not decline in a one-to-one fashion with chronological age. Numerous factors (e.g., medical history, educational level, lifestyle) can contribute to significant differences in cognitive abilities among individuals within the same age range. In one study, Arbuckle et al.[200] assessed the relative contributions of chronological age and social and personality factors to memory function in normal old people. Chronological age was found to be the least influential factor, accounting for only a small part of the total variance in memory performance.

Our own work has shown that environmental influences and psychological factors can significantly affect cognitive function in old age. In several studies,[79,80,124,201] groups of old people living in the community or in institutions were compared on a wide range of clinical and experimental neuropsychological tests. Despite being carefully matched for age, IQ, health, and other factors, the community group consistently outperformed their counterparts in residences. Subsequent experimentation showed that these differences could be attributed to poor adjustment to the demands of institutional life. For example, old people in institutions, who were as healthy as the community-dwelling individuals, were generally less active and perceived themselves as having little control over decisions that affected their lives. Within our institutionalized sample, performance on tests of learning and memory was found to correlate significantly with measures of psychosocial function. Further, in comparisons over time, changes in activity level and perceived control correlated with changes in cognitive performance.

We have since modified and extended this longitudinal study to another group of institutionalized older adults and also included a group that lives in the community. If anything, the results are even more striking and apply equally to institutionalized and community-dwelling older adults. Performance on psychosocial tests of control, optimism, and activity correlate highly with performance on neuropsychological tests of cognitive function, especially those that are sensitive to damage to prefrontal cortex. Even more interesting are the data related to the longitudinal aspect of the study. Changes in psychosocial well-being correlated with changes in cognition. Although it may not have been surprising to find such correlations as functions decline, it was unexpected to obtain these correlations as psychosocial well-being improved over time in some of the participants in the study.

The results from the psychosocial studies suggest that decline in cognitive function with age is not irreversible, even when the decline is gauged by performance on tests that purport to reflect the functional integrity of different brain structures. A possible interpretation of our results is that the viability of various neural structures depends not only on biological aging, but also on environmental and psychosocial factors whose effects on brain structures may be reversible. A significant feature of our results is that neuropsychological tests of prefrontal function were among the most sensitive both to biological aging and to psychosocial influences. It is hoped that by taking all these factors into consideration, future investigations on the neuropsychology of aging will be broader in scope and will provide an integrated account of how biological, environmental, and psychosocial variables interact.

MEMORY AND WORKING WITH MEMORY: A FRAMEWORK FOR UNDERSTANDING THE EFFECTS OF FRONTAL SYSTEM DETERIORATION WITH AGE

As is clear from this review, memory is not a unitary process. A number of separable components have been identified at both the functional and structural level. We have distinguished two broad classes of memory tests, explicit and implicit, performance on which is likely mediated by different neural structures. Explicit tests of memory such as recognition and recall depend on the conscious recollection of previously experienced events. On implicit tests, the subject is not required to refer intentionally to the past in performing the test; memory is inferred from the effects on behavior of experience or practice. Performance on implicit tests is likely mediated by perceptual and semantic input modules, located in the posterior neocortex, and by motor output modules in the basal ganglia (and probably other regions as well).[140,146]

Conscious recollection can also be separated into two components, associative and strategic. The associative component involves the mandatory and relatively automatic encoding, storage, and retrieval of information that is consciously apprehended. This process is dependent on the medial temporal lobe/hippocampus and its related cortical and subcortical structures.[135,140,202]

The associative system, with the hippocampus at its core, is a system that automatically encodes consciously apprehended information and, in response to the appropriate cue, automatically delivers aspects of the stored information back to consciousness as a memory. *Recovered consciousness* of a previously experienced event is a necessary aspect of recollection.[202] The system, however, lacks intelligence. Sometimes the memories that are delivered are veridical, sometimes they are not. How can one be distinguished from the other? Sometimes the memories are delivered in a haphazard fashion without temporal order or contextual information. How are they organized? Sometimes the initial cue is effective, at other times an appropriate cue must be found if the initial one fails. What guides this search?

Strategic processes associated with the prefrontal cortex are necessary to perform these functions and, thereby, confer "intelligence" and control on the associative system. These strategic processes coordinate, interpret, and elaborate the information in consciousness to provide the hippocampal-associative-memory system with the appropriate encoding information and retrieval cues that it takes as its input. Comparable processes are involved in evaluating the hippocampal system's output and placing those retrieved memories in a proper spatiotemporal context. In short, it is a *working-with-memory* system.[2,140] What makes us conscious of the various processes involved in memory search are not the operations of the hippocampal-associative system, but rather the operations of the strategic frontal system that occupy consciousness. We are aware of the questions we deliver to the hippocampus, the answers we get from it, and the evaluation of the answers, but we are not aware of the ecphoric operations of the hippocampus itself.[132,138,140]

As this brief account indicates, at least three distinguishable neurological components underlie performance on implicit and explicit tests of memory.[146,202] (1) A neocortical component that is involved in *registration* (engram formation) and reactivation and that mediates performance on some implicit tests of memory; (2) an associative/hippocampal component that operates only on consciously apprehended information by binding engrams (*cohesion*) that are associated with the conscious experience into a memory trace, and that delivers aspects of the memory traces back to consciousness in response to appropriate retrieval cues; and (3) a strategic/frontal system that operates on the input to the hippocampal component and the output from it. The frontal system may also be involved in engram formation and reactivation in the neocortex as the results of some recent studies on priming and procedural memory indicate. It is the *working-with-memory* component of the frontal lobes through which manipulations of strategies and cognitive resources exert their effect.

A working-with-memory deficit captures the essence of the impairment associated with frontal lesions. As we said at the beginning of the paper and have indicated throughout, what is impaired is not the memory itself but the uses to which memory is put, the inferences based on memory, the temporal ordering of remembered episodes, their placement in proper contexts, and the implementation of encoding and retrieval strategies with respect to particular events.[209] In other words, what is impaired is the application of remembered events to the organization of behaviors in a current context. Indeed, deficits on these types of tests are often striking and are found consistently in patients with frontal lesions and in elderly people with presumed frontal dysfunction, whereas performance on more traditional working memory tests such as backward digit span and reading span[203] is sometimes unimpaired (see Craik and Jennings,[129] Frisk and Milner,[204] and Petrides[8]).

Cognitive Resources and Frontal Functions

Based on our description of the distinguishing characteristics of hippocampal and frontal systems, it follows that it is the frontal system that should be more prone to depletion of cognitive resources. The hippocampal system, being modular,[135,136,205] operates in a relatively automatic fashion with little expenditure of cognitive resources. The advantage of a neuropsychological model of aging is that it has no need to appeal to the concept of cognitive resources (see Navon[206] and Salthouse,[207] for critiques of the concept of cognitive resources). It is sufficient, from a neuropsychological view, to ascribe memory decline in the elderly to deteriorating frontal and hippocampal functions. At the same time, the neuropsychological framework is capable of accommodating the concept of cognitive resources and of suggesting some counterintuitive, but neuropsychologically appealing, predictions about the type of deficits that might be observed if cognitive resources were reduced with age.

According to our model, an account of memory decline in the elderly that appeals to depletion of cognitive resources with age as a causal agent[107,108,129,207,208] should have its greatest effect in those memory functions that are mediated by the frontal lobes. As yet, we know of no direct evidence in favor or against this hypothesis in old people but a number of recent studies on divided attention and dual-task performance in young people support it. Moscovitch[227] found that the sequential finger-tapping task at encoding and retrieval lowers performance on the following, frontal-lobe–sensitive tests: release from PI, free recall of a categorized list of words, and phonemic or letter fluency.[228] Sequential finger-tapping had little or no noticeable effect on the nonrelease trials of PI, on rate of learning of a categorized list, and on category fluency, all of which are sensitive to hippocampal or temporal lobe damage. In a similar vein, Miyake et al.,[210] Dunbar and Sussman[211] and Roberts et al.[212] have shown that concurrent interfering tasks affect performance on tests of grammatical judgment, on WCST, and on antisaccade tasks presumably by depleting cognitive resources from aspects of working memory that are mediated by the frontal lobes. Consistent with the frontal-lobe interference hypothesis is the observation from PET studies that concurrent interfering tasks significantly reduce frontal-lobe activation necessary for encoding information in episodic memory.[213,214]

Working-with-Memory: Speculations on Mechanisms

In the introduction we noted that the frontal lobes are large, heterogeneous structures with distinct architectonic regions. Our view that working-with-memory describes a common underlying function of the frontal lobes can be interpreted in two ways. One is that each of the distinct regions of prefrontal cortex has the same function although the domain in which it executes this function varies from region to region. The strategic, organizational role of the frontal lobes in memory is no different from its role in problem-solving, ordering motor or linguistic sequences, and so on. Even with respect to memory, different regions of the frontal lobes may be allocated to handle information from different domains (e.g., spatial versus verbal[215,216]) or from different aspects of the same domain (upper or lower visual field[7,217]). However, in each case, the same type or types of underlying functions will be involved.

An alternative interpretation is that working-with-memory is comprised of different functional subcomponents, such as planning, retrieval, and monitoring, each of which is mediated by different regions of prefrontal cortex. Petrides[8] distinguishes among three major regions of prefrontal cortex: the ventrolateral, mid-dorsal lateral, and ventromedial frontal cortex. The ventrolateral frontal cortex constitutes the first stage of interaction between perceptual, semantic, and memory modules in the posterior lateral neocortex and medial temporal lobes. The ventrolateral frontal cortex is necessary for the active (voluntary) retrieval of information from the modules which is then put into the service of executive functions such as planning and decision making. The mid-dorsal lateral region is a second-order region that operates on information received from ventrolateral cortex and serves a monitoring function that is critical for planning and organization. The ventromedial frontal cortex is part of the basic limbothalamic system underlying episodic memory and may itself be important in initiating retrieval from that system and monitoring its output.[133,218] Consistent with Petrides' model is evidence he obtained from PET activation studies which showed that even when the stimuli are identical, these different regions of prefrontal cortex are differentially activated depending on the cognitive demands of the task.

The two interpretations of the working-with-memory function of the prefrontal cortex are not necessarily mutually exclusive. A fine-grained analysis of each of the regions may yet reveal that they themselves are further subdivided into smaller regions according to the type of domain-specific inputs they receive and process.

Future studies may also reveal the physiological mechanisms that are necessary for executing these frontal functions. A recurring suggestion is that initiation and maintenance of inhibitory processes is a hallmark of frontal-lobe function (for recent proponents of this view, see Dempster,[219] Diamond,[220] Hasher and Zacks,[108] and Shimamura[221]). According to this view, all the deficits associated with frontal-lobe deterioration or damage can be attributed wholly, or in part, to a breakdown of inhibitory processes necessary for suppressing irrelevant or erroneous information and for gating or biasing relevant or correct information. There is no doubt that loss of inhibitory control is an important component of the frontal-lobe syndrome. The inhibitory hypothesis also has some intuitive appeal and has been successful in accounting for disorders such as perseveration, response intrusions, and inattention associated with frontal-lobe damage. It is more difficult to see, however, how loss of inhibition can account for the type of deficits in memory for temporal order and frequency. No doubt, inhibition must play a role at some level because it is a ubiquitous aspect of interactions among elements in neural networks. To be truly effective, the inhibitory model would have to specify exactly at what level inhibition operates both in terms of the frontal lobes and in terms of the cognitive task to which inhibition is applied. Computational models such as those proposed by Dehaene and Changeux,[222] Kimberg and Farah,[223] and Levine and Prueitt[224] approach the necessary degree of specificity. By developing and testing such models, at both a cognitive and neurophysiological level, we will gain a clearer understanding of how the frontal lobes accomplish their working-with-memory function and how this function deteriorates with age.

REFERENCES

1. TULVING, E., S. KAPUR, F. I. M. CRAIK, M. MOSCOVITCH & S. HOULE. 1994. Hemispheric encoding/retrieval asymmetry in episodic memory: Positron emission tomography findings. Proc. Natl. Acad. Sci. USA **91:** 2016–2020.
2. MOSCOVITCH, M. & G. WINOCUR. 1992. The neuropsychology of memory and aging. *In* The Handbook of Aging and Cognition. F. I. M. Craik & T. A. Salthouse, Eds.: 315–372. Lawrence Erlbaum. Hillsdale, NJ.
3. JONES, E. G. & T. P. S. POWEL. 1970. An anatomical study of converging sensory pathways within the cerebral cortex of the monkey. Brain **93:** 793–820.

4. PANDYA, D. N. & C. L. BARNES. 1986. Architecture and connections of the frontal lobes. *In* The Frontal Lobes Revisited. E. Perecman, Ed.: 41–72. IRBN Press. New York.

5. MILNER, B. 1964. Some effects of frontal lobectomy in man. *In* The Frontal Granular Cortex and Behavior. J. M. Warren & K. Akert, Eds.: 313–331. McGraw Hill. New York.

6. MISHKIN, M. 1964. Preservation of central sets after frontal lesions in monkeys. *In* The Frontal Granular Cortex and Behavior. J. M. Warren & K. Akert, Eds. McGraw-Hill, New York.

7. GOLDMAN-RAKIC, P. S. 1987. Circuitry of primate prefrontal cortex and regulation of behavior by representational memory. *In* Handbook of Physiology—The Nervous System. F. Plum, Ed. Vol. 5. American Physiological Society. Bethesda, MD.

8. PETRIDES, M. 1994. Frontal lobes and working memory: Evidence from investigations of the effects of cortical excisions in nonhuman primates. *In* Handbook of Neuropsychology. F. Boller & J. Grafman, Eds. Vol. 9: 59–82. Elsevier. Amsterdam.

9. PETRIDES, M. & D. N. PANDYA. 1994. Comparative architectonic analysis of the human and the macaque frontal cortex. *In* Handbook of Neuropsychology. F. Boller & J. Grafman, Eds. Vol. 9: 17–57. Elsevier. Amsterdam.

10. FUSTER, J. M. 1989. The Prefrontal Cortex. 2nd edit. Raven Press. New York.

11. LURIA, A. R. 1966. Higher Cortical Functions in Man. Basic Books. New York.

12. PETRIDES, M. 1989. Frontal lobes and memory. *In* Handbook of Neuropsychology. F. Boller & J. Grafman, Eds. Vol. 3. Elsevier Science Publishers. Amsterdam.

13. STUSS, D. T. & D. F. BENSON. 1986. The Frontal Lobes. Raven Press. New York.

14. MILNER, B. 1963. Effects of different brain lesions on card sorting. Arch. Neurol. **9:** 90–100.

15. BENTON, A. L. 1968. Differential behavioral effects in frontal lobe disease. Neuropsychologia **6:** 53–60.

16. NEWCOMBE, F. 1969. Missile Wounds of the Brain. Oxford University Press. London.

17. JONES-GOTMAN, M. & B. MILNER. 1977. Design fluency: The invention of nonsense drawings after focal lesions. Neuropsychologia **15:** 653–674.

18. RUFF, R. M., C. C. ALLEN, C. E. FARROW, H. NIEMAN, *et al.* 1994. Differential impairment in patients with left versus right frontal lobe lesions. Arch. Clin. Psychol. **9:** 41–55.

19. MARTIN, R. C., D. W. LORING, K. J. MEADOR & G. P. LEE. 1990. The effects of lateralized temporal lobe dysfunction on formal and semantic word fluency. Neuropsychologia **28:** 823–829.

20. JOANETTE, Y. & P. GOULET. 1986. Criterion-specific reduction of verbal fluency in right brain-damaged right-handers. Neuropsychologia **24:** 875–879.

21. MICELI, G., C. CALTAGIRONE, G. GAINOTTI, C. MASULLO & M. C. SILVERI. 1981. Neuropsychological correlates of localized cerebral lesions in non-aphasic brain-damaged patients. J. Clin. Neuropsychol. **3:** 53–63.

22. PENDELTON, M. G., R. K. HEATON, R. A. W. LEHMAN & D. HULIHAN. 1982. Diagnostic utility of the Thurstone world fluency test in neuropsychological evaluations. J. Clin. Neuropsychol. **4:** 307–317.

23. HEATON, R. K. 1981. Wisconsin Card Sorting Test Manual. Psychological Assessment Resources, Inc. Odessa, FL.

24. ANDERSON, S. W., R. D. JONES, A. P. TRANEL, D. TRANEL & H. DAMASIO. 1990. Is the Wisconsin Card Sorting Test an index of frontal lobe damage? J. Clin. Exp. Neuropsychol. **12:** 80.

25. ROBINSON, A. L., R. K. HEATON, R. A. W. LEHMAN & D. W. STILSON. 1980. The utility of the Wisconsin Card Sorting Test in detecting and localizing frontal lobe lesions. J. Consult. Clin. Psychol. **48:** 605–614.

26. TEUBER, H. L., W. S. BATTERSBY & M. B. BENDER. 1951. Performance of complex visual tasks after cerebral lesions. J. Nerv. Ment. Dis. **114:** 413–429.

27. NELSON, H. E. 1976. A modified card sorting test sensitive to frontal lobe defects. Cortex **12:** 313–324.

28. RAZ, N., F. GUNNING, D. P. HEAD, S. D. BRIGGS, J. H. DUPUIS, J. McQUAIN, W. J.

LOKEN, A. E. THORNTON & J. D. ACKERS. 1995. In search of neuroanatomical substrates of memory and executive abilities: Aging as a model system. Soc. Neurosci. Abstr. **21:** 195–914.

29. RAZ, N., D. HEAD, F. GUNNING & J. D. ACKER. 1996. Neural correlates of working memory and strategic flexibility: A double dissociation study. Paper presented at meeting of the International Neuropsychological Society.

30. BENTON, A. L., P. J. ESLINGER & A. R. DAMASIO. 1981. Normative observations on neuropsychological test performance in old age. J. Clin. Neuropsychol. **3:** 33–42.

31. LEACH, L. R., C. M. WARNER, R. HOTZ-SUD, E. KAPLAN & M. FREEDMAN. 1991. The effects of age on Wisconsin Card Sorting variables. J. Clin. Exp. Neuropsychol. **13:** 28 (Abstr.).

32. STROOP, J. R. 1935. Studies of interference in serial verbal reactions. J. Exp. Psychol. **18:** 643–662.

33. MACLEOD, C. M. 1991. Half a century of research on the Stroop effect: An integrative review. Psychol. Bull. **109:** 163–203.

34. GOLDEN, C. J. 1978. Stroop color and word test. Stoelting Co. Chicago, IL.

35. PERRET, E. 1974. The left frontal lobe of man and the suppression of habitual responses in verbal categorical behavior. Neuropsychologia **12:** 323–330.

36. STUSS, D. T. 1991. Interference effects on memory functions in postleukotomy patients: An attentional perspective. *In* Frontal Lobe Function and Dysfunction. H. S. Levin, H. M. Eisenberg & A. L. Benton, Eds.: 157–172. Oxford University Press. New York.

37. COHN, N. B., R. E. DUSTMAN & D. C. BRADFORD. 1984. Age-related decrements in Stroop color test performance. J. Clin. Psychol. **40:** 1244–1250.

38. COMALLI, P. E., JR., S. WAPNER & H. WERNER. 1962. Interference effects of Stroop color-word test in childhood, adulthood, and aging. J. Gen. Psychol. **100:** 47–53.

39. MILNER, B. 1974. Hemispheric specialization: Scope and limits. *In* The Neurosciences: Third Research Program. F. O. Schmitt & F. G. Worden, Eds. MIT Press. Cambridge, MA.

40. MILNER, B., P. CORSI & G. LEONARD. 1991. Frontal-lobe contribution to recency judgements. Neuropsychologia **29:** 601–618.

41. SHIMAMURA, A. P., J. S. JANOWSKY & L. R. SQUIRE. 1990. Memory for temporal order in patients with frontal lobe lesions and patients with amnesia. Neuropsychologia **28:** 803–813.

42. McANDREWS, M. P. & B. MILNER. 1991. The frontal cortex and memory for temporal order. Neuropsychologia **29:** 849–859.

43. BUTTERS, M. A., A. W. KASZNIAK, E. L. GLISKY, P. J. ESLINGER & D. L. SCHACTER. 1994. Recency discrimination deficits in frontal lobe patients. Neuropsychology **8:** 343–353.

44. HUPPERT, F. A. & M. PIERCY. 1976. Recognition memory in amnesic patients: Effects of temporal context and familiarity of material. Cortex **4:** 3–28.

45. SQUIRE, L. R. 1982. Comparisons between forms of amnesia: Some deficits are unique to Korsakoff's syndrome. J. Exp. Psychol. Learn. Mem. Cogn. **8:** 560–571.

46. VRIEZEN, E. & M. MOSCOVITCH. 1990. Temporal ordering and conditional associative learning in Parkinson's disease. Neuropsychologia 1283–1294.

47. SAGAR, J. J., N. J. COHEN, E. V. SULLIVAN, S. CORKIN & J. H. GROWDEN. 1988a. Remote memory in Alzheimer's disease and Parkinson's disease. Brain **111:** 185–206.

48. SAGAR, J. J., E. V. SULLIVAN, J. D. E. GABRIELLI, S. CORKIN & J. H. GROWDEN. 1988b. Temporal ordering and short-term memory deficits in Parkinson's disease. Brain **111:** 525–540.

49. KINSBOURNE, M. 1973. Age effects on letter span related to rate and sequential dependency. J. Gerontol. **28:** 317–319.

50. NAVEH-BENJAMIN, M. 1990. Coding of temporal order information: An automatic process? J. Exp. Psychol. Learn. Mem. Cogn. **16:** 117–126.

51. VRIEZEN, E. 1988. Memory for temporal order and conditional associative learning

in patients with Parkinson's disease. M.A. thesis. University of Toronto. Toronto, Ontario.

52. McCORMACK, P. D. 1982. Temporal coding and study-phase retrieval in young and elderly adults. Bull. Psychon. Soc. **20:** 242–244.

53. McCORMACK, P. D. 1981. Temporal coding by young and elderly adults: A test of the Hasher-Zacks model. Dev. Psychol. **17:** 80–86.

54. PERLMUTTER, M., R. METZGER, T. NEZWORSKI & K. MILLER. 1981. Spatial and temporal memory in 20 and 60 year olds. J. Gerontol. **36:** 59–65.

55. LeFEVER, F. F. & E. I. KUMKOVA. 1995. The recency test: Clinical adaptations of an experimental procedure for studying frontal lobe functions with implications for lateral specialization and different modes of temporal judgment. Paper presented at TENNET, May, Montreal.

56. PARKIN, A. J., B. M. WALTER & N. M. HUNKIN. 1995. The relationship between normal aging, frontal lobe function, and memory for temporal and spatial information. Neuropsychology **9:** 304–312.

57. ESLINGER, P. J. & L. M. GRATTAN. 1993. Frontal lobe and frontal-striatal substrates for different forms of human cognitive flexibility. Neuropsychologia **31:** 17–28.

58. KAUSLER, D. H., W. LICHTY & T. M. DAVIS. 1985. Temporal memory for performed activities: Intentionality and adult age differences. Dev. Psychol. **211:** 1132–1138.

59. FREEDMAN, M. & M. OSCAR-BERMAN. 1986. Bilateral frontal lobe disease and selective delayed response deficits in humans. Behav. Neurosci. **100:** 332–342.

60. JACOBSEN, C. F. 1935. Functions of the frontal association in primates. Arch. Neurol. Psychiatry **33:** 558–569.

61. NISSEN, H. W., A. H. RIESEN & V. NOWLIS. 1938. Delayed response and discrimination learning by chipmanzees. J. Comp. Psychol. **26:** 361–386.

62. KOLB, B. 1984. Functions of the frontal cortex of the rat: A comparative review. Brain Res. Rev. **8:** 65–98.

63. WINOCUR, G. 1991a. Functional dissociation of the hippocampus and prefrontal cortex in learning and memory. Psychobiology **19:** 11–20.

64. WINOCUR, G. 1991b. A comparison of normal old rats and young adult rats with lesions to the hippocampus or prefrontal cortex on a test of matching-to-sample. Neuropsychologia **30:** 769–781.

65. DIAMOND, A., S. ZOLA-MORGAN & L. R. SQUIRE. 1989. Successful performance by monkeys with hippocampal lesions on A$\overline{\text{B}}$ and object retrieval, two tasks that work developmental changes in human infants. Behav. Neurosci. **103:** 526–537.

66. DIAMOND, A. & P. S. GOLDMAN-RAKIC. 1989. Comparison of human infants and rhesus monkeys on Piaget's A$\overline{\text{B}}$ task: Evidence for dependence on dorsolateral prefrontal cortex. Exp. Brain Res. **74:** 24–40.

67. BARTUS, R. T., D. FLEMING & H. R. JOHNSON. 1978. Aging in the rhesus monkey: Debilitating effects on short-term memory. J. Gerontol. **33:** 858–871.

68. WINOCUR, G. 1986. Memory decline in aged rats: A neuropsychological interpretation. J. Gerontol. **41:** 758–761.

69. PETRIDES, M. 1985. Deficits in conditional associative learning tasks after frontal- and temporal-lobe lesions in man. Neuropsychologia **23:** 249–262.

70. PETRIDES, M., B. ALIVISATOS, A. C. EVANS & E. MEYER. 1993. Dissociation of human mid-dorsal lateral from posterior dorsolateral frontal cortex in memory processing. Proc. Natl. Acad. Sci. USA **90:** 873–877.

71. PETRIDES, M., B. ALIVISATOS, E. MEYER & A. C. EVANS. 1993. Functional activation of the human frontal cortex during the performance of verbal working memory tasks. Proc. Natl. Acad. Sci. USA **90:** 878–883.

72. WINOCUR, G. 1992. Conditional learning in aged rats: Evidence of hippocampal and prefrontal cortex impairment. Neurobiol. Aging **13:** 131–135.

73. PETRIDES, M. & B. MILNER. 1982. Deficits on subject-ordered tasks after frontal and temporal-lobe lesions in man. Neuropsychologia **20:** 249–262.

74. PASSINGHAM, R. E. 1985. Memory of monkeys (*Macaca mulatta*) with lesions in prefrontal cortex. Behav. Neurosci. **U99:** 3–21.

75. KOLB, B., R. J. SUTHERLAND & I. WHISHAW. 1983. A comparison of the contributions

of the frontal and parietal association cortex to spatial localization in rats. Behav. Neurosci. **97:** 13–27.

76. DE TOLEDO-MORRELL, L. & F. MORRELL. 1984. Electrophysiological markers of aging and memory loss in rats. Ann. N. Y. Acad. Sci. **444:** 296–311.

77. BARNES, C. A. 1988. Aging in the physiology of spatial memory. Neurobiol. Aging **9:** 563–568.

78. INGRAM, D. K. 1988. Complex maze learning in rodents as a model of age-related memory impairment. Neurobiol. Aging **9:** 475–485.

79. WINOCUR, G. & M. MOSCOVITCH. 1990a. Hippocampal and prefrontal cortex contributions to learning and memory. Analysis of lesion and aging effects on maze learning in rats. Behav. Neurosci. **104:** 544–551.

80. WINOCUR, G. & M. MOSCOVITCH. 1990b. A comparison of cognitive function in institutionalized and community-dwelling old people of normal intelligence. Can. J. Psychol. **44:** 435–444.

81. CORKIN, S. 1965. Tactually-guided maze learning in man: Effects of unilateral cortical excisions and bilateral hippocampal lesions. Neuropsychologia **3:** 339–351.

82. SCHACTER, D. L., J. L. HARBLUCK & D. R. MCLACHLAN. 1984. Retrieval without recollection: An experimental analysis of source amnesia. J. Verb. Learn. Verb. Behav. **23:** 593–611.

83. SHIMAMURA, A. P. & L. R. SQUIRE. 1987. A neuropsychological study of fact memory and source amnesia. J. Exp. Psychol. Learn. Mem. Cogn. **13:** 464–473.

84. PARKIN, A. J., N. R. C. LENG & N. STANHOPE. 1988. Memory impairment following ruptured aneurysm of the anterior communicating artery. Brain & Cognition **7:** 231–243.

85. JANOWSKY, J. S., A. P. SHIMAMURA & L. R. SQUIRE. 1989a. Source memory impairment in patients with frontal lobe lesions. Neuropsychologia **27:** 1043–1056.

86. MCINTYRE, J. S. & F. I. M. CRAIK. 1987. Age differences in memory for item and source information. Can. J. Psychol. **41:** 175–192.

87. DYWAN, J. & L. L. JACOBY. 1990. Effects of aging on source monitoring: Differences in susceptibility to false fame. Psychol. & Aging **5:** 379–387.

88. BARTLETT, J. C., L. STRATER & A. FULTON. 1991. False recency and false fame of faces in young adulthood and old age. Memory & Cognition **19:** 177–188.

89. SCHACTER, D. L., A. W. KASZNIAK, J. F. KIHLSTROM & M. VALDISERRI. 1991. On the relation between source memory and aging. Psychol. & Aging **6:** 559–568.

90. SCHACTER, D. L., D. OSOWIECKI, A. W. KASZNIAK, J. F. KIHLSTROM & M. VALDISERRI. 1994. Source memory: Extending the boundaries of age-related deficits. Psychol. & Aging **9:** 81–89.

91. KAUSLER, D. H. & J. M. PUCKETT. 1980. Adult age differences in recognition memory for a nonsemantic attribute. Exp. Aging Res. **6:** 349–355.

92. LIGHT, L. L., D. LAVOIE, D. VALENCIA-LAVER, S. A. A. OWENS & G. MEAD. 1992. Direct and indirect measures of memory for modality in young and older adults. J. Exp. Psychol. Learn. Mem. Cogn. **18:** 1284–1297.

93. MITCHELL, D. B., R. R. HUNT & F. A. SCHMITT. 1986. The generation effect and reality monitoring: Evidence from dementia and normal aging. J. Gerontol. **41:** 79–84.

94. RABINOWITZ, J. C. 1989. Judgments of origin and generation effects: Comparisons between young and elderly adults. Psychol. & Aging **4:** 259–268.

95. HASHTROUDI, S., M. K. JOHNSON, N. VNEK & S. A. FERGUSON. 1994. Aging and the effects of affective and factual faces on source monitoring and recall. Psychol. & Aging **9:** 160–169.

96. COHEN, G. & D. FAULKNER. 1989. Age differences in source forgetting: Effects on reality monitoring and eyewitness testimony. Psychol. & Aging **4:** 10–17.

97. GUTTENTAG, R. E. & R. R. HUNT. 1988. Adult age differences in memory for imagined and performed actions. J. Gerontol. Psychol. Sci. **43:** P107–108.

98. HASHTROUDI, S., M. K. JOHNSON & L. D. CHROSNIAK. 1989. Aging and source monitoring. Psychol. & Aging **4:** 106–112.

99. KORIAT, A., H. BEN-ZUR & D. SHCEFFER. 1988. Telling the same story twice: Output monitoring and age. J. Mem. Lang. 27: 23–39.
100. LIGHT, L. L. 1991. Memory and aging: Four hypotheses in search of data. Ann. Rev. Psychol. 42: 333–376.
101. CRAIK, F. I. M., L. W. MORRIS, R. G. MORRIS & E. R. LOEWEN. 1990. Relations between source amnesia and frontal lobe functioning in older adults. Psychol. Aging 5: 148–151.
102. SPENCER, W. & N. RAZ. 1994. Memory for facts, source and context: Can frontal lobe dysfunction explain age-related differences? Psychol. & Aging 9: 149–158.
103. FERGUSON, S. A., S. HASHTROUDI & M. K. JOHNSON. 1992. Age differences in using source-relevent cues. Psychol & Aging 1: 443–452.
104. KLIEGL, R. & U. LINDENBERGER. 1988. A mathematical model of proactive interference in cued recall: Localizing adult age differences in memory functions. Paper presented at the Cognitive Aging Conference, Atlanta, Georgia.
105. GLISKY, E. L., M. R. POLSTER & B. C. ROUTHIEAUX. 1995. Double dissociation between item and source memory. Psychol. & Aging 9: 229–235.
106. SMITH, M. L. & B. MILNER. 1988. Estimation of frequency of occurrence of abstract designs after frontal or temporal lobectomy. Neuropsychologia 26: 297–306.
107. HASHER, L. & R. T. ZACKS. 1979. Automatic and effortful processes in memory. J. Exp. Psychol. Gen. 108: 356–388.
108. HASHER, L. & R. T. ZACKS. 1988. Working memory, comprehension, and aging: A review and a new view. In The Psychology of Learning and Motivation. G. H. Bower, Ed. Vol. 22: 193–225. Academic Press. New York.
109. FREUND, J. L. & K. L. WITTE. 1986. Recognition and frequency judgments in young and elderly adults. Am. J. Psychol. 99: 81–102.
110. KAUSLER, D. H., M. K. HAKAMI & R. WRIGHT. 1982. Adult age differences in frequency judgments of categorical representations. J. Gerontol. 37: 365–371.
111. KAUSLER, D. H., W. LICHTY & M. K. HAKAMI. 1984. Frequency judgments for distractor items in a short-term memory task: Instructional variations and adult age differences. J. Verb. Learn. Verb. Behav. 23: 660–668.
112. ATTIG M. & L. HASHER. 1980. The processing of frequency of occurrence information by adults. J. Gerontol. 35: 66–69.
113. ELLIS, N. R., R. L. PALMER & C. L. REEVES. 1988. Developmental and intellectual differences in frequency processing. Devel. Psychol. 24: 38–45.
114. CERMAK, L. S., N. BUTTERS & J. MOREINES. 1974. Some analyses of the verbal encoding deficit of alcoholic Korsakoff patients. Brain & Lang. 1: 141–150.
115. WINOCUR, G., M. KINSBOURNE & M. MOSCOVITCH. 1981. The effect of cuing on release from proactive interference in Korsakoff amnesic patients. J. Exp. Psychol. Hum. Learn. Mem. 7: 56–65.
116. MOSCOVITCH, M. 1982. Multiple dissociations of function in amnesia. In Human Memory and Amnesia. L. S. Cermak, Ed. Lawrence Erlbaum. Hillsdale, NJ.
117. JANOWSKY, J. S., A. P. SHIMAMURA, M. KRITCHEVSKY & L. R. SQUIRE. 1989. Cognitive impairment following frontal lobe damage and its advance to human amnesia. Behav. Neurosci. 103: 548–560.
118. FREEDMAN, M. & L. S. CERMAK. 1986. Semantic encoding deficits in frontal lobe disease and amnesia. Brain & Cognition 5: 108–114.
119. ELIAS, C. S. & N. HIRASUNA. 1976. Age and semantic and phonological encoding. Dev. Psychol. 12: 497–503.
120. PUGLISI, J. T. 1981. Semantic encoding in older adults as evidence by release from proactive inhibition. J. Gerontol. 36: 743–745.
121. DOBBS, A. R., J. B. AUBREY & B. G. RULE. 1989. Age-associated release from proactive interference: A review. Can. Psychologist 30: 588–595.
122. MOSCOVITCH, M. & G. WINOCUR. 1983. Contextual cues and release from proactive inhibition in old and young people. Can. J. Psychol. 37: 331–344.
123. WINOCUR, G. 1982. The amnesic syndrome: A deficit in cue utilization. In Human Memory and Amnesia. L. S. Cermak, Ed.: 139–166. Erlbaum. Hillsdale, NJ.
124. WINOCUR, G., M. MOSCOVITCH & J. FREEDMAN. 1987. An investigation of cognitive

function in relation to psychosocial variables in institutionalized old people. Can. J. Psychol. **41:** 257–269.

125. PARKIN, A. J. & A. LAWRENCE. 1994. A dissociation in the relation between memory tasks and frontal lobe tests in the normal elderly. Neuropsychologia **32:** 1523–1532.

126. BUTTERFIELD, E. C., T. O. NELSON & V. PECK. 1988. Developmental aspects of the feeling of knowing. Dev. Psychol. **24:** 654–663.

127. LACHMAN, J. L., R. LACHMAN & C. THRONESBERY. 1979. Metamemory through the adult life span. Dev. Psychol. **15:** 543–545.

128. CALEV, A. 1984. Recall and recognition in mildly disturbed schizophrenics: The use of matched-tasks. J. Abnorm. Psychol. **93:** 172–177.

129. CRAIK, F. I. M. & J. M. JENNINGS. 1992. Human memory. *In* The Handbook of Aging and Cognition. F. I. M. Craik & T. A. Salthouse, Eds.: 51–110. Erlbaum. Hillsdale, NJ.

130. CRAIK, F. I. M. 1983. On the transfer of information from temporary to permanent storage. Philos. Trans. R. Soc. Lond. B. **302:** 341–359.

131. CRAIK, F. I. M. 1986. A functional account of age differences in memory. *In* Human Memory and Cognitive Capabilities. F. Klix & H. Hagendorf, Eds.: 409–422. Elsevier. Amsterdam.

132. TULVING, E. 1983. Elements of Episodic Memory. Clarendon Press. Oxford, UK.

133. MOSCOVITCH, M. 1989. Confabulation and the frontal system: Strategic vs. associative retrieval in neuropsychological theories of memory. *In* Varieties of Memory and Consciousness: Essays in Honor of Endel Tulving. H. L. Roediger III & F. I. M. Craik, Eds. Erlbaum. Hillsdale, NJ.

134. MOSCOVITCH, M. & C. UMILTÀ. 1990. Modularity and neuropsychology: Implications for the organization of attention and memory in normal and brain-damaged people. *In* Modular Processes in Dementia. M. E. Schwartz, Ed. MIT/Bradford. Cambridge, MA.

135. MOSCOVITCH, M. & C. UMILTÀ. 1991. Conscious and nonconscious aspects of memory: A neuropsychological framework of modules and central systems. *In* Perspectives on Cognitive Neuroscience. R. G. Lister & H. J. Weingartner, Eds. Oxford University Press. Oxford.

136. HIRST, W., M. K. JOHNSON, E. A. PHELPS & B. T. VOLPE. 1988. More on recognition and recall in amnesics. J. Exp. Psychol. Learn. Mem. Cogn. **14:** 758–762.

137. MAYES, A. R. 1988. Human Organic Memory Disorders. Cambridge University Press. Cambridge, MA.

138. GRADY, C. L., A. R. McINTOSH, B. HORWITZ, J. M. MAISOG, L. G. UNGERLEIDER, M. J. MENTIS, P. PIETRINI, M. B. SCHAPIRO & J. V. HAXBY. Age-related reductions in human recognition memory involve altered cortical activation during encoding. Science **269:** 218–221.

139. WHEELER, M. A., D. T. STUSS & E. TULVING. Frontal lobe damage produces episodic memory impairment. J. Int. Neuropsychol. Soc. In press.

140. MOSCOVITCH, M. 1992. Memory and working-with-memory: A component process model based on modules and central systems. J. Cognit. Neurosci. **4:** 257–267.

141. INCISA DELLA ROCHETTA, A. 1986. Classification and recall of pictures after unilateral frontal or temporal lobectomy. Cortex **22:** 189–211.

142. INCISA DELLA ROCHETTA, A. & B. MILNER. 1993. Strategic search and retrieval inhibition: The role of the frontal lobes. Neuropsychologia **31:** 503–524.

143. PARKIN, A. J. & B. M. WALTER. 1992. Recollective experience, normal aging and frontal dysfunction. Psychol. & Aging **7:** 290–298.

144. ROEDIGER, H. L. & K. B. McDERMOTT. 1993. Implicit memory in normal human subjects. *In* Handbook of Neuropsychology. H. Spinnler & F. Boller, Eds. Vol. 8: 63–131. Elsevier. Amsterdam.

145. MOSCOVITCH, M., E. VRIEZEN, & Y. GOSHEN-GOTTSTEIN. 1993. Implicit tests of memory in patients with focal lesions and degenerative brain disorders. *In* Handbook of Neuropsychology. H. Spinnler & F. Boller, Eds. Vol. 8: 133–173. Elsevier. Amsterdam.

146. MOSCOVITCH, M. 1994. Memory and working-with-memory: Evaluations of a compo-

nent process model and comparisons with other models. *In* Memory Systems. D. L. Schacter & E. Tulving, Eds.: 269–310. MIT/Bradford. Cambridge, MA.

147. SCHACTER, D. L. 1990. Perceptual representational systems and implicit memory: Toward a resolution of the multiple memory systems debate. Ann. N. Y. Acad. Sci. **608:** 543–571.

148. SCHACTER, D. L. 1992. Priming and multiple memory systems: Perceptual mechanisms of implicit memory. J. Cognit. Neurosci. **4:** 244–256.

149. SQUIRE, L. R. 1987. Memory and Brain. Oxford University Press. New York.

150. TULVING, E. & D. L. SCHACTER. 1990. Priming and human memory systems. Science **247:** 301–306.

151. SHALLICE, T. 1982. Specific impairments of planning. Philos. Trans. R. Soc. Lond. **B298:** 199–209.

152. SAINT-CYR, J. A., A. E. TAYLOR & A. E. LANG. 1988. Procedural learning and neostriatal function in man. Brain **111:** 941–959.

153. WILSON, B. & A. BADDELEY. 1988. Semantic, episodic, and autobiographical memory in a post meningitic amnesic patient. Brain & Cognition **8:** 31–46.

154. ROEDIGER, H. L. 1990. Implicit memory. Retention without remembering. Am. Psychologist **45:** 1043–1056.

155. TARDIF, T. & F. I. M. CRAIK. 1989. Reading a week later: Perceptual and conceptual factors. J. Mem. & Lang. **28:** 107–125.

156. MARTONE, M., N. BUTTERS, M. PAYNE, J. T. BECKER & D. S. SAX. 1984. Dissociation between skill learning and verbal recognition in amnesia and dementia. Arch. Neurol. **41:** 965–970.

157. MAYES, A. R. & P. GOODING. 1989. Enhancement of word completion priming in amnesics by cueing with previously novel associates. Neuropsychologia **27:** 1057–1072.

158. HOWARD, D. V., A. F. FRY. & C. M. BRUNE. 1991. Aging and memory for new associations: Direct versus indirect measures. J. Exp. Psychol. Mem. Learn. Cogn. **17:** 779–792.

159. GRAF, P. 1990. Life-span changes in implicit and explicit memory. Bull. Psychon. Soc. **28:** 353–358.

160. HOWARD, D. V. & J. H. HOWARD, JR. 1989. Age differences in learning serial patterns: Direct versus indirect measures. Psychol. & Aging **4:** 357–364.

161. HOWARD, D. V. 1991. Implicit memory: An expanding picture of cognitive aging. Annu. Rev. Gerontol. Geriatr. **11:** 1–22.

162. LIGHT, L. L. & D. LAVOIE. 1993. Direct and indirect measures of memory in old age. *In* Implicit Memory: New Directions in Cognition, Development, and Neuropsychology. P. Graf & M. E. J. Masson, Eds.: 207–230. Erlbaum. Hillsdale, NJ.

163. MOSCOVITCH, M. 1982b. A neuropsychological approach to perception and memory in normal and pathological aging. *In* Aging and Cognitive Processes. F. I. M. Craik & S. Trehub. Eds. Plenum Press. New York.

164. MITCHELL, D. B. 1989. How many memory systems? Evidence from aging. J. Exp. Psychol. Learn. Mem. Cogn. **15:** 31–49.

165. MITCHELL, D. B., A. S. BROWN & D. R. MURPHY. 1990. Dissociations between procedural and episodic memory: Effects of time and aging. Psychol. & Aging **5:** 264–276.

166. MOSCOVITCH, M., G. WINOCUR & D. McLACHLAN. 1986. Memory as assessed by recognition and reading time in normal and memory impaired people with Alzheimer's disease and other neurological disorders. J. Exp. Psychol. Gen. **115:** 331–347.

167. RABBITT, P. M. A. 1982. How do old people know what to do next? *In* Aging and Cognitive Processes. F. I. M. Craik & S. Trehub, Eds. Plenum Press. New York.

168. LIGHT, L. L., A. SINGH & J. L. CAPPS. 1986. Dissociation of memory and awareness in young and older adults. J. Clin. Exp. Neuropsychol. **8:** 62–74.

169. LIGHT, L. L. & A. SINGH. 1987. Implicit and explicit memory in young and older adults. J. Exp. Psychol. Learn. Mem. Cogn. **13:** 531–541.

170. SNODGRASS, J. G. & J. CORWIN. 1988. Pragmatics of measuring recognition memory: Applications to dementia and amnesia. J. Exp. Psychol. Gen. **117:** 34–50.

171. HOWARD, D. V. 1988. Implicit and explicit assessment of cognitive aging. *In* Cognitive

Development in Adulthood: Progress in Cognitive Development Research. M. L. Howe & C. J. Brainerd, Eds.: 3–37. Springer-Verlag. New York.

172. ROSE, T. L., J. A. YESAVAGE, R. D. HILL & G. H. BOWER. 1986. Priming effects and recognition memory in young and elderly adults. Exp. Aging Res. **12**: 31–37.

173. DAVIS, H. P., A. COHEN, M. GUNDY, P. COLOMBO, G. VAN DUSSELDORP, N. SIMOLKE & J. ROMANO. 1990. Lexical priming deficits as a function of age. Behav. Neurosci. **104**: 288–297.

174. LIGHT, L. L. & S. A. ALBERTSON. 1989. Direct and indirect tests of memory for category exemplars in young and older adults. Psychol. & Aging **4**: 487–492.

175. JELICIC, M., F. I. M. CRAIK & M. MOSCOVITCH. Submitted.

176. WIGGS, C. L. 1990. Aging and memory for frequency of occurrence of novel visual stimuli: Direct and indirect measures. Unpublished Ph.D. dissertation. Georgetown University. Washington, D.C.

177. REES-NISHIO, M. 1984. Memory, emotion, and skin conductance responses in young and elderly normal and memory-impaired people. Unpublished Ph.D. dissertation. University of Toronto. Toronto, Ontario.

178. MOSCOVITCH, M. 1985. Memory from infancy to old age: Implications for theories of normal and pathological memory. Ann. N.Y. Acad. Sci. **444**: 78–96.

179. HASHTROUDI, S., L. D. CHROSNIAK & B. L. SCHWARTZ. 1991. A comparison of the effects of aging on priming and skill learning. Psychol. & Aging **6**: 605–615.

180. WRIGHT, B. M. & R. B. PAYNE. 1985. Effects of aging on sex differences in psychomotor reminiscence and tracking proficiency. J. Gerontol. **40**: 179–181.

181. BUTTERS, N., W. C. HEINDEL & D. P. SALMON. 1990. Dissociation of implicit memory in dementia: Neurological implications. Bull. Psychon. Soc. **28**: 359–366.

182. CHIARELLO, C. & W. J. HOYER. 1988. Adult age differences in implicit and explicit memory: Time course and encoding effects. Psychol. & Aging **3**: 358–366.

183. HULTSCH, D. F., M. E. J. MASSON & B. J. SMALL. 1991. Adult age differences in direct and indirect tests of memory. J. Gerontol.

184. WINOCUR, G., M. MOSCOVITCH & D. T. STUSS. A neuropsychological investigation of explicit and implicit memory in institutionalized and community-dwelling old people. Neuropsychology. In press.

185. NISSEN, M. J. & P. C. BULLEMER. 1987. Attentional requirements of learning: Evidence from performance measures. Cogn. Psychol. **19**: 1–32.

186. HOWARD, D. V., & J. H. HOWARD, JR. 1992. Adult age differences in the rate of learning serial patterns: Evidence from direct and indirect tests. Psychol. & Aging **7**: 232–241.

187. JACKSON, G. M. & S. R. JACKSON. Serial reaction time learning: Sequence or probability learning? J. Exp. Psychol. Learn. Mem. Cogn. In press.

188. STADLER, M. A. 1992. Statistical structure and implicit learning. J. Exp. Psychol. Learn. Mem. Cogn. **18**: 318–327.

189. COHEN, A., R. I. IVRY & S. W. KEELE. 1990. Attentional structure in sequence learning. J. Exp. Psychol. Learn. Mem. Cogn. **16**: 17–30.

190. DOYON, J., A. M. OWEN, M. PETRIDES, V. SZIKLAS & A. C. EVANS. 1994. Functional anatomy of visuomotor skill learning using positron emission tomography. Soc. Neurosci. Abstr. **20**: 154.12.

191. FERRARO, F. R., D. A. BALOTA & L. T. CONNOR. 1992. Implicit memory and the formation of new associations in nondemented Parkinson's disease individuals and individuals with senile dementia of the Alzheimer type: A serial reaction time (SRT) investigation. Brain & Cognition **21**: 163–180.

192. KNOPMAN, D. S. & M. J. NISSEN. 1991. Procedural learning is impaired in Huntington's disease: Evidence from the serial reaction time task. Neuropsychologia **29**: 245–254.

193. WILLINGHAM, D. B. & W. J. KOROSHETZ. 1990. Evidence for dissociable motor skills in Huntington's disease patients. Psychobiology **21**: 173–182.

194. PASCUAL-LEONE, A., J. GRAFMAN & M. HALLETT. 1995. Procedural learning and prefrontal cortex. Ann. N.Y. Acad. Sci. This volume.

195. JACKSON, G. M. & S. R. JACKSON. 1992. Sequence structure and sequential learning:

The evidence from ageing reconsidered. Tech. Rep. No. 92-9. Institute of Cognitive and Decision Sciences, University of Oregon. Eugene, OR.

196. JACKSON, G. M., S. R. JACKSON, J. HARRISON, L. HENDERSON & D. KENNARD. 1995. Serial reaction time learning and Parkinson's disease: Evidence for a procedural learning deficit. Neuropsychologia 33: 577–593.

197. KAY, H. & M. SIME. 1962. Discrimination with old and young rats. J. Gerontol. 17: 75–80.

198. WINOCUR, G. 1984. The effects of retroactive and proactive interference on learning and memory in old and young rats. Dev. Psychobiol. 17: 537–545.

199. CAMPBELL, B. A. & V. HAROUTUNIAN. 1981. Effects of age on long-term memory: Retention of fixed-interval responding. J. Gerontol. 36: 338–341.

200. ARBUCKLE, T. Y., D. GOLD & D. ANDRES. 1986. Cognitive functioning of older people in relation to social and personality variables. Psychol. & Aging 1: 55–62.

201. WINOCUR, G., M. MOSCOVITCH & D. WITHERSPOON. 1987. Contextual cuing and memory performance in brain-damaged amnesics and old people. Brain & Cognition 6: 129–141.

202. MOSCOVITCH, M. 1995a. Models of consciousness and memory. In The Cognitive Neurosciences. M. S. Gazzaniga, Ed.: 1341–1356. MIT Press. Cambridge, MA.

203. DANEMAN, M. & P. A. CARPENTER. 1980. Individual differences in integrating information between and within sentences. J. Exp. Psychol. Learn. Mem. Cogn. 9: 561–584.

204. FRISK, V. & B. MILNER. 1990. The role of the left hippocampal region in the acquisition and retention of story content. Neuropsychologia 28: 349–359.

205. FODOR, J. 1983. The Modularity of Mind. MIT Press. Cambridge, MA.

206. NAVON, D. 1984. Resources—A theoretical soup stone? Psychol. Rev. 91: 216–234.

207. SALTHOUSE, T. A. 1982. Adult Cognition. Springer-Verlag. New York.

208. CRAIK, F. I. M. & M. BYRD. 1982. Aging and cognitive deficits: The role of attentional resources. In Aging and Cognitive Processes. F. I. M. Craik & S. Trehub, Eds. Plenum Press. New York.

209. MOSCOVITCH, M. 1995b. Confabulation: A neuropsychological perspective. In Memory Distortion. D. L. Schacter et al., Eds. Harvard University Press. Cambridge, MA.

210. MIYAKE, A., P. A. CARPENTER & M. A. JUST. 1995. A capacity approach to syntactic comprehension disorders: Making normal adults perform like aphasic patients. Cogn. Neuropsychol. 11: 671–717.

211. DUNBAR, K. & D. SUSSMAN. 1995. Toward a cognitive account of frontal lobe function: Simulating frontal lobe deficits in normal subjects. Ann. N. Y. Acad. Sci. This volume.

212. ROBERTS, R. J., JR., L. D. HAGAR & C. HERON. 1994. Prefrontal cognitive processes: Working memory and inhibition in the antisaccade task. J. Exp. Psychol. Gen. 23: 374–393.

213. SHALLICE, T., P. FLETCHER, C. D. FRITH, P. M. GRASBY, R. S. J. FRACKOWIAK & R. J. DOLAN. 1994. Brain regions associated with acquisition and retrieval of verbal episodic memory. Nature 368: 633–635.

214. FLETCHER, P. C., C. D. FRITH, P. M. GRASBY, T. SHALLICE, R. S. J. FRACKOWIAK & R. J. DOLAN. 1995. Brain systems for encoding and retrieval of auditory-verbal memory: An in vivo study in humans. Brain 118: 401–416.

215. MILNER, B., M. PETRIDES & M. L. SMITH. 1985. Frontal lobes and the temporal organization of memory. Hum. Neurobiol. 4: 137–142.

216. WILSON, F. A. W., S. P. O. SCALAIDHE & P. S. GOLDMAN-RAKIC. 1993. Dissociation of object and spatial processing domains in primate prefrontal cortex. Science 260: 1955–1958.

217. GOLMAN-RAKIC, P. S. 1991. The circuitry of working memory revealed by anatomy and metabolic imaging. In Frontal Lobe Function and Injury. H. Levin & H. M. Eisenberg, Eds. Oxford University Press, Oxford.

218. DELUCA, J. & B. J. DIAMOND. 1995. Aneurysm of the anterior communicating artery: A review of neuroanatomical and neuropsychological sequelae. J. Clin. Exp. Neuropsychol. 17: 100–121.

219. DEMPSTER, F. N. 1992. The rise and fall of the inhibitory mechanisms: Toward a unified theory of cognitive development and aging. Dev. Rev. **12:** 45–75.
220. DIAMOND, A. 1990. Developmental progression in human infants and infant monkeys, and the neural basis of the inhibitory control of reaching. Ann. N. Y. Acad. Sci. **608:** 394–426.
221. SHIMAMURA, A. P. 1995. Memory and frontal lobe function. *In* The Cognitive Neurosciences. M. S. Gazzaniga, Ed. The MIT Press. Cambridge, MA.
222. DEHAENE, S. & J. P. CHANGEUX. 1989. A simple model of prefrontal cortex function in delayed-response tasks. J. Cognit. Neurosci. **1:** 244–261.
223. KIMBERG, D. Y. & M. J. FARAH. 1993. A unified account of cognitive impairments following frontal lobe damage: The role of working memory in complex, organized behavior. J. Exp. Psychol. Gen. **122:** 411–428.
224. LEVINE, D. S. & P. S. PRUEITT. 1989. Modelling some effects of frontal lobe damage: Novelty and perseveration. Neural Networks **2:** 103–116.
225. STUSS, D. T., M. P. M. ALEXANDER, C. L. PALUMBO, L. BUCKLE, L. SAYER & E. J. POGUE. 1994. Organizational strategies of patients with unilateral or bilateral frontal lobe injury in word list learning. Neuropsychology **8:** 355–373.
226. SHIMAMURA, A. P., F. B. GERSHBERG, P. J. JURICA, J. A. MANGELS & R. KNIGHT. 1992. Intact implicit memory in patients with frontal lobe lesions. Neuropsychologia **30:** 931–937.
227. MOSCOVITCH, M. 1994. Cognitive resources and dual task interference effects at retrieval in normal people: The role of the frontal lobes and medial temporal cortex. Neuropsychology **8:** 524–534.
228. MARTIN, A., C. L. WIGGS, F. L. LALONDE & C. MACK. 1994. Word retrieval to letter and semantic cues: A double dissociation in normal subjects using interference tasks. Neuropsychologia **32:** 1487–1494.

Memory and the Prefrontal Cortex[a]

ARTHUR P. SHIMAMURA

Department of Psychology
University of California, Berkeley
Berkeley, California 94720-1650

The prefrontal cortex has been associated with a variety of memory functions, including delayed response, conditional learning, immediate memory, free recall, memory for temporal order, and metamemory.[1-4] Neuropsychological studies of brain-injured patients and lesion studies using primate models have provided key findings concerning the contribution of prefrontal cortex to memory. The pattern of memory disorders associated with prefrontal lesions suggests an impairment in *working memory,* which is associated with organizing and monitoring information retrieved from memory. The role of the prefrontal cortex as a working memory or executive control process has been exemplified in various theories of frontal lobe function.[1,5-8]

This paper briefly reviews the contribution of the prefrontal cortex to human memory performance. Topics include new learning capacity, remote memory, memory for temporal order, and metamemory. Findings suggest that memory disorders associated with prefrontal lesions may be related to problems in controlling and monitoring information processing. In particular, the prefrontal cortex may be involved in filtering or inhibiting irrelevant or extraneous neural activity in posterior cortex.

NEW LEARNING ABILITY

Patients with prefrontal lesions do not exhibit gross impairment on clinical tests of new learning ability. For example, Janowsky *et al.*[9] demonstrated that patients with prefrontal lesions perform within the normal range on the Wechsler Memory Scale-Revised (WMS-R), a clinical test battery that assesses both verbal and non-verbal memory on measures of recall, recognition memory, and paired-associate learning. Generally good performance on tests of new learning ability in patients with prefrontal lesions can be contrasted with the severe learning impairment associated with lesions involving the medial temporal lobe (e.g., hippocampus) or diencephalic midline (e.g., thalamic nuclei). These lesions produce organic amnesia, in which patients have extreme difficulty remembering information and events encountered since the onset of amnesia.[10,11]

Despite relatively good performance on clinical tests of new learning capacity, patients with prefrontal lesions exhibit moderate impairment on standard tests of new learning. In particular, these patients exhibit impairment on tests of free

[a] This work was supported by grants from the National Institute on Aging (AG09055) and the National Institute of Mental Health (MH48757).

recall.[9,12-16] On these tests, a list of items (e.g., words or pictures) are presented, and subjects are asked to recollect as many items from the list as possible. Tests of free recall place heavy demands on internally generated memory strategies because no cues are presented during testing other than a simple command to recall the information.

Recent findings suggest that the prefrontal cortex contributes to memory organization both at the time of learning and at the time of retrieval. During learning, patients with prefrontal lesions are less likely to engage in useful organizational strategies, such as subjective organization or category clustering.[12,14,16] Moreover, patients are benefited by providing category cues at the time of learning[14] or simply by providing instructions that a list contains semantically related words.[17] Category cues and information about the structure of a word list provide semantic organization of new information that patients with prefrontal lesions apparently cannot glean by themselves.

The prefrontal cortex also appears to contribute significantly to the retrieval of information in memory. Patients with prefrontal lesions are benefited by the provision of category cues at the time of retrieval.[14] Also, patients exhibit significant impairment on tests of verbal fluency in which subjects must retrieve well-learned information from semantic memory.[9] Positron emission tomography (PET) findings suggest that individuals engaged in a memory task involving retrieval of general semantic knowledge show a preponderance of left prefrontal activity, whereas a task involving retrieval of episodic or autobiographical knowledge show a preponderance of right prefrontal activity.[18]

A prominent feature of working memory is the control or filtering of extraneous information processing. Several studies suggest a problem in increased susceptibility of interfering information during tests of new learning ability. Shimamura et al.[19] presented three study-test learning trials of a list of 12 related paired-associates (e.g., thief–crime; lion–hunter). Following the three learning trials, subjects were asked to learn a second list in which each cue word used in the first list was paired with a new target word (e.g., thief–bandit; lion–circus). This memory test paradigm is called AB-AC paired-associate learning. Although patients appeared to learn the first list nearly as a well as control subjects, they exhibited disproportionate impairment when they were required to ignore the first associations and learn new ones (FIG. 1).

Findings from studies of new learning ability suggest that the prefrontal cortex is involved in working memory processes associated with organizational strategies. Deficits in these processes influence new learning ability, but they do not produce the profound and selective amnesic disorder associated with medial temporal or diencephalic lesions. Instead, prefrontal lesions appear to affect memory strategies that become important when few retrieval cues are present at test. For example, patients with prefrontal lesions exhibit greater impairment on tests of free recall than tests of recognition memory. Also, this impairment in working memory produces greater susceptibility to interference. Increased interference has been observed on tests of paired-associate learning as well as on other tests in which extraneous or irrelevant cues are provided.[13,19]

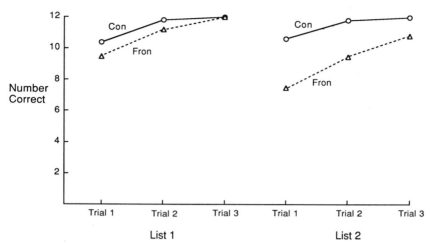

FIGURE 1. Performance by patients with prefrontal lesions and control subjects on a test of AB-AC paired-associate learning. Subjects were given three study-test learning trials of a list of 12 related paired-associates (*lion–hunter*) and then another three study-test learning trials using another list in which the cue word was the same but the target word was different (*lion–circus*). Performance on the second list by patients with prefrontal lesions was particularly affected, presumably because of the increased interference from the first list. Con, control subjects; Fron, frontal patients.

REMOTE MEMORY AND RETRIEVAL STRATEGIES

The prefrontal cortex contributes to working memory processes important for both learning and retrieval. As a result, studies of new learning ability are unable to disambiguate disruptions that occur at the time of learning from those that occur at the time of retrieval. Tests of remote memory (e.g., past public events, past famous faces), however, can assess the specific impairment associated with retrieval deficits because memory can be tested for information learned well before brain damage.

The role of the prefrontal cortex in memory for remote information has not been tested extensively. Some studies have suggested that the remote memory impairment (i.e., retrograde amnesia) that is observed in patients with Korsakoff's syndrome is related to general cortical atrophy or specifically to frontal lobe damage.[20,21] In particular, Kopelman[21] found that remote memory performance of patients with Korsakoff's syndrome was correlated with performance on tasks sensitive to frontal lobe pathology (e.g., verbal fluency, card sorting, cognitive estimation). Yet, computerized tomography (CT) measures of frontal lobe atrophy in patients with Korsakoff's syndrome were not significantly correlated with performance on tests of remote memory.[21]

Della Sala *et al.*[22] assessed memory for remote autobiographical information in patients with prefrontal lesions. Subjects were asked to recollect memories from various time periods (e.g., "Can you remember anything in particular that

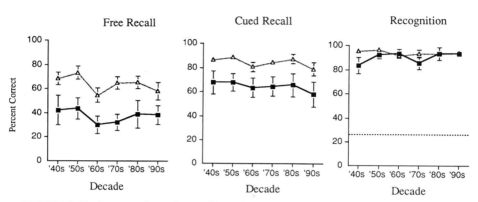

FIGURE 2. Performance by patients with prefrontal lesions and control subjects on a test of remote memory. Subjects were presented photographs of individuals ("famous faces") who became famous during various time periods between 1940 and 1995. Free and cued recall performance was significantly impaired in patients with prefrontal lesions, whereas recognition memory was less affected. ▬■▬ Frontal patients; ···△··· Control subjects.

happened to you or to a member of your family before you reached the age of 15?"). The four patients with bilateral frontal lobe lesions exhibited impairment on this test of autobiographical memory. However, only two of 12 patients with unilateral frontal lobe lesions exhibited impairment on this test. Across all 16 patients, performance on the autobiographical test was correlated with performance on tests of executive working memory (e.g., verbal fluency, sorting, digit cancellation). The authors suggest that the frontal lobes are important in mediating search strategies that facilitate retrieval of autobiographical memory.

Recently, we assessed patients with unilateral prefrontal lesions on tests of memory for public events and famous faces.[23] We used tests previously used to assess retrograde amnesia in patients with severe memory disorders.[24–26] For each test, measures of free recall and recognition memory were obtained for public events that spanned from the 1940s to 1990s (e.g., Who shot John Lennon? Chapman) and famous faces (e.g., Michael Dukakis, Meryl Streep). Additionally, for the famous faces test, we assessed the benefits of semantic and phonemic cues during retrieval. Patients with prefrontal lesions exhibited impairment on free recall measures of remote public events and famous faces (FIG. 2). Recognition memory was not impaired, although memory performance in certain decades was affected. On the famous faces test, cued recall was impaired and thus did not completely ameliorate retrieval deficits.

Findings of impaired remote memory extend the array of memory deficits observed in patients with prefrontal lesions. They suggest an impairment in retrieval processes because in many instances the information tested was learned many years prior to brain injury. The disproportionate impairment of free recall compared to recognition memory observed on these tests of remote memory is similar to that observed on tests of new learning and suggests that prefrontal cortex facilitates the implementation of retrieval strategies.

MEMORY FOR TEMPORAL ORDER

Milner[27] was the first to report that patients with prefrontal lesions exhibit an impairment in memory for temporal order. She reported a study of recency judgments, in which subjects are shown a series of stimuli (e.g., words, pictures) and are asked to judge which one of two stimuli was presented more recently.[28] In another test of temporal order memory,[29] subjects were presented a list of 15 words one at a time and then asked to reconstruct the list order from a random display of the words. Memory for temporal order was assessed by correlating a subject's judged order with the actual presentation order of the words. Patients with prefrontal lesions exhibited impaired memory for temporal order on this test.

In everyday experiences, one often forgets the context in which some information was encountered. Such instances represent a loss of source or contextual memory. Findings of specific "source amnesia" suggest a distinction between memory for facts and memory for contextual memory.[30–32] Neuropsychological analyses of *source amnesia* suggest that memory for spatial-temporal context may be a disorder related to prefrontal lesions and not a disorder associated with damage to the medial temporal or diencephalic areas that cause amnesia.[33,34]

Janowsky et al.[34] assessed source memory in patients with prefrontal lesions, age-matched control subjects, and younger control subjects. Subjects learned a set of 20 trivia facts that could not be previously recalled (e.g., the name of the dog on the Cracker Jacks box is Bingo). After a 6–8-day retention interval, fact recall was tested for the 20 learned facts (e.g., What is the name of the dog on the Cracker Jacks box?) and for 20 new facts. When subjects correctly answered a fact question, they were asked to recollect the source of the information ("Can you tell me where you learned the answer?" "When was the most recent time you heard that information?"). Source memory ability was significantly impaired in patients with prefrontal lesions. Interestingly, source memory impairment also occurs in normal aging, as indicated by the finding that older control subjects (mean age, 63.9 years) made more source errors than younger control subjects (mean age, 49.4 years).[34,35] Neuronal cell loss associated with normal aging does occur prominently in the frontal lobes,[36] which suggests that source memory impairment in normal aging may also be related to subtle frontal lobe dysfunction.

METAMEMORY

Interference in retrieval can produce "memory blocking" effects, which can be commonly observed when information is on the "tip of the tongue." Indeed, patients with anomic deficits experience inordinate occasions of this annoying lapse of memory. Metamemory refers to knowledge about one's memory capabilities and knowledge about strategies that can aid memory.[37] Patients with prefrontal lesions exhibited metamemory deficits when they were asked to evaluate their memory capabilities or "feeling of knowing." In one test, subjects were given 24 sentences to learn (e.g., Patty's garden was full of marigolds). After a delay, cued recall was assessed for the last word in each sentence (e.g., Patty's garden was full of _____). If the correct answer to a question could not be recalled, then subjects rated their feeling of knowing—that is, they rated on a four-point scale how likely they would be able to recognize the answer if some choices were given (e.g., very likely to recognize the answer, not very likely to recognize the answer). To verify the accuracy of these feeling-of-knowing judgments, the ratings were correlated with performance on an subsequent recognition test. Patients with prefrontal lesions exhibited deficits in feeling-of-knowing accuracy. That is, they were poor at assessing what they knew and what they did not know.

The feeling-of-knowing impairment exhibited by patients with prefrontal lesions may be related to deficits in other tasks that involve memory retrieval and inferential reasoning. One such example is the finding that patients with prefrontal lesions have difficulty making estimates or inferences from everyday experiences (e.g., How tall is the average English woman?).[38] Answers to such questions are not readily available and typically require search-and-retrieval strategies. Similarly, patients with prefrontal lesions have difficulty estimating the price of objects.[39] All these deficits—that is, deficits in cognitive estimation as well as in feeling-of-knowing judgments—might be construed as deficits in metamemory (i.e., knowing about what is stored in memory).

PREFRONTAL CORTEX AS A DYNAMIC FILTERING MECHANISM

The variety of memory deficits associated with prefrontal lesions suggests an impairment in working memory.[5–8, 40] Patients with prefrontal lesions are not able to control or monitor inadvertent information processing. This problem affects memory performance as a result of poor initiation of memory strategies and increased interference from recently activated memories. One possibility is that the prefrontal cortex controls information processing by filtering irrelevant or extraneous neural processing. Specifically, the prefrontal cortex may act to gate or inhibit activity in posterior cortical regions. Based on this view, the array of cognitive disorders associated with prefrontal cortex lesions can be explained by a problem in selecting and organizing neural activity.

Some physiological evidence suggests that the prefrontal cortex is involved in the control of posterior cortical activity. Knight and colleagues studied scalp-evoked potentials in patients with prefrontal lesions. In one study,[41] the amplitude of middle latency auditory evoked potentials, which are presumed to be generated in primary auditory cortex, was *potentiated* as a result of prefrontal lesions. Thus, there appeared to be a *disinhibition* of posterior cortical activity as a result of prefrontal lesions. In a PET study of normal individuals,[42] *increases* in activity in the dorsolateral prefrontal cortex were related to *decreases* in activity in posterior cortical regions. Thus, as a result of the extensive reciprocal connections between the prefrontal cortex and other cortical areas, it may be that inhibitory control of many aspects of mental function is provided by this proposed filtering mechanism. Based on this view, a multitude of cognitive disorders would occur as a result of prefrontal lesions, not because different areas of the prefrontal cortex are serving different functions, but because these areas are inhibiting different posterior cortical regions, which themselves serve different cognitive functions. This view extends an earlier view of *response competition* as the mediator of frontal lobe dysfunction,[43,44] a view which was presumed limited and did not adequately account for many findings from human and animal lesion studies.

CONCLUSION

In recent years, a plethora of research findings about human prefrontal function has accumulated. Both neuropsychological and neuroimaging studies have contributed to our understanding of the prefrontal cortex. Memory functions associated with prefrontal cortex appear to be related to the control and organization of memory—that is, working memory. Damage to the prefrontal cortex impairs a variety of memory functions, including aspects of new learning, remote memory, memory for temporal order, and metamemory. Deficits appear to be most pronounced when performance depends upon self-initiated encoding and organizational strategies, such as observed on tests of free recall. Also, tests involving extensive search and retrieval processes, such as tests of source memory and metamemory, are susceptible to prefrontal lesions. These memory deficits may be part of a broader cognitive impairment associated with problems in controlling extraneous or irrelevant information processing. That is, the prefrontal cortex may be involved in filtering or gating neural activity in posterior cortex which enables more efficient information processing.

REFERENCES

1. FUSTER, J. M. 1989. The Prefrontal Cortex, 2nd edit. Raven Press. New York.
2. MILNER, B., M. PETRIDES & M. L. SMITH. 1985. Frontal lobes and the temporal organization of memory. Hum. Neurobiol. 4: 137–142.
3. SHIMAMURA, A. P. & P. J. JURICA. 1994. Memory interference effects and aging: Findings from a test of frontal lobe function. Neuropsychology 8: 408–412.
4. STUSS, D. T., G. A. ESKES & J. K. FOSTER. 1994. Experimental neuropsychological studies of frontal lobe functions. In Handbook of Neuropsychology. F. Boller & J. Grafman, Eds.: 149–185. Elsevier. Amsterdam.
5. BADDELEY, A. 1986. Working Memory. Oxford University Press. Oxford, UK.
6. GOLDMAN-RAKIC, P. S. 1987. Circuitry of primate prefrontal cortex and regulation of behavior by representational memory. In Handbook of Physiology: The Nervous System, Vol. 5. F. Plum, Ed.: 373–417. American Physiological Society. Bethesda, MD.
7. MOSCOVITCH, M. 1994. Cognitive resources and dual-task interference effects at retrieval in normal people: The role of the frontal lobes and medial temporal cortex. Neuropsychology 8: 524–534.
8. SHIMAMURA, A. P. 1994a. Memory and frontal lobe function. In The Cognitive Neurosciences. M. S. Gazzaniga, Ed.: 803–813. MIT Press. Cambridge, MA.
9. JANOWSKY, J. S., A. P. SHIMAMURA, M. KRITCHEVSKY & L. R. SQUIRE. 1989. Cognitive impairment following frontal lobe damage and its relevance to human amnesia. Behav. Neurosci. 103: 548–560.
10. SHIMAMURA, A. P. 1989. Disorders of memory: The cognitive science perspective. In Handbook of Neuropsychology. F. Boller & J. Grafman, Eds.: 35–73. Elsevier Sciences Publishers. Amsterdam.
11. SQUIRE, L. R. 1992. Memory and the hippocampus: A synthesis from findings with rats, monkeys, and humans. Psychol. Rev. 99: 195–231.

12. ESLINGER, P. J. & L. M. GRATTAN. 1994. Altered serial position learning after frontal lobe lesion. Neuropsychologia **32:** 729–739.
13. DELLA ROCCHETTA, A. I. 1986. Classification and recall of pictures after unilateral frontal or temporal lobectomy. Cortex **22:** 189–211.
14. GERSHBERG, F. B. & A. P. SHIMAMURA. The role of the frontal lobes in the use of organizational strategies in free recall. Neuropsychologia. In press.
15. JETTER, W. *et al.* 1986. A verbal long term memory deficit in frontal lobe damaged patients. Cortex **22:** 229–242.
16. STUSS, D. T., M. P. ALEXANDER, C. L. PALUMBO & L. BUCKLE. 1994. Organizational strategies of patients with unilateral or bilateral frontal lobe injury in word list learning tasks. Neuropsychology **8:** 355–373.
17. HIRST, W. & B. T. VOLPE. 1988. Memory strategies with brain damage. Brain & Cognition **8:** 379–408.
18. TULVING, E. *et al.* 1994. Hemispheric encoding/retrieval asymmetry in episodic memory: Positron emission tomography finding. Proc. Natl. Acad. Sci. USA **91:** 2016–2020.
19. SHIMAMURA, A. P., P. J. JURICA, J. A. MANGELS, F. B. GERSHBERG & R. T. KNIGHT. 1995. Susceptibility to memory interference effects following frontal lobe damage: Findings from tests of paired-associated learning. J. Cognit. Neurosci. **7:** 144–152.
20. SHIMAMURA, A. P. & L. R. SQUIRE. 1986. Korsakoff syndrome: A study of the relation between anterograde amnesia and remote memory impairment. Behav. Neurosci. **100:** 165–170.
21. KOPELMAN, M. D. 1989. Remote and autobiographical memory, temporal context memory and frontal atrophy in Korsakoff and Alzheimer patients. Neuropsychologia **27:** 437–460.
22. DELLA SALA, S., M. LAIACONA, H. SPINNLER & C. TRIVELLI. 1993. Autobiographical recollection and frontal damage. Neuropsychologia **31:** 823–839.
23. MANGELS, J. A., F. B. GERSHBERG, A. P. SHIMAMURA & R. T. KNIGHT. Impaired retrieval from remote memory in patients with frontal lobe lesions. Neuropsychology. In press.
24. ALBERT, M. S., N. BUTTERS & J. LEVIN. 1979. Temporal gradients in the retrograde amnesia of patients with alcoholic Korsakoff's disease. Arch. Neurol. **36:** 211–216.
25. COHEN, N. J. & L. R. SQUIRE. 1981. Retrograde amnesia and remote memory impairment. Neuropsychologia **19:** 337–356.
26. SQUIRE, L. R., F. HAIST & A. P. SHIMAMURA. 1989. The neurology of memory: Quantitative assessment of retrograde amnesia in two groups of amnesic patients. J. Neurosci. **9:** 828–839.
27. MILNER, B. 1971. Interhemispheric differences in the localization of psychological processes in man. Br. Med. Bull. **127:** 272–277.
28. MILNER, B., P. CORSI & G. LEONARD. 1991. Frontal-lobe contribution to recency judgements. Neuropsychology **29:** 601–618.
29. SHIMAMURA, A. P., J. S. JANOWSKY & L. R. SQUIRE. 1990. Memory for the temporal order of events in patients with frontal lobe lesions and amnesic patients. Neuropsychologia **28:** 803–813.
30. HIRST, W. 1982. The amnesic syndrome: Descriptions and explanations. Psychol. Bull. **91:** 435–460.
31. MAYES, A. R., P. R. MEUDELL & A. PICKERING. 1985. Is organic amnesia caused by a selective deficit in remembering contextual information? Cortex **21:** 167–202.
32. TULVING, E. 1983. Elements of Episodic Memory. Clarendon Press. Oxford, UK.
33. SCHACTER, D. L., J. HARBLUK & D. McLACHLAN. 1984. Retrieval without recollection: An experimental analysis of source amnesia. J. Verb. Learn. Verb. Behav. **23:** 593–611.
34. JANOWSKY, J. S., A. P. SHIMAMURA & L. R. SQUIRE. 1989. Source memory impairment in patients with frontal lobe lesions. Neuropsychologia **27:** 1043–1056.
35. McINTYRE, J. S. & F. I. M. CRAIK. 1987. Age differences in memory for item and source information. Can. J. Psychol. **42:** 175–192.
36. HAUG, H. *et al.* 1983. Anatomical changes in aging brain: Morphometric analysis of

the human prosencephalon. *In* Brain Aging: Neuropathology and Neuropharmacology. J. Cervos-Navarro & H. I. Sarkander, Eds.: 1–12. Raven Press. New York.

37. METCALFE, J. & A. P. SHIMAMURA, EDS. 1994. Metacognition: Knowing About Knowing. MIT Press. Cambridge, MA.

38. SHALLICE, T. & M. E. EVANS. 1978. The involvement of the frontal lobes in cognitive estimation. Cortex **14:** 294–303.

39. SMITH, M. L. & B. MILNER. 1984. Differential effects of frontal-lobe lesions on cognitive estimation and spatial memory. Neuropsychologia **22:** 697–705.

40. JONIDES, J. *et al.* 1993. Spatial working memory in humans as revealed by PET. Nature **363:** 623–625.

41. KNIGHT, R. T., D. SCABINI & D. L. WOODS. 1989. Prefrontal gating of auditory transmission in humans. Brain Res. **504:** 338–342.

42. FRITH, C. D. *et al.* 1991. A PET study of word finding. Neuropsychologia **29:** 1137–1148.

43. BRUTKOWSKI, S., M. MISHKIN & H. E. ROSVOLD. 1963. Positive and inhibitory motor conditioned reflexes in monkeys after ablation of orbital or dorso-lateral surface of the frontal cortex. *In* Central and Peripheral Mechanisms of Motor Function. E. Gutmann & P. Hnik, Eds.: 133–141. Czechoslovak Academy of Sciences. Prague.

44. LURIA, A. R. 1973. The Working Brain. Basic Books. New York.

Dual-Task Paradigm: A Means To Examine the Central Executive

SERGIO DELLA SALA,[a,b] ALAN BADDELEY,[c]
COSTANZA PAPAGNO,[d] AND HANS SPINNLER[d]

[a]Department of Psychology
University of Aberdeen
Old Aberdeen, United Kingdom

[c]MRC Applied Psychology Unit
Cambridge, United Kingdom

[d]III Department of Neurology
S. Paolo Hospital
University of Milan
Milan, Italy

INTRODUCTION

Dual-Task Experiments in Alzheimer's Disease

In previous work[1] we have shown that when patients affected by dementia of the Alzheimer disease (AD) type are required to perform two tasks simultaneously, they are particularly impaired, even when pains are taken to ensure that the level of performance on the individual tasks is equated with that of age-matched controls.

A follow-up longitudinal study showed that this disadvantage became more pronounced with the progression of the disease, whereas performance on the single task did not show this same degree of sensitivity.[2] A further longitudinal experiment[2] varied difficulty within a single task. The results showed no interaction between task difficulty and progressive deterioration in performance. These findings mitigated the possibility that the rate of deterioration is dependent simply on the level of task difficulty.

The outcome of this series of experiments supports the view that patients with AD may suffer from a deficit in their ability to cope with the cognitive processing necessary for carrying out two tasks simultaneously, irrespective of the difficulty of each of the single tasks.

The Central Executive Deficit Interpretation of the Dual-Task Findings in Alzheimer's Disease

The data summarized above cannot easily be accounted for by a model based on partial reallocation of available activation (see ref. 3), but are not inconsistent

---

[b] Address correspondence to Prof. Sergio Della Sala, Department of Psychology, University of Aberdeen, King's College, AB9 2UC Old Aberdeen, UK.

161

with the hypothesis of a deficit in a cognitive resource independent of those required to perform either the digit span or the tracking task on their own, which is responsible for the coordination of dual-task performance. Within the frame of reference of Baddeley and Hitch's[4] working memory model two active subsystems were postulated: a system involved in the maintenance of verbal information and a system responsible for the manipulation of visuospatial images. A central executive has also been proposed in the model, the role of which is that of coordinating information from the two (or more) slave systems (see refs. 1 and 5). Therefore, the impairment in dual-task performance found in patients with AD has been attributed to a deficit of the central executive component of working memory.[5,6]

Toward a Cognitive Architecture of the Central Executive

Among the different components of working memory, the central executive has been the least investigated. Until very recently its specification has been so vague to be equated to a ragbag.[7] Many cognitive models contain at least one (literally) cloudy area. Indeed, the cloudy central executive concept is still open to the criticism of being just a convenient homunculus, a sort of assertive little god that in some enigmatic way manages and supervises all the substantial decisions. It is certainly in need of a more defined cognitive architecture, and perhaps a further fractionation (for a discussion see ref. 8). The dual-task paradigm seems to be a promising way of tackling this issue more analytically because it provides a convenient means of directly testing the central executive hypothesis.

Aims of the Present Investigation

The computerized version of the dual-task paradigm employed in the series of studies reported above was somewhat inconvenient logistically and impractical for everyday clinical use. The aim of this paper is to report a replication of the previous findings with a paper and pencil version of the dual-task we developed and validated. Moreover, because it has been postulated that the anatomical locus of the central executive lies within the frontal lobes,[1] the possible relationship between the executive task (dual-task) and frontal damage remains open. To address this theoretical question, some experimental data drawn from a recent study of ours in which we tested a group of patients with a lesion limited to the prefrontal areas of the brain will also be discussed.

PAPER AND PENCIL VERSION OF THE DUAL-TASK PARADIGM

The aim of this experiment was to replicate the findings of Baddeley[9] using a paper and pencil version of the dual-task test.

Subjects

Patients with AD. Twelve patients (9 females and 3 males, mean age 65.7 ± SD 8.3 years, with 7.2 ± SD 3.9 years of formal education) participated in the study. They were diagnosed as patients with AD according to standardized criteria[10,11] broadly in line with those of the NINCDS-ARDA[12] and the DSM IV.[13] In all but one case (where the patient had a normal CT scan), the patients showed signs of mild cortical atrophy. Neurological examination was uneventful for 10 of them, while eliciting paratonia in one and bradykinesia and tonic grasping in another. The presenting symptom was amnesia in six cases, behavioral disturbances in five, and acalculia in one.

During a series of pilot studies it became clear that patients with AD showing severe cognitive impairment were unable to accomplish the task. Therefore, an inclusion criterion was set, using a psychometric tool, the Milan Overall Dementia Assessment (MODA), that measures severity of dementia,[14] hence ensuring the inclusion of only mildly deteriorated patients. All patients included in the study scored higher than 40 out of a total score of 100 in the MODA, and performed above 70% on its questionnaire investigating everyday coping abilities.[14]

Controls. Twelve normal subjects, matched individually with the patients for sex, age, and educational level, also took part in the experiment. Their mean age was 65.5 ± SD 5.9 years and their mean formal education 7.3 ± SD 4.3 years. They had no physical handicaps and were free of detectable present or past diseases of the central nervous system that could impair their performance.

METHODS

Memory Span

Baseline digit span. Subjects were first tested using a standard procedure to measure digit span. They were presented with a list of digits read aloud by the examiner at one digit per second and were asked for immediate ordered recall. The number of digits was gradually increased by one item. Three lists at each length were given. Span was taken as the maximum length at which the subject performed all three lists without error. This rather conservative measure of span was chosen after a series of pilot studies demonstrated that it was better suited for our experimental conditions.

Single-task condition. The subjects were then presented continuously with lists of digits at their own span for a period of two minutes. The number of lists presented in two minutes varied across individuals, because it was dependent on the subject's span. Performance was therefore measured by the percentage of correct sequences.

Dual-task condition. Subjects were again presented for two minutes with lists of sequences at their own span, while concomitantly being required to perform the tracking task. Once again performance was measured as the percentage of completely correct sequences that were recalled.

Tracking

Single-task condition. Subjects were required to cross out, using a felt pen, 1 sq cm boxes linked to form a path laid out on an A4 sheet of paper. All subjects first performed practice trials using a 10-box path, until the examiner was reassured that they had understood the task. Each experimental sheet had 80 boxes. The subjects were asked to start at one end of the chain and place a cross in each successive box as rapidly as possible. If subjects managed to cross all the boxes before the time limit of two minutes had elapsed, then a second sheet was presented. The total number of crossed boxes was taken as the score.

Dual-task condition. Subjects performed the same test simultaneously with digit span, for two minutes.

RESULTS

In agreement with most of the previous literature (for a review see ref. 6), patients with AD performed more poorly on digit span than matched controls. Their scores were respectively $3.75 \pm$ SD 0.62 and $5.17 \pm$ SD 1.03, $t(\text{df} = 22) = 4.08$, $p < 0.001$.

More interesting for our purpose are the data derived from comparison between the single and dual task performance in the continuous task paradigm. The performance of the patients with AD and that of the normal controls is shown in TABLE 1. The measure taken for span is the mean percentage of correct sequences as a function of subject group, both for the single task condition (span performed alone for two minutes) and the dual task condition (effect of concurrent tracking). The measure of tracking is the number of boxes crossed in two minutes. FIGURE 1 shows the scatterograms of individual performance in the single and dual task condition for (A) percentage of correct span sequences and (B) tracking (number of boxes).

TABLE 1. Effect of Dual Task on Memory Span and Tracking Performance

	AD Patients ($n = 12$)	Controls ($n = 12$)
Span[a]		
Single	87.6 (9.9)[c]	92.0 (7.9)[c]
Dual	50.0 (21.5)	92.0 (9.0)
Tracking[b]		
Single	42.2 (16.2)	58.0 (12.1)
Dual	36.0 (13.9)	59.9 (11.8)

[a] Span measure is the percentage of correct sequences as a function of subject group—patients with Alzheimer's disease (AD) and their matched controls.
[b] Tracking score is the total number of crossed out boxes within the allotted time.
[c] Standard deviations in parentheses.

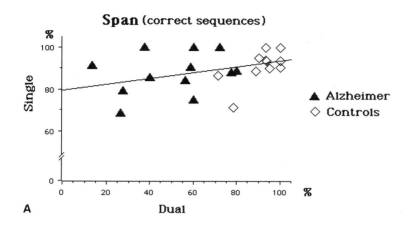

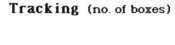

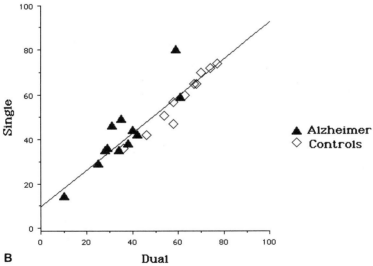

FIGURE 1. Individual performance of patients with Alzheimer's disease (*filled triangles*) and matched controls (*open diamonds*) in the single- and dual-task conditions as a function of the percentage of correct span sequences (**A**) and the number of boxes in the tracking task (**B**).

Analysis of variance suggested that the patients with AD made significantly more errors in the span task that did the control group [F(1,22) = 28.97, $p <$ 0.001]. The effect of condition was also significant [F(1,22) = 37.98, $p < 0.001$] as was the interaction between groups and the dual-task effect [F(1,22) = 38.05, $p < 0.001$]. The results concerning the tracking performance mirrored those of the span. An analysis of variance demonstrated an effect of group [F(1,22) = 12.90, $p < 0.002$], a marginal effect of condition [F(1,22) = 4.40, $p < 0.05$], and a significant interaction [F(1,22) = 15.63, $p < 0.001$].

The correlation between the severity of the cognitive impairment as measured by the MODA[14] and the decrement in performance of the two tasks when performed within the dual-task paradigm (single–dual) was respectively 0.59 for the span and 0.08 for the tracking. This suggests that patients with AD may have been treating tracking as the more important of the two tasks and protecting tracking performance at the expense of increasing memory errors. Greene et al.[15] also reported dual-task impairment in patients with AD; however, their patients showed a decrement in performance in the tracking task rather than in the memory span. The issue of trade-off between tasks is further discussed below.

DISCUSSION

Our paper and pencil adaptation of the dual-task paradigm suggests that our original finding[9] was robust and of some generality. Such a conclusion is strengthened by the results of the recent study by Greene et al.,[15] which also used the paper and pencil version of the task to study patients with AD. They not only observed that the performance was impaired in their patients, but also found significant correlation ($r = 0.49$) between performance of this test and on a quite different dual-task performance measure. This was taken from Robertson et al.'s[16] Test of Everyday Attention, involving what were superficially very different tasks, namely, scanning a telephone directory for pairs of symbols at the same time as counting auditory tones.

The paper and pencil version of the dual-task paradigm proved to be suitable for use with cognitively impaired patients, which suggests possible practical implications. Because the memory deficit is so characteristic of the neuropsychological profile of patients with AD understanding its nature is likely to be important in analyzing the functional deficit occurring in AD, which in turn may lead to the development of tests for early diagnosis. The dual-task approach reported here seems promising in this respect because it combines considerable sensitivity to the effect of AD while being relatively impervious to the effect of normal aging. At the same time it avoids the inherent complexity of most dual-task techniques. Therefore, this paradigm is probably a useful tool for screening out patients with AD at an early stage of their cognitive derangement.

However, although our new version of the test appears promising, if it is to be readily used in the clinic, it is important to have a simple way of combining tracking and memory scores. Without such a combined score, interpretation is complicated by the fact that different subjects may choose to distribute their attention differentially across the two subtests. We are at present in the process of collecting norms which should allow scaled scores to be developed in the hope that it will be possible to combine the two scaled scores to produce a unitary measure. This in turn will allow researchers and clinicians to evaluate performance of individual patients and thereby employ a multiple single-case approach.

A second issue concerns the anatomical localization of the executive processes underlying dual-task performance. It has been suggested[2,5,6,9,17–20] that a deficit in the controlling central executive component of working memory may be characteristic of AD, and that it may lie at the root of many of the cognitive processing deficits.[2] The present results are consistent with the hypothesis that patients with AD are particularly impaired in the operation of a system devoted to the integration of performance of two (or more) concurrent tasks.

However, these findings still leave some major theoretical questions unanswered. Although the concept of a central executive is purely a functional one,[21] it has been suggested that executive processes may be closely associated with frontal lobe function.[1,22,23] Our data, showing a clear impairment in dual-task performance in AD, are not easily interpreted in these terms. In fact the traditional lesions (plaques, tangles, amyloid deposits) described in pathological studies of AD are more numerous and appear earlier in the temporal (and parietal) than in the frontal lobes.[24–27] This yielded some circumvolutions in the attempts to account for the data.[2,28] However, it has recently been hypothesized that the degenerative process in AD might be initiated by a loss of synapses[29] paramount in the frontal cortex,[30] which correlates highly with the measures of cognitive impairment.[31] This new evidence might help to elucidate the biological substrate of our findings.

Be this as it may, we decided to test directly the hypothesis applying the dual-task technique to the study of a sample of patients with frontal lobe lesions (Baddeley *et al.*, in preparation), combining it with three other measures of executive function. Two of these were standard neuropsychological tests, namely, the modified version[32] of the Wisconsin Card Sorting Test (WCST),[33] whereas the second was a measure of verbal fluency in which the subject was required to generate as many words as possible beginning with a specified initial letter,[34] the letters in question being *F, P,* and *L*.[35] The third estimate of executive function was based on the behavior of the patients, assessed in two ways. The purpose of the assessments was to detect signs of behavioral disturbance, whether in the form of inertia and apathy or of euphoric/moriatic type. One source of such information came from a clinical interview with the patients and their relatives, and the other was based on an assessment by a second neurologist of the behavior as reported in the patients' clinical notes. Of 27 patients assessed, the two assessors agreed on 24, with the remaining three dropped from the analysis. This left 12 subjects who showed dysexecutive behavior, and 12 subjects who did not.

The two groups did not differ in their digit span performance when performed alone, but whereas the addition of the box tracking task had no effect on the nondysexecutive subjects, the dysexecutive group showed significant impairment. The pattern for concurrent tracking was similar though less marked.

Although the patients tended to show impaired performance on both verbal fluency (20 of 24 scored below the cutoff) and WCST (14 out of 24 successfully achieved three or fewer categories), neither of these two tests differentiated between those subjects who showed behavioral disturbance and those who did not.

The anatomical site of the lesion also did not prove to be a good marker to differentiate the two groups. In fact the number of unilateral, right and left, and bilateral lesions was almost identical in the dysexecutive and nondysexecutive subgroups.

Our results therefore suggest an association between dual-task impairment and behavioral disturbances. Although this finding was somewhat serendipitous, it is not an isolated observation. Alderman[36] reports a study of brain-damaged patients who present with severe behavioral problems and who are treated using a rehabilitation program based on the principle of reinforcement, delivered through a token economy system. In some of his patients these methods failed to work, leading Alderman to explore the possible differences between the successful "responders" and the "nonresponders." He used a range of standard neuropsychological tests such as verbal fluency and WCST without finding any substantial difference between the two groups. However, when he employed the dual-task methodology based on our earlier studies,[2,9] Alderman successfully discriminated between the two groups showing that the nonresponders were consistently impaired in the capacity to combine two tasks.

Why should poor dual-task performance be associated with behavioral disturbances? At this point one can only speculate, but one possibility is that social behavior requires the subject to balance his or her own desires and needs against those of other people. Failure to perform this particular dual task is likely to lead to behavior that is socially unacceptable.

Although we have indeed observed failure to combine tasks in patients with damage to the frontal lobes, it is important to note that such dual-task impairment is not an inevitable consequence of frontal lobe damage. Evidence currently available gives few clues to more precise localization, but does support earlier claims of an association between the frontal lobes and executive control.

Although our results are consistent with the assumption of some form of central executive, they argue against the idea of a unitary holistic executive and in favor of a fractionation of the system into subcomponents. The observation, for example, that our frontal patients show impaired performance on WCST and verbal fluency, but that these are not strongly associated with behavioral signs argues for such a fractionation. The picture emerging from several studies using a wider range of conventional neuropsychological tests points in the same direction.[8] For example, Burgess and Shallice,[37] and Duncan et al. (in preparation) both studied the performance of brain-damaged patients on a wide range of conventional "frontal" tests, with both finding only low intercorrelations between the various measures of frontal function. Della Sala et al. (in preparation) studied some 50 brain-damaged patients with a focal lesion in the frontal lobes using a series of tests that are classically associated with executive dysfunction. As predicted, many subjects performed below the cutoff score on some of the tests. However, several different double dissociations emerged from this set of data, giving little support to the view of a single executive structure located within the frontal lobes. Broadly similar dissociations among executive tasks and between executive tasks and behavioral derangement have been reported also in single case studies.[38,39]

The results described above suggest a multicomponent executive system. This is not of course a new idea.[40,41] However, abandoning the idea of a unitary executive is only a first step. There is, furthermore, a danger of simply labeling the various tasks with hypothetical executive capacities such as maintaining set, controlling serial order or judging recency. Unless there is a clear attempt to separate the concept from its instantiation in a particular test, then little progress is likely to be made.

An alternative approach that we ourselves have adopted is to specify particular executive functions on an *a priori* basis. In the case of the present dual-task study, the function proposed was a necessary component of the working memory model.[4] Having demonstrated that one instantiation of the concept was fruitful in attempting to understand the cognitive deficit in AD, we have pressed on to change the surface characteristics of the task on the grounds that if the concept is genuinely useful, then it will generalize beyond the tasks on which it was initially developed. We would argue that dual-task performance has so far fulfilled this promise and, as such, provides an encouraging precedent for attempting to explore other executive processes.

In the meantime, our paper and pencil version of the dual-task paradigm appears to have considerable promise as a useful clinical tool. It appears to tap an important component of executive function that is impaired, not only in Alzheimer's disease but also in a subset of frontal patients with a susceptibility to behavioral disturbance. If the test is to realize its potential, however, it is still necessary to collect norms and to solve the problem of combining the constituent measures into a single index. We hope to report work on this in the near future.

ACKNOWLEDGMENT

We thank Dr. Annalena Venneri for her help in preparing some of the material for this paper.

REFERENCES

1. BADDELEY, A. D., R. H. LOGIE, S. BRESSI, S. DELLA SALA & H. SPINNLER. 1986. Dementia and working memory. Q. J. Exp. Psychol. **38A:** 603–618.
2. BADDELEY, A. D., S. BRESSI, S. DELLA SALA, R. H. LOGIE & H. SPINNLER. 1991. The decline of working memory in Alzheimer's disease: A longitudinal study. Brain **114:** 2521–2542.
3. LOGIE, R. H. 1995. Working Memory in Human Cognition. J. Richardson, Ed. Oxford University Press. Oxford, UK.
4. BADDELEY, A. D. & G. I. HITCH. 1974. Working memory. *In* The Psychology of Learning and Motivation. G. H. Bower, Ed. Vol. **8:** 47–90. Academic Press. New York.
5. BADDELEY, A. D. 1992. Working memory. Science **255:** 556–559.
6. DELLA SALA, S., R. LOGIE & H. SPINNLER. 1993. Is primary memory deficit of Alzheimer patients due to a "central executive" impairment? J. Neurolinguistics **7:** 325–346.
7. BADDELEY, A. Exploring the central executive. Q. J. Exp. Psychol. In press.
8. DELLA SALA, S. & R. H. LOGIE. 1993. When working memory does not work: The role of working memory in neuropsychology. *In* Handbook of Neuropsychology. F. Boller & H. Spinnler, Eds. Vol. **8:** 1–62. Elsevier Science Publisher B.V. Amsterdam.
9. BADDELEY, A. D. 1986. Working Memory. Clarendon Press. Oxford, UK.

10. DELLA SALA, S., P. NICHELLI & H. SPINNLER. 1986. An Italian series of patients with organic dementia. Ital. J. Neurol. Sci. 7: 27–41.
11. SPINNLER, H. & S. DELLA SALA. 1988. The role of clinical neuropsychology in the neurological diagnosis of Alzheimer's disease. J. Neurol. 235: 258–271.
12. MCKANN, G., D. DRACHMAN, M. FOLSTEIN, R. KATZMAN, D. PRICE & E. M. STADLAN. 1984. Clinical diagnosis of Alzheimer's disease: Report of the NINCDS-ADRDA work group under the auspices of the Department of Health and Human Services task force on Alzheimer's disease. Neurology 34: 939–944.
13. AMERICAN PSYCHIATRIC ASSOCIATION. 1994. Diagnostic and Statistical Manual of Mental Disorders, DSM-III-R. 4th edit. American Psychiatric Association. Washington, DC.
14. BRAZZELLI, M., E. CAPITANI, S. DELLA SALA, H. SPINNLER & M. ZUFFI. 1994. A neuropsychological instrument adding to the description of patients with suspected cortical dementia: The Milan overall dementia assessment. J. Neurol. Neurosurg. Psychiatry 57: 1510–1517.
15. GREENE, J., A. D. BADDELEY & J. HODGES. 1995. Autobiographical memory and executive function in early dementia of Alzheimer type. Neuropsychologia. In press.
16. ROBERTSON, I. H., T. WARD & V. RIDGEWAY. 1994. The Test of Everyday Attention. Thames Valley Test Company. Flempton, UK.
17. MORRIS, R. G. 1986. Short-term forgetting in senile dementia of the Alzheimer's type. Cogn. Neuropsychol. 3: 77–97.
18. SPINNLER, H., S. DELLA SALA, R. BANDERA & A. D. BADDELEY. 1988. Dementia and the structure of human memory. Cogn. Neuropsychol. 5: 193–211.
19. MORRIS, R. G. & A. D. BADDELEY. 1988. Primary and working memory functioning in Alzheimer-type dementia. J. Clin. Exp. Neuropsychol. 10: 279–296.
20. BECKER, J. T. 1988. Working memory and secondary memory deficits in Alzheimer's disease. J. Clin. Exp. Neuropsychol. 10: 739–753.
21. BADDELEY, A. D. & B. WILSON. 1988. Frontal amnesia and the dysexecutive syndrome. Brain & Cognition 7: 212–230.
22. SHALLICE, T. 1982. Specific impairments of planning. Philos. Trans. R. Soc. Lond. B 298: 199–209.
23. SHALLICE, T. 1988. From Neuropsychology to Mental Structure. Cambridge University Press. Cambridge, UK.
24. TERRY, R. D. & R. KATZMAN. 1983. Senile dementia of the Alzheimer type. Ann. Neurol. 14: 497.
25. KHACHATURIAN, Z. S. 1985. Diagnosis of Alzheimer's disease. Arch. Neurol. 42: 1097.
26. YAMAGUCHI, H., S. HIRAI, M. MORIMATSO, M. SHOJI & Y. IHARA. 1988. A variety of cerebral amyloid deposits in the brains of Alzheimer-type dementia demonstrated by beta-protein immunostaining. Acta Neuropathol. 76: 541.
27. BRAAK, H. & E. BRAAK. 1991. Neuropathological staging of Alzheimer-related changes. Acta Neuropathol. 82: 239.
28. SPINNLER, H. 1991. The role of attentional disorders in the cognitive deficits of dementia. In Handbook of Neuropsychology. F. Boller & J. Grafman, Eds. Vol. 5: 79–122. Elsevier. Amsterdam.
29. MASLIAH, E., A. MILLER & R. D. TERRY. 1993. The synaptic organization of the neocortex in Alzheimer's disease. Med. Hypotheses 41: 334–340.
30. DE KOSKY, S. T. & S. W. SCHEFF. 1990. Synapse loss in frontal cortex biopsies in Alzheimer's disease: Correlation with cognitive severity. Ann. Neurol. 27: 457.
31. TERRY, R. D., E. MASLIAH, D. P. SALMON et al. 1991. Physical basis of cognitive alterations in Alzheimer disease: Synapse loss is the major correlate of cognitive impairment. Ann. Neurol. 30: 572.
32. NELSON, H. E. 1976. A modified card sorting test sensitive to frontal lobe defects. Cortex 12: 313–324.
33. GRANT, D. & E. A. BERG. 1948. A behavioural analysis of degree of reinforcement and ease of shifting to new responses in a Weigl-type card sorting problem. J. Exp. Psychol. 38: 404–411.

34. BENTON, A. L. & K. D. S. HAMSHER. 1978. Multilingual aphasia examination. University of Iowa. Iowa City, IA.
35. NOVELLI, G., C. PAPAGNO, E. CAPITANI, M. LAIACONA, G. VALLAR & S. F. CAPPA. 1986. Tre Test Clinici di ricerca e produzione lessicale: taratura su soggetti normali. Arch. Psicol. Neurol. Psichiatr. **47:** 477–406.
36. ALDERMAN, N. Maximizing the learning potential of brain injured patients. PhD thesis. In preparation.
37. BURGESS, P. W. & T. SHALLICE. Fractionnement du syndrome frontale. Rev. Neuropsychol. In press.
38. ESLINGER, P. J. & A. R. DAMASIO. 1985. Severe disturbance of higher cognition after bilateral frontal ablation: Patient EVR. Neurology **35:** 1731–1741.
39. BRAZZELLI, M., N. COLOMBO, S. DELLA SALA & H. SPINNLER. 1994. Spared and impaired cognitive abilities after bilateral frontal damage. Cortex **30:** 27–51.
40. MILNER, B. & M. PETRIDES. 1984. Behavioural effects of frontal lobe lesions in man. Trends Neurosci. **7:** 403–407.
41. MCCARTHY, R. A. & E. K. WARRINGTON. 1990. Cognitive Neuropsychology: A Clinical Introduction. Academic Press. London.

Temporal Processing

JOAQUIN M. FUSTER[a]

Department of Psychiatry and
Brain Research Institute
School of Medicine
University of California at Los Angeles
Los Angeles, California 90024

INTRODUCTION

The role of the prefrontal cortex in temporal processing coincides with its role in the temporal organization of behavior. It is a role of cognitive *processing in time,* not processing of time. The distinction is important: here time is treated as a Kantian category, in other words, time relative to the experiences and behavior of the organism. So I shall not deal with measurements or discriminations of time, which are demonstrably not prefrontal functions. Rather I shall deal with temporal order, timeliness (in behavioral terms) and the temporal syntax of behavior, which very much seem to fall within the physiological purview of the prefrontal cortex.

In this paper I will attempt to substantiate the following two fundamental aspects of prefrontal involvement in temporal processing: (1) The prefrontal cortex is the highest stage in the neural hierarchy of motor memory; it represents the temporally extended schemes, programs, and plans of behavioral action. (2) The prefrontal cortex, in cooperation with other cortical regions, performs a syntactic function on behavioral actions. The essential elements of this syntactic function are working memory and preparatory set.

PREFRONTAL CORTEX AND MOTOR MEMORY

The most convincing evidence of the role of prefrontal cortex in the representation of motor memory comes from human neuropsychology. Patients with large injuries of dorsolateral prefrontal cortex are unable to construe elaborate plans of prospective action. In fact, the inability to plan is probably the most characteristic and least disputed of all prefrontal dysfunctions.[1-4] The patient with prefrontal damage may execute long and even complex routines, but is incapable of formulating new plans for future behavior. Thus, habits and procedural memory appear preserved, while the formation of elaborate and novel representations of behavior is defective.

There is also relevant indirect evidence to that effect from nonhuman primates. It is well known that monkeys with dorsolateral prefrontal lesions have difficulty *learning* new behaviors with substantial temporal dimensions and order, such as

[a] Address correspondence to J. M. Fuster, M.D., Ph.D., UCLA Neuropsychiatric Institute, 760 Westwood Plaza, Los Angeles, CA 90024.

delay tasks.[5] Of course, they also have difficulty performing such tasks correctly after having learned them, but this is because of failure of the temporal syntactic property of the prefrontal cortex (see below), which normally allows the bridging of time delays in a behavioral "gestalt."

Thus, human and animal data point to dorsolateral prefrontal cortex as the highest level in a hierarchy of motor structures that extends from the spinal cord to the cortex, with intermediate levels, *inter alia,* in the cerebellum and the basal ganglia. The most primitive, instinctual, and automated—or reflex—movements would be represented in the spinal cord, brain stem, hypothalamus, and other subcortical formations, whereas the most novel, voluntary, and temporally extended structures of behavior—the schemes, programs and plans of action—would be represented in the cortex of the frontal lobe.

Within the dorsolateral cortex of the frontal lobe it is possible to distinguish three separate but interlinked stages of motor memory: prefrontal, premotor, and motor cortex—in descending hierarchical order. In addition to neuropsychological evidence such as noted above to support the prefrontal formation and storage of action plans, electrophysiological data support the role of premotor and motor regions in the formation and storage of more limited schemes of action (see refs. 5 and 6 for reviews). Thus, according to these data, the premotor region—Brodmann's area 6, including supplementary motor area (SMA)—participates in the representation of actions defined by goal and trajectory, whereas the motor cortex—area 4—represents the most concrete movements in terms of direction and muscle groups involved to accomplish them.

Linguistic structures are represented at all three levels of the frontal motor hierarchy.[6] Schemes of propositional speech are presumably represented in prefrontal cortex because that kind of speech is commonly affected by prefrontal lesions. Syntactic speech at its most elementary level is represented in Broca's area, and to some extent in premotor cortex. The pronunciation of words, which is dependent on the oropharyngeal musculature, is represented in primary motor cortex.

PREFRONTAL CORTEX AND TEMPORAL ORGANIZATION

One of the most pervasive problems in cognitive neuroscience is the anatomical separation of the substrate for representation from the substrate for processing of memory, whether it be perceptual or motor memory. Evidence is rapidly accumulating, however, that the two are the same: the very same neural structure that represents a perceptual memory or a motor act serves to process sensory data or the motor act. In either case, in perception or in motion, we know that the representational and processing substrates consist in, or at least include, vast and overlapping cortical networks. The available neuropsychological and neurophysiological data from both monkeys and humans strongly support this general principle (see ref. 6 for review), and there seems to be a total absence of convincing evidence to contradict it. From a functional point of view, the principle makes much sense, because the dynamics of perception and movement depend very closely on memory. Memory makes perception and movement, much as these two make memory.

The key to understanding the interplay of representational substrates in sequential behavior and, more specifically, the role of the prefrontal cortex in it, lies in the consideration of the perception-action cycle. This is the flow of neural and environmental information that takes place in the execution of any sequence, or gestalt, of behavior. It is the neural apparatus by which perception translates into action. By way of an anatomically well-known array of connections, structures in the sensory and motor hierarchies interact with one another in a cybernetic flow of information that includes the environment (FIG. 1). It is important to note that at all hierarchical levels the interactions are bidirectional, including feedforward as well as feedback.

At the highest stage of the perception-action cycle, the prefrontal cortex, interacting with posterior cortex—that is, coordinating perceptual networks with motor networks—exerts its temporal syntactic function. This is essentially a function of bridging temporally separate elements of a behavioral gestalt, which is a structure of behavior with a specific and well-defined goal. That gestalt can vary widely; it can be as diverse as a sentence of speech, a single trial in a conventional delay task, or an orderly plan of action.

How does the dorsolateral prefrontal cortex reconcile cross-temporal contingencies to unify the behavioral gestalt? How does it perform temporal syntax? The best evidence available indicates that the dorsolateral prefrontal cortex does so by supporting two basic functions of sensory and motor integration across time: short-term working memory and preparatory motor set. These two cognitive functions, in essence, bridge time at the top of the perception-action cycle. Later I will discuss possible mechanisms by which the prefrontal cortex supports these two cognitive functions. But first, let me summarize the evidence demonstrating that, indeed, the dorsolateral prefrontal cortex mediates cross-temporal contingencies and supports working memory and "working set."

The first and best such evidence comes from the study of the effects of dorsolateral prefrontal lesions on performances of delay tasks, tasks that require the reconciling of events separated by time. The literature on this score goes back to Jacobsen.[7] Here, I will simply refer to our studies demonstrating that, in the monkey, the cooling of dorsolateral prefrontal cortex, that is, the area of the sulcus principalis, induces a reversible deficit in performance of active short-term memory tasks that demand the temporary retention of visual,[8] tactile,[9] or auditory[10] information, whether that information is defined in spatial coordinates or not (FIG. 2).

Other evidence comes from electrophysiological studies of the frontal lobe with microelectrodes, also in the monkey. The first such studies in delay tasks using substantial delay intervals (>10 s) were conducted in our laboratory.[11] Here I shall limit myself to referring to a study[12] that points to the interplay of two classes of neurons, in dorsolateral prefrontal cortex, that seem to support the two above-mentioned functions of short-term memory and short-term set: One class of neurons is attuned to a perceptual cue, the other to the motor response the cue predicts. Both types of cells probably help mediate the cross-temporal contingency between the two (FIG. 3).

More recent evidence of the involvement of prefrontal cortex in working mem-

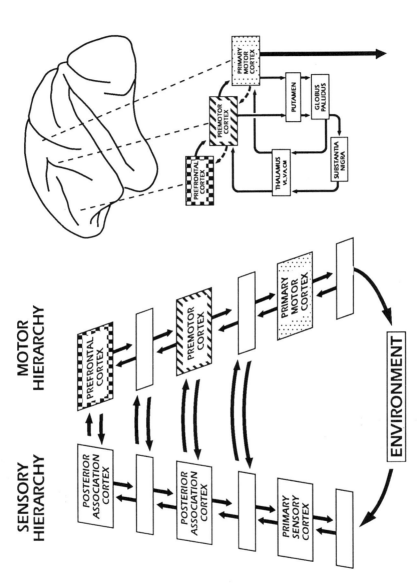

FIGURE 1. Connective anatomy of the perception-action cycle. (*Right*) The cortical motor hierarchy and its subcortical connective loops. (From Fuster.[6] Reproduced with permission of MIT Press.)

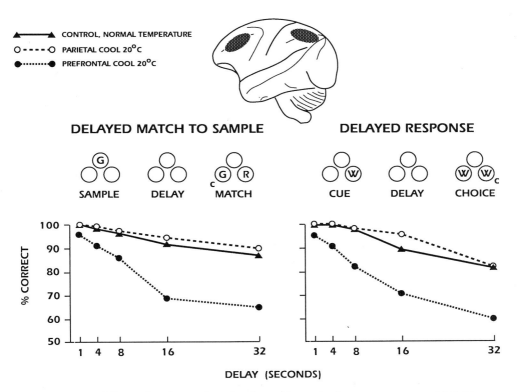

FIGURE 2. Effects of cooling prefrontal and posterior parietal cortex on a nonspatial (*left*) and a spatial (*right*) visual delay task. (From Fuster.[6] Reproduced with permission of MIT Press.)

ory and motor set comes from imaging studies in the human. In one such study by PET, with Swartz and others,[13] we were able to observe the activation of prefrontal areas 9 and 46 in a short-term memory task with abstract visual pictures. In accord with microelectrode data from the monkey during the delay of visual memory tasks, we also observed the activation of motor and premotor areas. Probably the activation of these frontal areas during that period is related to the preparation for motor response (FIG. 4).

COOPERATIVE INTERACTION BETWEEN POSTERIOR
AND FRONTAL CORTEX

The mediation of cross-temporal contingencies involves the dorsolateral prefrontal cortex in close cooperation with areas of posterior (post-central, postrolandic) cortex. In this manner, the preparation for prospective action is coordi-

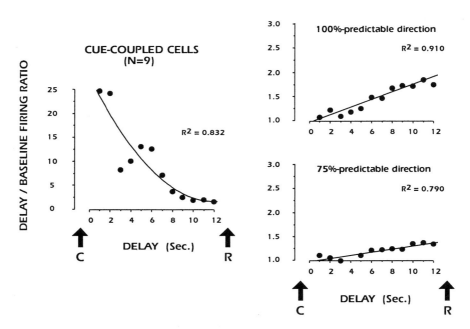

FIGURE 3. Average firing of prefrontal cells during the delay of a delayed-response task with varying degrees of contingency between a visual cue (color) and the direction of the delayed motor response. Note that motor-coupled cells show direction-selective acceleration of firing as that response grows near; the slope of acceleration is steeper as the monkey can predict with 100% certainty the direction of the response. (From Quintana and Fuster.[12] Reproduced, with permission, from *NeuroReport.*)

nated with the temporary retention—that is, the working memory—of the information on which that action is contingent. This is probably accomplished by some kind of tonic feedback from prefrontal cortex on the area or areas that represent that information. The possibility of reverberating activity between prefrontal and posterior areas cannot be excluded. Some time ago we obtained evidence of interactions between prefrontal and inferotemporal cortex in visual short-term memory.[14] Monkeys trained to perform a visual memory task (delayed matching to sample) were equipped with cooling probes over inferotemporal cortex and a microelectrode recording rig over prefrontal cortex, or vice versa. Cooling of either cortex induced a deficit in memory performance and, in addition, cellular activity changes in the other cortex. Excitations as well as inhibitions of discharge were observed during the period of presentation of the memorandum (sample), as well as during the subsequent delay (FIG. 5). Probably the most significant finding was a diminution in the ability of cells to differentiate by firing rate the behaviorally critical physical property (color) of the memorandum. Importantly, the cells af-

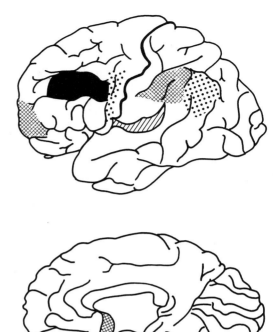

FIGURE 4. Areas in which FDG-activation during the memory task (delayed matching to sample) exceeds activation during a control no-memory task (immediate matching to sample). Shading pattern reflects result of discriminant analysis: black, F ratio >11.0; cross-hatching, F, 5.0–11.0; dotted, F, 4.0–5.0.

fected by distant cooling were predominantly situated in supragranular layers, a finding that is in agreement with the common observation that cortico-cortical connections originate and terminate in those layers. More recently, also by use of microelectrode and cooling methods, functional interactions have been demonstrated between parietal and prefrontal cortex in working memory.[15,16]

Another indicator, albeit more indirect, of the functional interaction between prefrontal and posterior cortex is the finding of slow oscillations (0.1–0.5 Hz) in the discharge of cells in both cortices during short-term memory tasks.[17] Possibly those oscillations of discharge reflect the reverberation of activity, at the service of working memory, between prefrontal and posterior regions.

CONCLUDING COMMENT: PREFRONTAL CORTEX AND THE SYNTAX OF ACTION

In conclusion, I have outlined experimental evidence indicating that the dorsolateral prefrontal cortex is essential for the mediation of cross-temporal contingen-

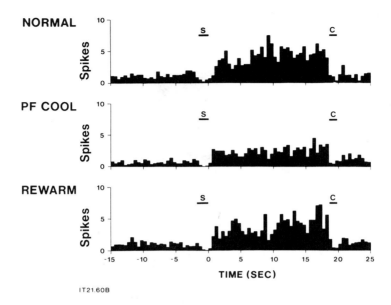

FIGURE 5. Firing of a cell in inferotemporal cortex during a delayed matching to sample task. (*Top*) Normal temperature. (*Middle*) Bilateral prefrontal (PF) cooling to 20 °C. (*Bottom*) Prefrontal cortex rewarmed to normal temperature. S, sample period; C, choice period. (From Fuster *et al.*[14] Reproduced, with permission, from *Brain Research*.)

cies.[18] Some of that evidence, especially the one that derives from microelectrode recording, implicates prefrontal cortex in working memory and preparatory set, two cognitive functions that appear critical for the mediation of cross-temporal contingencies. Furthermore, microelectrode and cooling studies of the functional relationships between cortical areas suggest that cross-temporal mediation and its supporting functions (memory and set) rely on the interaction of dorsolateral prefrontal cortex with sectors of posterior cortex.

Thus, in the light of the empirical data gathered so far in our and other laboratories, it seems increasingly evident that the prefrontal cortex is the neural structure that provides our actions with their syntax across time. We may be almost ready to answer the challenge posed by Karl Lashley when he wrote:

> The problems of the syntax of action are far removed from anything which we can study by direct physiological methods today, yet in attempting to formulate a physiology of the cerebral cortex we cannot ignore them. . . . We can, perhaps, postpone the fatal day when we must face them, by saying they are too complex for present analysis, but there is danger here of constructing a false picture of those processes that we believe to be simpler.[19]

It may be too soon to specify the mechanisms by which the prefrontal cortex accomplishes the syntax of action, but it seems that these mechanisms apply to an enormous range of actions: from sequences of skeletal movement to sequences of logical reasoning, from motor behavior to language. Only now can we begin to speculate and to experiment on those mechanisms as they involve vast areas of the neocortex that become sequentially and reciprocally activated in that syntactic process with a temporal dimension.

Basically that process would be the same and in all instances would involve the dorsolateral prefrontal cortex, whether the syntax is between the cue and the delayed response, between two mutually contingent actions in procedural learning, between premises and conclusions in logical reasoning, or between the subject and the predicates in propositional language.

REFERENCES

1. WALSH, K. W. 1978. Neuropsychology. Churchill Livingstone. Edinburgh.
2. MILNER, B. 1982. Some cognitive effects of frontal-lobe lesions in man. Phil. Trans. R. Soc. Lond. B 298: 211–226.
3. SHALLICE, T. 1982. Specific impairments of planning. Phil. Trans. R. Soc. Lond. B 298: 199–209.
4. OWEN, A. M., J. J. DOWNES, B. J. SAHAKIAN, C. E. POLKEY & T. W. ROBBINS. 1990. Planning and spatial working memory following frontal lobe lesions in man. Neuropsychologia 28: 1021–1034.
5. FUSTER, J. M. 1989. The Prefrontal Cortex. 2nd edit. Raven Press. New York.
6. FUSTER, J. M. 1995. Memory in the Cerebral Cortex: An Empirical Approach to Neural Networks in the Human and Nonhuman Primate. MIT Press. Cambridge, MA.
7. JACOBSEN, C. F. 1935. Functions of the frontal association area in primates. Arch. Neurol. Psychiatry 33: 558–569.
8. BAUER, R. H. & J. M. FUSTER. 1976. Delayed-matching and delayed-response deficit from cooling dorsolateral prefrontal cortex in monkeys. J. Comp. Physiol. Psychol. 90: 293–302.
9. SHINDY, W. W., K. A. POSLEY & J. M. FUSTER. 1994. Reversible deficit in haptic delay tasks from cooling prefrontal cortex. Cereb. Cortex 4: 443–450.
10. SIERRA-PAREDES, G. & J. M. FUSTER. 1993. Auditory-visual association task impaired by cooling prefrontal cortex. Soc. Neurosci. Abstr. 19: 801.
11. FUSTER, J. M. & G. E. ALEXANDER. 1971. Neuron activity related to short-term memory. Science 173: 652–654.
12. QUINTANA, J. & J. M. FUSTER. 1992. Mnemonic and predictive functions of cortical neurons in a memory task. NeuroReport 3: 721–724.
13. SWARTZ, B. E., E. HALGREN, F. SIMPKINS, M. GEE & M. MANDELKERN. 1995. Cortical metabolic activation in humans during a visual memory task. Cereb. Cortex. 5: 205–214.
14. FUSTER, J. M., R. H. BAUER & J. P. JERVEY. 1985. Functional interactions between inferotemporal and prefrontal cortex in a cognitive task. Brain Res. 330: 299–307.
15. QUINTANA, J., J. M. FUSTER & J. YAJEYA. 1989. Effects of cooling parietal cortex on prefrontal units in delay tasks. Brain Res. 503: 100–110.
16. CHAFFEE, M. & P. S. GOLDMAN-RAKIC. 1994. Prefrontal cooling dissociates memory- and sensory-guided oculomotor delayed response functions. Soc. Neurosci. Abstr. 20: 808.
17. BODNER, M., Y.-D. ZHOU & J. M. FUSTER. 1994. Temporal structure in the spike discharge of parietal neurons during a tactile memory task. Soc. Neurosci. Abstr. 20: 357.
18. FUSTER, J. M. 1985. The prefrontal cortex, mediator of cross-temporal contingencies. Hum. Neurobiol. 4: 169–179.
19. LASHLEY, K. S. 1951. The problem of serial order in behaviour. In Cerebral Mechanisms in Behaviour. The Hixon Symposium. L. A. Jeffress, Ed.: 112–136. John Wiley & Sons. New York.

Duration Processing after Frontal Lobe Lesions[a]

PAOLO NICHELLI,[b-d] KIMBERLY CLARK,[b]
CAROLINE HOLLNAGEL,[b] AND JORDAN GRAFMAN[b]

bCognitive Neuroscience Section
Medical Neurology Branch
National Institute of Neurological Disorders and Stroke
National Institutes of Health
Bethesda, Maryland 20892

cClinica Neurologica
Università degli Studi
Modena, Italy

INTRODUCTION

Grafman and colleagues[1-3] have proposed that in prefrontal cortex knowledge is represented in the form of Structured Event Complexes (SECs) that hierarchically link a set of events, actions, or ideas to form a knowledge unit (e.g., a schema). Similarly, Kien[4] described a hierarchic model of motor organization that allows nested levels of representation to operate simultaneously at different time scales. He also showed that simple elaborations of this model can allow its application to human memory and planning. An essential part of the information that is coded at each time-frame level is the order and duration of its content. Single movement, routines, and complex behaviors are coded within a frame as having a specific duration. The frontal cortex is involved at a superordinate level of motor control, planning and programming movement routines and complex behaviors. One could therefore argue not only that the frontal cortex is involved in timing those routines and those behaviors but also that it could serve as a neural substrate for discriminating durations in the same time range.

Single-unit recording studies done with monkeys provide some evidence of a role of prefrontal cortex in timing. Niki and Watanabe[5] reported neurons that show increased firing through the delay interval with abrupt cessation of the increase just preceding response initiation. Fuster[6] demonstrated that some cells in monkey prefrontal cortex show patterned, sustained activity during tasks with cross-temporal contingencies (i.e., in tasks where there is a dependent relationship between temporally separate events). These delay-related neural discharges might be involved in timing or, in more general terms, could serve as a basis for representing durations. According to an alternative view, the role of prefrontal cortex is not

[a] This work was supported in part by Grant No. 95-3-586 from the Italian National Research Council to P.N.

[d] Address correspondence to Paolo Nichelli, M.D., Clinica Neurologica, Università di Modena, Via Del Pozzo, 71, 41100 Modena, Italy.

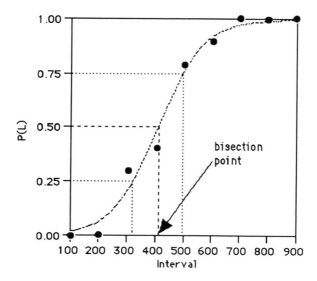

FIGURE 1. Plotting of an individual bisection performance at the short-interval discrimination task.

dependent on temporal coding per se, but rather on maintaining a complex relational mapping in working memory.[7,8]

Studies with brain-damaged patients provide only indirect support to the notion that the frontal lobe might be involved in duration processing. Patients with frontal lobe lesions typically show defective memory for temporal information, such as serial order reconstruction[9] and relative recency judgments.[10] Although these tasks assess memory for temporal relationships among items, they do not test explicitly memory for the duration of temporal intervals. However, current models of temporal coding suggest that memory for temporal order and temporal duration are strictly related.[11,12]

The present study examines the hypothesis that the temporal deficits of patients with frontal lobe lesions extend to perception of temporal duration. To tackle this issue we used a perceptual-timing task known as "time bisection". Bisection tasks require subjects to classify intermediate temporal intervals as more similar to a short- or long-reference interval. The proportion of intervals judged to be long is then plotted as a function of interval duration. An ogive curve usually is obtained (FIG. 1).

This allows the experimenter to compute: (1) *The bisection point* (i.e., the duration classified as "long" on 50% of trials). In FIGURE 1 the bisection point is the value on the abscissa corresponding to $P(L) = 0.5$. Lower bisection points indicate that the subject tended to classify short stimuli as more similar to the long rather than to the short standard, whereas larger bisection points suggest the opposite tendency. (2) *The difference limen* (i.e., half the difference of the duration classified as "long" on 75% of trials and that classified as "long" on 25% of

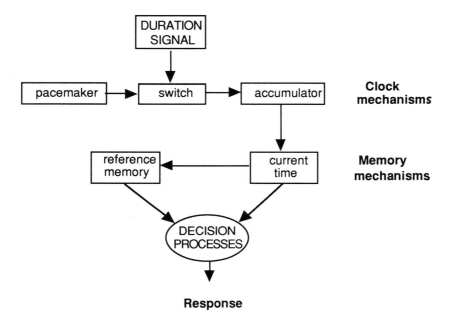

FIGURE 2. Schematic representation of the Scalar Timing Theory model for duration processing. (Modified from Allan and Gibbon.[19])

trials). In FIGURE 1 the difference limen is half of the difference between values on the abscissa corresponding to P(L) = 0.75 and to P(L) = 0.25. (3) *The Weber ratio* (i.e., the difference limen divided by the bisection point). According to the Weber law, the difference limen is expected to vary as a function of the bisection point. Thus, the ability of the system to discriminate time intervals is better measured by the value of the Weber ratio than by the difference limen. Finally, from the proportion of unexplained variance, one can measure (4) the subject's *precision* (i.e., evaluate the consistency over repeated trials in adopting the same decisional criterion[13]).

We analyzed these data in the framework of the Scalar Timing Theory.[14] According to this model (FIG. 2), a duration signal activates a switch that gates impulses emitted at a steady rate by a pacemaker. An accumulator counts the pulses and store the result in a "current time" working memory. Finally, a decision process compares current time values with those in a reference memory system.

Although only a few studies using time bisection procedure have been done in humans,[15] studies with animals after either focal brain lesions[16] or selective pharmacological manipulations,[17] based on the recorded changes of the time bisection parameters, allow sensitive prediction about the computing level that is damaged in a given subject. For instance, a decay of the memory trace in the "current time" working memory mechanism would cause intervals to be judged shorter than the corresponding ones stored in the reference memory system. As a consequence, the bisection function would shift to the right and the bisection point would increase. Forgetting from the reference system might cause an opposite leftward shift of the bisection function. However, if forgetting were to cause the short- and long-reference intervals to be less distinct from each other, a flattening of the bisection plot with a corresponding increase of both the difference limen and the Weber fraction would also be expected. An impairment of the switch that gates pulses from the pacemaker to the accumulator would also cause a flattening of the curve. Finally, changing the decisional bias during the test (as might occur for an attentional disorder) would possibly both flatten the curve and increase the proportion of variance unexplained by the logistic regression (i.e., decreased precision).

We have used a time-bisection procedure to test time discrimination in patients with frontal lobe damage. Because current hypotheses emphasize the possibility that different neural structures might susbserve time discrimination depending on the time range, we tested patients both in the range of hundreds of milliseconds and in the range of seconds. To rule out any general perceptual deficit and to control for more general inconsistencies in the decisional bias, we also included a test of classification of segments (spatial bisection), where subjects were required to classify lines of different length as more similar to a standard short- or long-reference segment.

METHODS

Subjects

We examined 11 patients with focal frontal lesions (FL, mean age = 43.2 years) and compared their performance with that of 13 normal controls (NC, mean age = 41.5). Educational level was 14.2 years in FL and 15.2 in NC subjects. Age and educational level were not significantly different in the two groups. Two patients had a lesion restricted to the left frontal lobe. In six patients the right frontal lobe was lesioned. The remaining three patients had a bilateral frontal lesion.

Bisection Tasks

We administered the following time bisection and spatial bisection tasks.

Time Bisection

Short-interval discrimination. Standard short and standard long intervals were 100 and 900 ms, respectively. Subjects were asked to classify nine different time durations (from 100 to 900 ms, at 100-ms increments) as more similar to the short or to the long standard.

Long-interval discrimination. Standard short and standard long intervals were 8 and 32 s, respectively. Subjects were asked to classify nine different durations (from 8 to 32 s, at 4-s increments). To avoid time estimates obtained by overt counting, during the intervals numbers were presented at a random rate in the center of the screen and we asked subjects to read them aloud.

Spatial Bisection

Line-length discrimination. Stimuli were horizontal lines displayed in the center of the screen. Standard short and standard long lines were 6 and 54 mm, respectively. Subjects were asked to classify nine different durations (from 6 to 54 mm, at 6-mm increments).

Bisection Procedure

Each subject was exposed to five presentations both of a standard short and of a standard long stimulus. Temporal intervals were marked at the beginning and at the end of each interval by a 10-ms 900-Hz tone. Either a small square (for the short-interval discrimination task) or numbers (for the long-interval discrimination task) appeared in the center of the computer screen during each interval. Each standard long and standard short stimulus was preceded by a visual warning stating either "This is the short interval (line)" or "This is the long interval (line)." Then, a six-trial practice session followed, where subjects were required to classify as short or long only the longest and the shortest stimuli. Finally, subjects were asked to classify either time durations or line lengths as being more similar to the short or to the long stimulus. Stimuli were presented in a random order. There were 10 blocks for each subject: on each block of trials all possible time durations (or lines) were examined once. Therefore the short-interval and the line-length discrimination tasks consisted of 90 trials, whereas the long-interval discrimination task consisted of 70. At the beginning of each block of trials the standard short and long stimuli were presented as reference values. Two computer keys were assigned respectively for the "short" and for the "long" response.

Bisection Scoring

The number of times each subject classified an interval (or a line) as long was plotted against stimulus duration (see FIG. 1). Then, the proportion of long responses [P(L)] were analyzed by iterative least-square fitting to an unbiased logistic regression for interval duration. For each subject we computed the function:

$$P(L) = \frac{e^{(\beta 0 + \beta 1)}}{1 + e^{(\beta 0 + \beta 1)}}$$

Based on each individual function, we computed the *bisection point*, the *difference limen*, the *Weber ratio*, and the subject's *precision*. "Precision" was defined as the complement to 1 of the ratio between unexplained and total variance, or more precisely:

$$1 - \frac{SSE}{SST} \times 100$$

where SSE is the sum of squares of the error, and SST is the total sum of squares.

RESULTS

The variables we measured in this study were either not normally distributed in the two groups or had unequal variance. Therefore we chose to compare the two experimental groups with a rank statistical analysis. Accordingly, unless stated differently, p values reported henceforth refer to the nonparametric Mann-Whitney U test. Average group performances are always followed by ± standard error values.

Short-Interval Discrimination Task

Data from 11 FL patients and 13 NC were available for this analysis. The average bisection point was 409 ± 26.2 ms in FL patients and 443 ± 24.7 ms in NC subjects (n.s.). The Weber ratio was larger in FL patients (0.206 ± 0.014) than in NC (0.159 ± 0.018 ms; $p = 0.03$). Precision was 97.2 ± 0.6% in FL patients and 97.7 ± 0.5% in NC (n.s.). Thus, discrimination accuracy was impaired in the range from 100 to 900 ms, but precision of the performance (i.e., consistency of classification criteria over repeated trials) was remarkably unaffected.

Long-Interval Discrimination Task

Data from 7 FL patients and 13 NC subjects were available for this analysis. The data of one FL patient was lost due to a computer hard-disk failure. Two remaining FL patients refused to be tested with this task. B.S. became very agitated and tense in the training phase, commenting he was completely lost. R.R. only completed the first block: he could not pay attention to the task and reported he was feeling disoriented and frustrated. However, the outcome of the rank statistical analysis did not change when we repeated it after having awarded these two FL patients the scores of the second worst performing subject.

The average bisection point was 14.54 ± 1.48 s in FL patients and 17.76 ± 0.71 s in NC subjects (n.s.). The Weber ratio was significantly larger in FL patients (0.280 ± 0.041) than in NC subjects (0.139 ± 0.019; $p = 0.013$). Precision also was impaired in FL patients within this time range: 89.6% ± 2.7 in FL patients and 97.5% ± 1.1 in NC subjects ($p = 0.009$).

Line-Length Discrimination Task

All subjects' performance could be fitted by a logistic regression. The bisection point was 28.4 ± 1.4 mm in FL patients and 24.2 ± 1.3 mm in NC subjects. The

Weber ratio was 0.1 ± 0.01 in FL and 0.07 ± 0.02 in NC (n.s.). Precision values were $99.6\% \pm 0.2\%$ in NC subjects and 99.1% 0.2% in FL patients. The performances of both groups were at peak. As a consequence, the NC's greatest precision, as revealed by Mann-Whitney U test ($p = 0.04$), was a possible ceiling-effect artifact. In summary, FL patients could carry out a segment classification task as accurately as normal subjects. No firm conclusion can be reached about their precision. However, they were fairly good in maintaining the same decisional criterion throughout the task.

CONCLUSION

The data we presented in this paper support the notion that patients with lesion of the frontal lobe are impaired in discriminating time durations. While bisecting short durations, FL patients showed impaired accuracy (i.e., increased Weber fraction) without a corresponding impairment in precision. In the framework of the Scalar Timing Theory, such a finding is possibly due either to a random error at the switch level or to a dysfunction in the reference memory system. We favor the hypothesis of damage at the level of the reference memory system. This hypothesis is consistent with the idea that durations are represented in the prefrontal cortex, possibly where the movements or behavioral routines of corresponding time frames are stored.

Mangels *et al.*[18] recently found a normal discrimination threshold for short intervals in a group of six patients with frontal lobe lesions. However, they used a different, possibly less sensitive, procedure to test time discrimination. Also, their group of patients included only subjects with unilateral frontal lobe lesions, whereas most of our patients had extensive frontal lesions and three of them had a bilateral involvement of the frontal lobe. At the long interval discrimination task, FL patients showed both decreased accuracy and impaired precision of performance. This association points to a deficit in sustaining attention and/or in maintaining the same decisional criterion through the whole task.

Our sample of patients was too small and lesion location was too heterogeneous to allow comparing the effect of different frontal regions on duration discrimination. Based on the hypothesis that durations are represented where frames of knowledge of a corresponding time length are represented, we would argue that lesions critical in determining an impairment of the reference memory system for time intervals are located in the dorsolateral frontal cortex. Our hypothesis also implies that temporal discrimination might be selectively affected in a different range of durations depending on the site of the lesion.

Further studies will be needed to test this hypothesis and to disentangle attentional deficits and decisional bias from intrinsic deficits of duration processing.

REFERENCES

1. GRAFMAN, J. 1989. Plans, actions, and mental sets: Managerial knowledge units in the frontal lobe. *In* Integrating Theory and Practice in Clinical Neuropsychology. E. Perecman, Ed. Erlbaum. Hillsdale, NJ.

2. GRAFMAN, J. & J. HENDLER. 1991. Planning and the brain. Behav. Brain Sci. **14:** 563–564.

3. GRAFMAN, J., A. SIRIGU, L. SPECTOR & J. HENDLER. 1993. Damage to the prefrontal cortex leads to decomposition of structured event complexes. J. Head Trauma Rehabil. **8:** 73–87.

4. KIEN, J. 1992. Remembering and planning: A neuronal network model for the selection of behavior and its development for use in human language. *In* The Evolution of Information Processing Systems. K. Haefner, Ed.: 229–255. Springer. Berlin.

5. NIKI, H. & M. WATANABE. 1979. Prefrontal and cingulate activity during timing behavior in the monkey. Brain Res. **171:** 213–224.

6. FUSTER, J. M., 1984. Behavioral electrophysiology of the frontal cortex. Trends Neurosci. **7:** 408–414.

7. ROSENKILDE, C. E., H. E. ROSVOLD & M. MISKIN. 1981. Time discrimination with positional responses after selective prefrontal lesions in monkeys. Brain Res. **210:** 129–144.

8. GOLDMAN-RAKIC, P. S. 1990. Cellular and circuit basis of working memory in prefrontal cortex of nonhuman primates. *In* Progress in Brain Research 85. The Prefrontal Cortex: Its Structure, Function and Pathology. H. B. M. Uylings, C. G. Van Eden, J. P. De Bruin, M. A. Corner & M. G. Feenstra, Eds.: 325–336. Elsevier. New York.

9. SHIMAMURA, A. P., J. S. JANOWSKY & L. R. SQUIRE. 1990. Memory for the temporal order of events in patients with frontal lobe lesions and amnesic patients. Neuropsychologia **28:** 803–813.

10. MILNER, B., P. CORSI & G. LEONARD. 1991. Frontal-lobe contribution to recency judgments. Neuropsychologia **29:** 601–618.

11. BOLTZ, M. G. 1993. The remembering of auditory event durations. J. Exp. Psychol. Learn. Mem. Cogn. **18:** 938–956.

12. MILLER, R. R. & R. C. BARNET. 1993. The role of time in elementary associations. Curr. Dir. Psychol. Sci. **2:** 106–110.

13. NICHELLI, P. 1993. The neuropsychology of temporal information processing. *In* Handbook of Neuropsychology, Vol. 8. F. Boller & J. Grafman, Eds.: 339–371. Elsevier Science Publishers. Amsterdam.

14. GIBBON, J., R. M. CHURCH & W. H. MECK. 1984. Scalar timing in memory. Ann. N.Y. Acad. Sci. **423:** 52–77.

15. WEARDEN, J. H. 1991. Human performance on an analogue of an interval bisection task. Q. J. Exp. Psychol. **43B:** 59–81.

16. MECK, W. H., R. M. CHURCH, G. L. WENK & D. S. OLTON. 1987. Nucleus basalis magnocellularis and medial septal area lesions differently impair temporal memory. J. Neurosci. **7:** 3505–3511.

17. MECK, W. H. 1983. Selective adjustment of speed of internal clock and memory processes. J. Exp. Psychol. Anim. Behav. Processes **9:** 171–201.

18. MANGELS, J. A., B. B. IVRY & L. L. HELMUTH. 1994. The perception of long and short temporal durations in patients with frontal lobe or cerebellar lesions. First Annual Cognitive Neuroscience Society Meeting. San Francisco, CA.

19. ALLAN, G. A. & J. GIBBON. 1991. Human bisection at the geometric mean. Learn. Motiv. **22:** 39–58.

A Multidisciplinary Approach to Anterior Attentional Functions[a]

D. T. STUSS,[b,c] T. SHALLICE,[b,d] M. P. ALEXANDER,[e,f]
AND T. W. PICTON[b,c]

[b] Rotman Research Institute of Baycrest Centre
3560 Bathurst Street
North York, Ontario M6A 2E1, Canada

[c] Departments of Medicine (Neurology) and Psychology
University of Toronto
Toronto, Canada

[d] University College, London WCIE 6BT, UK
SISSA, Trieste

[e] Braintree Rehabilitation Hospital
Braintree, Massachusetts 02184

[f] Boston University School of Medicine
Boston, Massachusetts

INTRODUCTION

Understanding the functions of the human prefrontal cortex is essential to any understanding of human cognition. This region, which comprises between a quarter and a third of the human cerebral cortex,[1,2] is what most readily distinguishes a primate brain from the brains of other mammals.[3] Unfortunately, understanding the cognitive processes carried out by the prefrontal cortex is hampered by several factors: the complexity of these processes; the extensive connections between the frontal lobes and other regions of the brain; the absence of clear animal homologues for many hypothesized prefrontal processes; and the relative rarity of patients with exclusively frontal lesions.

Although the neuropsychological approach has been quite successful in the study of posterior brain functions, several factors have impeded its effectiveness in evaluating frontal lobe function. First, theories of prefrontal functions have used terms or concepts that derive from everyday language and are not easily operationalized into experimental paradigms. Second, the clinical tests that show deficits in patients with frontal lobe lesions generally involve multiple components and lack performance measures specific to particular cognitive processes, making a detailed functional analysis of these processes virtually impossible. A third problem is the absence of clinical conditions with specific anatomical relations to the prefrontal cortex, like Korsakoff's psychosis to the mammillary bodies or Parkinson's disease to the basal ganglia.

[a] This work was supported by grants from the Ontario Mental Health Foundation (to D.T.S.) and the Medical Research Council of Canada (to D.T.S. and T.W.P.).

191

A fourth and more subtle problem arises from the way that theoretical inferences in neuropsychology depend upon the pattern of associations and dissociations across different tasks. The correlation between different tasks held to be sensitive to frontal lobe lesions has been low (e.g., ref. 4). One possible reason is that tests demonstrating selective frontal lobe deficits may not show the same results from one session to the next. Performance on a particular task may depend upon learning or adopting an effective strategy, and this can vary from one test session to the next. Indeed, variability of performance is probably characteristic of patients with frontal lesions.[5] A second possibility is that any two frontal tests may each be individually sensitive to frontal lesions but heavily loaded on other nonfrontal processes that differ between the tests.[6] A final possibility for why frontally sensitive tests correlate weakly with each other is that they evaluate anatomically and functionally separate systems within the frontal lobes.[7,8] Proper assessment of this possibility will require detailed anatomical information for each patient.

A NEW APPROACH

In this paper we present a new approach to the study of frontal lobe functioning. We start with the assumption that there is no single basic frontal process.[9,10] There are five steps in the approach. The first is to determine a set of putative frontal processes that are closely related and that are used in many different tasks. The second is to select a set of tasks, each of which loads differently on the different processes. The third is to describe the tasks in the context of a theory of frontal lobe function that provides predictions about underlying cognitive processes and cerebral mechanisms. The fourth is to test individual subjects more than once to estimate reliability and variability. The fifth is to use different experimental methods to provide converging evidence for interpreting distinct frontal processes. The methods we suggest are anatomical (lesion location), neuropsychological (behavioral tests), and physiological (event-related potentials or ERPs).

ERPs are used to illustrate the physiological approach. Other techniques, such as those measuring cerebral blood flow, are also important sources of convergence. Recent developments in source analysis[11] should allow us to localize ERP components generated in the frontal lobes, thereby providing a physiological basis for psychological theories of frontal function. Because extensive ERP evaluations of frontal lobe patients have not yet been made, our ERP discussion is more hypothetical than for the neuropsychological methods.

The theoretical framework by which we characterize the component processes is the Supervisory System model of Norman and Shallice.[6,12,13] The framework is represented diagrammatically in a simplified form in FIGURE 1. The theory follows the basic tenet of other theories of executive abilities—the separation between routine and nonroutine activities. The theory translates some of Luria's concepts[14] into cognitive psychology and information-processing theory. Four components for cognitive processing are postulated: (1) cognitive units or modules, (2) schemata, (3) contention scheduling, and (4) supervisory (attentional) system. The first three components are related to routine activities. Basic cogni-

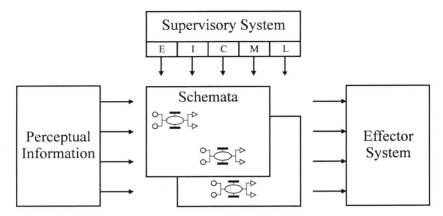

FIGURE 1. Supervisory Systems in human attention. This diagram derives from earlier representations (e.g., ref. 12). The interface between incoming information and behavior occurs through schemata. Their hierarchical arrangement is suggested by the overlapping levels. Schemata are controlled by a Supervisory System and by mechanisms intrinsic to the connectivity of the schema level. The Supervisory System consists of many component processes. This diagram indicates five of these processes that are particularly important in attention: Energization of schemata, Inhibition of schemata, adjustment of Contention scheduling, Monitoring of schema activity, and control of "if-then" Logical processes. The neuroanatomical basis of the different processes represented in the diagram is unknown. Schemata are probably mainly located in parietal and temporal association areas. The Supervisory System probably involves the prefrontal cortices. The diagram is highly simplified.

tive operations are carried out in modules or units. Such units are controlled by schemata, which are routine programs for the control of overlearned skills (FIG. 2). Even when complex, schemata are still standard and routine. Hierarchies of schemata allow component schemata to be recruited into more complex routine activities. Contention scheduling is the term used to describe the lateral inhibitory mechanisms that control competition between schemata. Schemata are activated by triggers, which can be perceptions or the output of other schemata. The fourth unit is the general executive component, labeled the Supervisory System. This system acts to handle nonroutine behaviors and functions primarily under four circumstances: when there is no known solution to the task at hand; when weakly activated schemata are evoked; when specific selection among schemata is necessary; and when inappropriate schemata must be inhibited. It functions by top-down activation or inhibition of schemata.

The Supervisory System has in the past been considered in terms of a general unitary process. Research in recent years has, however, suggested that the Supervisory System can be fractionated into component processes.[2,9,10,15] These findings show the importance of looking for associations and/or dissociations among hypothesized processes related to the frontal lobes. FIGURE 1 includes at least five independent supervisory processes: energizing schemata, inhibiting schemata, adjusting contention-scheduling, monitoring the level of activity in schemata, and control of "if-then" logical processes.

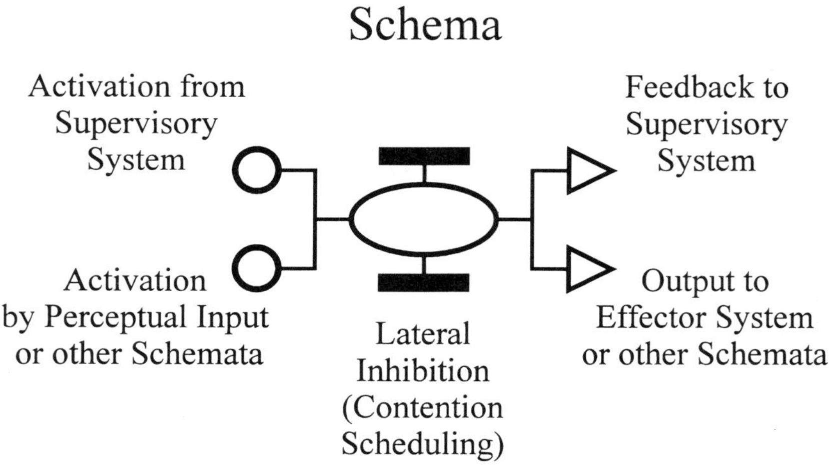

Schema

Activation from
Supervisory
System

Feedback to
Supervisory
System

Activation
by Perceptual Input
or other Schemata

Lateral
Inhibition
(Contention
Scheduling)

Output to
Effector System
or other Schemata

FIGURE 2. Schema interactions. A schema is a network of connected neurons that can be activated by sensory input, by other schemata, or by the Supervisory System. In turn, it can recruit other schemata to control cognitive processing systems so as to produce its required response(s). In addition, we propose it provides feedback to the Supervisory System about its level of activity. Different schemata compete for the control of thought and behavior by means of contention scheduling, which is probably mediated by lateral inhibition. The representation is highly simplified. A schema contains multiple internal connections, some of which provide internal feedback. One major characteristic of a schema that cannot be represented in a static diagram is the time-course of its activity. Once activated, a schema remains active for a period of time depending upon its goals and processing characteristics. In straightforward reaction-time tasks this can be assumed to be a few seconds (unless further stimuli arrive). More prolonged activity without triggering input requires repeated energization from the Supervisory System.

ATTENTION

The utility of this approach is illustrated by the example of attention. Recent views of attention have proposed that attention is a system with different components related to distinct anatomical or physiological bases. This has led to the differentiation of an anterior attentional system centered in the frontal lobe, and a posterior attentional system centered in the parietal lobe.[16–18] The posterior system appears to be responsible for the spatial allocation of attention, whereas the anterior attentional system is concerned with the executive control of attention. The nature of this executive control remains unclear.

We postulate that the control of attention is shown in the following seven types of tasks: sustaining, concentrating, sharing, suppressing, switching, preparing, and setting of attention (see TABLE 1). We define and characterize the processes involved in each task in terms of the Supervisory System model, and then consider the neuropsychological, anatomical, and electrophysiological evidence supporting the existence of these separate supervisory processes. Several of the tasks are considered diagrammatically in terms of the Supervisory System model (FIGS. 3–5).

TABLE 1. Tasks, Tests, Processes, and Converging Evidence

Attentional Task	Neuro-psychological Tests	Main Component Processes	Possible Anatomical Basis	Possible ERP Concomitants
Sustaining	Vigilance Numerosity	Monitoring Energizing Inhibiting	Right frontal	Frontal components of sensory ERP
Concentrating	Serial choice RT	Inhibiting Energizing Adjustment of contention-scheduling	Cingulate	P300-RT relations
Sharing	Dual-task performance	Energizing Monitoring	Cingulate Orbitofrontal	Allocation of processing negativity and P300 to shared tasks
Suppressing	Stroop	Logic Inhibiting	Dorsolateral	No-go P300
Switching	Wisconsin Card Sort	Inhibiting Energizing	Dorsolateral Medial frontal	Slow parietal positivities
Preparing	Warned RT	Energizing	Dorsolateral	CNV, particularly E-wave
Setting	Redundant information RT task	Energizing Monitoring	Left dorsolateral frontal	CNV, particularly O-wave

Abbreviations: ERP, event-related potentials; RT, reaction time; CNV, contingent negative variation.

We consider the role of the frontal lobes in controlling attention from two main perspectives. The first concerns the set of "processes" active during various attentional tasks. The other concerns the set of cerebral "mechanisms" necessary for carrying out these different tasks. Thus, the task of sustaining attention requires different processes to energize task-schemata, to inhibit conflicting schemata, to monitor the level of activation of schemata, and to control the application of if-then logic on the output of these schemata. A process refers to a specific functional subcomponent of carrying out the task successfully. The cerebral mechanisms are the specific material substrata that realize the processes. The distinction is analogous to that given by Marr[19] for different levels of explanation of the functioning of the nervous system.

Sustaining attention is required when relevant events occur at a relatively slow rate over prolonged periods of time (vigilance). If a response to an event utilizes only well-learned processes, it will theoretically be controlled by a schema or set of schemata. If it is not continually used, a selected schema will gradually lose activation over several seconds, thereby decreasing its power to activate its lower-level component schemata. This can occur by intrinsic decay of activation or by the selection of some irrelevant competing schema, which then inhibits the task-

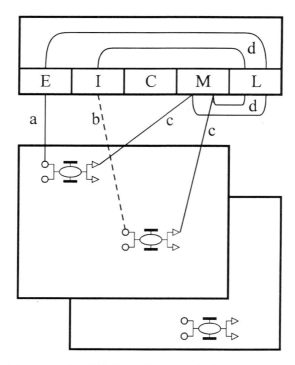

FIGURE 3. Sustaining attention. This figure diagrammatically represents what appears to be necessary for the process of sustaining attention. The Supervisory System must continuously reactivate (**a**) the target schemata required for detecting occasional stimuli or for performing occasional motor acts in order to counteract the internal tendency for these schemata to become quiescent in the absence of input. Also, the system must ensure that other schemata do not capture behavior. This diagram suggests that this is done by monitoring (**c**) the output of other schemata and inhibiting (**b**) these schemata if they become active. The monitoring system must also monitor the target schemata and continually re-energize these as they become inactive. The if-then logical analysis (**d**) connects the monitored information back to the control of the schemata.

schema. To prevent this situation, four Supervisory System processes are required. The first two are the explicit monitoring of the activation of the task-relevant schema and then re-energizing of this schema when the activation is low. The third is the inhibiting of an irrelevant schema if it has become inappropriately selected. The re-energization and inhibition processes are activated by feedback loops controlled by the if-then logical analysis (see FIG. 3).

Several lines of evidence suggest that the prefrontal cortex is involved in sustained attention (e.g., ref. 20). Posner and Petersen[18] describe a right lateral midfrontal system involved in sustained attention—their "vigilance" network—which they hold to be involved when "one needs to suspend activity while waiting for low probability events." In a task in which subjects counted the number

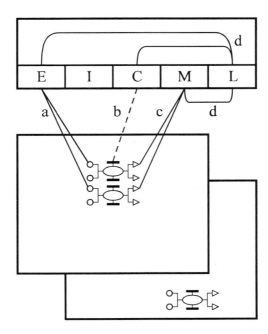

FIGURE 4. Concentrating attention. This figure represents what could be occurring in a task such as the serial choice reaction-time test. The Supervisory System must energize (**a**) several similar target schemata. In addition, the system must ensure that one of these schemata does not inappropriately capture behavior by inhibiting the others. This might in part be done by preventing more weakly active schemata from being strongly inhibited by their more active counterparts (**b**). The monitoring system (**c**) must monitor the target schemata to ensure that there are few if any incorrect responses, and use if-then logic (**d**) to cue other processes.

of stimuli occurring within a period of time ("numerosity" task), Wilkins *et al.*[21] demonstrated that patients with right frontal lesions had a significant deficit in sustaining attention (impaired performance at a slow presentation rate), despite an intact basic ability to do the task (normal performance at the fast rate). Similarly, patients with anterior brain lesions are impaired in simple continuous performance tests but not complex ones.[22] Cohen *et al.*[23] and Pardo *et al.*[24] also found greater right dorsolateral prefrontal activation in PET studies of vigilance tasks.[25] Turning to more complex tasks, Petrides[26] has reinterpreted the subject-ordered pointing task[27,28] as demanding on-line monitoring and being specifically related to dorsolateral areas 9 and 46 of the frontal lobes. In contrast to the earlier reports suggesting left frontal dominance, the recent work of his group with human PET-scan investigations suggests a right frontal dominance for monitoring of working memory.[29] However, it should be noted that subject-ordered pointing is a complex multicomponent task, and the different lateralizations may reflect different sub-processes involved. Our recent work on word-list learning also revealed a significant right dorsolateral frontal impairment on a measure of intra-list repetition

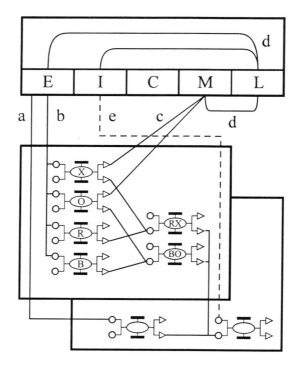

FIGURE 5. Suppressing attention. This figure represents what might be happening in a task that requires the subject to suppress attention to stimulus characteristics that are salient but not appropriate to the task requirements. The diagram is based on the task described in the text: a subject must respond as quickly as possible to a red "X" or a blue "O" as targets and to any other letter-color combinations as nontargets. The blue "X" and red "O" stimuli are associated with long reaction times and high error rates. The diagram shows "respond as quickly as possible" schemata **(a)** on the lower level and the stimulus processing schemata **(b)** on the upper level. At the beginning of the task the subject must monitor **(c)** responses and perform a controlled if-then logical analysis **(d)** on the Xs and Os (e.g., if it is an "X," is it also red?). In order to prevent incorrect target-response the Supervisory System must suppress **(e)** the responses (to X and O) until the if-then logic can be performed. As the subject becomes practiced in the task a new set of schemata for the conjunction of stimulus-features may develop, making unnecessary any intervention by the Supervisory System in the logic of the analysis. The Supervisory System must still energize the schemata and suppress the response schemata although to a lesser degree than before.

(double recalls), which was also interpreted as a deficit in on-line monitoring.[10] Although the experimental evidence is consistent, it remains unclear whether the explicit monitoring process alone is in the right dorsolateral frontal region, or whether both the monitoring and the activating/inhibiting processes are localized there, or even just the latter ones.

The stimulus-initiated activation of schemata and the monitoring of their activity may also be reflected in the later waves of the sensory evoked potentials. Thus, for the auditory system the N1-P2 waves appear to be generated by concurrent activity in both the auditory areas of the brain and the frontal lobes.[30] Moreover, frontal components are particularly prominent at slow rates of stimulation and during attention.[31-34] We predict that the frontal components of the sensory evoked potentials will be specifically related to monitoring processes in the frontal lobes.

Concentrating attention is needed when the required task is demanding and the required responses are occurring too quickly rather than too slowly. Theoretically, the activation of one schema within contention scheduling will lead to the inhibition of most others, especially those schemata that share processing resources with the activated schema. However, over-rapid use may lead to the key schemata themselves becoming increasingly refractory. Moreover, when a task has not been tackled frequently, a set of schema may have to be performed together which has not been integrated securely so that each must be separately triggered from higher levels. In such situations the Supervisory System will be needed to keep more than one schema active (see FIG. 4). In either of these cases additional energizing or activating supervisory input would be required. Another possibility is that the lateral inhibition between competing or even the newly cooperating schemata might need to be attenuated. The if-then logical analysis would be activated by the monitoring process to cue the energization and contention-scheduling processes.

From an anatomical perspective the anterior cingulate[18] has been associated with concentrating attention. Pandya *et al.*[35] have considered the anterior cingulate part of the prefrontal cortex. The primary evidence for frontal involvement in concentrating attention derives from PET studies. Tasks that lead to activation of the anterior cingulate on PET-CBF measures appear to have as a common denominator the need for concentrating attention on a demanding as opposed to a relatively undemanding task.[36-41] There are two possible cerebral mechanisms by which multiple schemata can be maintained, or refractory schemata reactivated. The first occurs via the extensive reciprocal connections of the anterior cingulate with the dorsolateral frontal cortices.[35] The second would relate to the role of the anterior cingulate in a midline thalamo-cingulate–supplementary motor area (SMA) circuit for motor activation. Projections between the cingulate and the dorsolateral cortex have also been evoked for activation of behaviors such as language.[42]

The basic test of concentrated attention is the serial reaction time (RT) task. Normal subjects should show a P300 wave closely related to the RT.[43,44] One hypothesis is that the patients with frontal lobe disorders will not show the same close connection between the P300 and RT in the serial RT task. The normal close connection indicates that the response schemata are tightly linked to the perceptual input. In patients with frontal lobe damage these links may not be as effectively maintained. Other response schemata can then take control of behavior, and task performance becomes variable. This type of ERP study does not look so much at the frontal functions that act on the schemata as on the links between schemata that are maintained by frontal processes.

Sharing attention is required when two or more unrelated tasks have to be carried out at the same time. If the two tasks are being carried out by unrelated sets of schemata, then there may be less mutual inhibition than in concentrating attention. However, activation will still be reduced so that the same type of activating/energizing process within the Supervisory System would be required. In addition, it may be necessary for explicit monitoring of task activation to occur especially if the input streams do not naturally lead to frequent triggering of each set of schemata. One effective strategy to maintain the balance of activation between the two task-schemata is to monitor the activity of one and to activate the second in proportion to the activity level of the first.

Although the performance of patients with frontal lesions in classic dual-task paradigms has to our knowledge not been published, indirect evidence suggests that the frontal lobes may play some role in this ability. Patients with frontal leukotomies and aneurysms of the anterior communicating artery (ACoA) have difficulty holding facts in memory while performing a second task such as counting backwards.[5,45] Moscovitch[46] demonstrated impairment in normal subjects in a list-learning task when they perform a concurrent task at encoding and retrieval. Moreover, a PET study has shown significantly increased anterior cingulate activation in a difficult compared with an easy dual-task condition.[47] These findings indirectly implicate the orbitofrontal and/or anterior cingulate regions in sharing attention.

Sharing attention between tasks causes ERP changes. Sensory-evoked potentials to attended stimuli show an extra superimposed processing negativity.[33] This processing negativity is smaller if attention has to be paid to more than one set of stimuli.[48] This demonstrates the allocation of attentional resources to different sensory demands. Target effects can be studied with the P300 wave.[49,50] The general finding is that the amplitude of the P300 wave in the response to a target reflects the amount of attentional resources allocated to a task. If two tasks share similar resources the competition between them shows up in the decreased amplitude of the P300. These ERP studies do not assess the frontal control processes directly, but look at their effects on schemata that are active in more posterior regions of the brain.

Suppressing attention is required when automatic processes select schemata that are inappropriate to task requirements. Tasks related to the Stroop give rise to such situations. FIGURE 5 illustrates an example derived from the work of Toth (personal communication) where a subject must respond to a red "X" or a blue "O" but not to other red or blue letters and not to either a red "O" or a blue "X." Subjects come to the task with a general schema for making fast motor responses to targets. Simply incorporating the positive values of the relevant target dimensions (e.g., "X" and "O") will allow effective use of the schemata for most stimuli, and this can be done with little training.[51] However, this will lead to false positive detection when the critical cross-dimensional stimuli occur. Until a considerable degree of training has taken place, such stimuli would require a process controlled by the Supervisory System, namely, a sequential if-then test based on a conditional association.[26] Such a process would be elicited by the occurrence of a positive value on either relevant dimension. In addition, the supervisory process inhibiting schemata would be needed to inhibit the output of the rapid-response schema while the if-then process was in operation.

Tasks such as the Stroop require suppressing attention to a salient dimension and attending to a nonsalient target dimension. Salient stimulus features are those that by dint of intensity, recent occurrence, reflex or prolonged learning elicit strong automatic responses, that is, have schemata that are rapidly and strongly triggered. Some patients with frontal-lobe pathology may be significantly impaired in the Stroop test.[52] Patients with bilateral orbitofrontal leukotomies are not impaired,[53] but patients with dorsolateral lesions have shown Stroop deficits.[54] A variety of phenomena that can arise with medial frontal lesions may be caused by a failure to inhibit or suppress responses: grasp reflex;[55] disorders of ocular fixation and control;[56,57] the alien hand syndrome;[58] the action disorganization syndrome;[59] and incidental utilization behavior.[60] The possibility of hemispheric asymmetry for suppressing attention should be examined. For example, left frontal involvement might be maximal for the commonly used language-dependent version of the Stroop test.

Although Stroop-like paradigms have been extensively studied in cognitive psychology, they have been only occasionally evaluated with ERPs. In these ERP experiments[61] no difference was found between the evoked potentials recorded when the stimuli are incompatible with the responses from when they are compatible. This suggests that the basic sensory processing of the stimuli is unchanged between the two conditions. However, it does not show what occurs in the brain to delay the responses to stimuli that are incompatible with the required response. Part of the problem may have been due to the limited number of recording channels in the early ERP studies. Other ERP studies have suggested that the inhibition of a response is associated with a very distinct frontal positive wave.[62,63] This finding is obtained in very simple paradigms wherein the subject has to respond quickly to one type of stimulus ("go") and not to respond to the other ("no-go"). It would seem that in a Stroop-like paradigm a subject would have to inhibit an incorrect automatic response in order to allow the correct response to occur. This should be associated with a similar frontal positive wave.

Switching attention is a component in well-known frontal lobe tasks such as the Wisconsin Card Sorting Test (WCST),[64] and in other tasks such as the Visual-Verbal Learning task requiring shifting from one concept to another within one set of stimuli.[65] The area of frontal lobe most likely to lead to impaired performance on the WCST is the dorsolateral frontal region of either hemisphere.[64] The WCST has many processing subcomponents. However, tasks that principally require just the detecting of a shift in the dimension which is relevant also show a frontal localization.[66] It remains to be determined if this is true for shifting attentional set when the relevant dimensions are already known. Switching attention occurs in a pure form in cognitive psychology paradigms that involve shifting between tasks requiring different stimulus-response mappings.[67] For instance, Meiran (manuscript submitted) uses a display in which a circle appears in one of the squares in a four-square grid. Two tasks are possible. In one, horizontal arrows direct the subject to decide whether the circle is within the left or the right pair of squares. In the other, vertical arrows require a top or bottom pair response.

There are three main findings. First, it takes longer to perform the tasks when the subject has to switch from one task to another within a block of trials rather than when the subject performs the same task over the whole block. This indicates that the switching takes time. Second, the earlier the occurrence of the arrows the less the difference between the switch and nonswitch trials in a switching block. This indicates that the subject can switch and prepare to perform the task prior to the stimuli being presented. The third and counterintuitive finding is that there is a definite cost for switching between tasks even when the subject knows about the upcoming task ahead of time by means of the warning cue (Meiran, submitted) or the ordering of the stimuli.[67] It is as though the processors cannot be fully reconfigured until a new stimulus arrives. Theoretically, switching attention will primarily require the specific activation of the less active schema which, through the operation of mutually inhibitory processes in contention scheduling, will lead to the deactivation of the currently selected schema. However, because of the need to return to these schemata on a later trial, contention-scheduling should be adjusted so as not to completely inhibit these unused schemata.

Switching attention has not been studied extensively in the ERP literature. Courchesne et al.[68] have studied a paradigm wherein the subject shifts attention from stimuli in the visual modality to concurrently presented stimuli in the auditory modality and vice versa. The ERPs associated with the signal to shift attention contain a large positive wave maximally recorded in the parietal regions. Stuss and Picton[69] also found a late parietal P4 wave associated with switching criteria during a concept-learning task. Thus, one has a striking contrast between ERP studies suggesting a posterior location, and neuropsychological tasks implicating frontal processes. Source analysis might be able to demonstrate both the frontal processes that initiate the switching and the posterior changes in the schemata that result from switching. In tasks that require the relevant dimensions to be determined (such as the WCST) the frontal processes may be more prominent than in tasks where simple switching occurs between known task dimensions.

Preparatory attention arises when an operation must be carried out later in time. A schema needs to be submaximally activated so that when the critical stimulus arrives a response can be optimally elicited. If the delay is more than a second, a preparatory schema may be used (e.g., counting) prior to activating the specific response schema. However, for very short intervals immediate activation of the schema prior to the occurrence of the stimulus will occur.

Few neuropsychological studies have been done in patients with frontal system lesions on preparatory attention. In some studies of patients with Parkinson's disease,[70–74] deficits in simple RT were observed when choice RT was unimpaired. This has been attributed to impairments of preparatory processes that are more critical in simple RT situations (see ref. 71). A deficit in the use of preparatory information has also been reported in patients with focal frontal lesions.[75] Moreover, Harrison et al.[76] have argued that only patients with Parkinson's disease with frontal involvement show this effect. Deficits in preparing a response, then, seem to occur maximally after dorsolateral lesions of either hemisphere, or their connecting regions.

The key measurement of preparing attention is the difference in RT between tasks with and without a preparatory signal. ERP recordings should demonstrate a frontally based contingent negative variation (CNV) in normal subjects which is reduced in patients with frontal lesions.[77] The CNV is a sustained frontal negative wave that occurs between two stimuli (S1–S2) when S2 requires a motor or perceptual response and when the subject understands that S2 bears some probabilistic relation (contingency) to S1. The CNV probably represents a combination of three processes: orientation to S1 (O-wave); preparation to respond to

S2 (E-wave); and some supervisory process maintaining attention between the stimuli.[78] The Bereitschaftspotential or "readiness potential" may contribute to the CNV when the response to S2 is motor, but a preparatory CNV still occurs when there is no motor response, as when expecting feedback.[69,79] The E-wave of the CNV should be a specific ERP sign of the preparatory processes that occur in the frontal lobes.

Setting attention relates to the consistent mobilization of the most appropriate schemata across testing sessions (see ref. 4). If a number of schemata have previously been used by a subject for a given task, then whichever schema is initially selected on a particular session will tend to remain selected with consistent use. This might not, however, be optimal. The Supervisory System can contain explicit representations of how the task has been carried out and how well it was executed in a previous session. Explicit monitoring of task operations will allow current task performance to be checked against these representations, and if a mismatch occurs then an alternative schema can be activated. Tasks that require active top-down processing cause particularly variable performance in head-injured patients.[15,80] Since these patients are likely to have frontal-lobe pathology, it is plausible that lack of stability reflects a disturbed frontal lobe attentional process. The evidence for localization of task-setting is tenuous. The published reports on verbal regulation of behavior, in which self-talk is used by a subject to maintain effective behavior, point to a possible association of this attentional process with the left dorsolateral frontal region.[14,81] It might be possible to evaluate task-setting in the early parts of the CNV when the subject decides how to prepare for the upcoming task.

ANATOMICAL RELATIONS

One reason for the weak correlation among frontal lobe tests considered earlier is that they involve separate anatomical systems within the frontal lobe. The review of the literature suggests that specific anatomical localizations for the different attentional processes can be postulated and this hypothesis directly examined. The possibility of hemispheric asymmetry for components of the Supervisory System should also be examined. For example, left frontal involvement might be maximal for the commonly used language-dependent version of the Stroop test.

Accurate documentation of lesion location is essential for testing any hypothesis of specific systems in the brain. However, investigating lesion-behavior relationships after frontal injury may be more complicated than after injury to other brain regions. First, although the frontal lobes are larger than the other lobes, few gyrus-specific localizations have been proposed. Thus, lesion size may be a critical variable in behavioral research. Second, analysis of lesions by standard gyral divisions is rarely concordant with the apparent regional organization of the frontal lobes.[82] Thus, lesion localization may only be informative if based on a priori nongyral regional distinctions within the frontal lobe. Third, lateralization of function is less robust for polar and orbital frontal regions than for posterior cortex.[42,83,84] Thus, for some behaviors simple analysis of right versus left may be less appropriate than comparing bilateral anterior versus posterior. Fourth, subcortical structures have highly specific connections with the frontal lobes. Thus, lesion studies may be incomplete without consideration of striatal lesions, particularly the dorsolateral caudate,[85] thalamic lesions, and the white matter connecting these regions.[7] Fifth, assembling patient groups that adequately represent all frontal structures cannot be accomplished if only patients with single infarctions are used. The use of nonstroke patients or patients with more than one stroke may create pathophysiological differences among subgroups of frontal cases. Almost all research with human frontal lesions has had to deal with this problem. The exception is the study of patients who have had surgery to control epilepsy, and this population has its own clinical and theoretical limitations. Despite these problems, in our prior work we were able to demonstrate specific effects of brain regions on memory and to demonstrate that etiology was not a significant factor in the results.[10]

Lesion analysis can be completed as follows. First, size can be measured planometrically (described in ref. 10) and adjusted for total brain size. This approach allows the use of CT/MRI studies performed on different machines using different scales. Second, the frontal lobe can be divided into several regions derived from the association maps of Mesulam and the connections with the striatum of Alexander et al.[85] The proposed regional divisions—cortical, subcortical white matter, and striatal—are outlined in FIGURE 6A and B. Third, past experience indicates that etiology will interact with lesion site to produce a few highly predictable groups. Dorsolateral lesion patients will mostly have had unilateral infarctions. Among the dorsolateral cortical lesions there will be a few unilateral traumatic contusions; among the deep lesions there will be a few spontaneous intracerebral hemorrhages. Patients with paramedian lesions will have more mixed etiologies, with a higher proportion of patients with bilateral lesions and a broader range of lesion sites. Patients with resected meningiomas or benign gliomas will be scattered in all groups (see TABLE 2 for a summary of the anticipated patient groups when studying frontal lobe deficiencies).

Patients can be analyzed by side of lesion (in patients with unilateral lesions), or by region of involvement (dorsolateral versus paramedial/polar) with or without regard to laterality. Regional involvement should be defined by the primary region involved. Most comparisons will be between groups with or without a particular region of involvement regardless of lesion distribution outside the region of interest. Right/left groupings should be maintained until no effects of side are demonstrated.

SUMMARY

The neuropsychological investigation of frontal lobe functioning requires a new approach. We have presented one possible framework. The focus of study should be defined categories of tasks that allow measurement of the component processes necessary for successful task completion. Our hypotheses derive from previous investigations showing dissociations of behaviors. Our approach is rooted in cognitive theory. Converging investigations from anatomy, neuropsychology, and physiology can be used to provide congruent evidence to demonstrate dissociable human prefrontal functions.

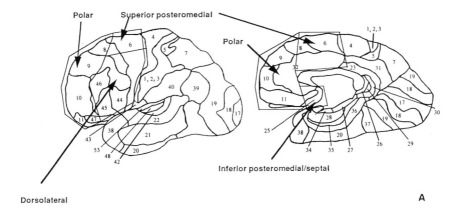

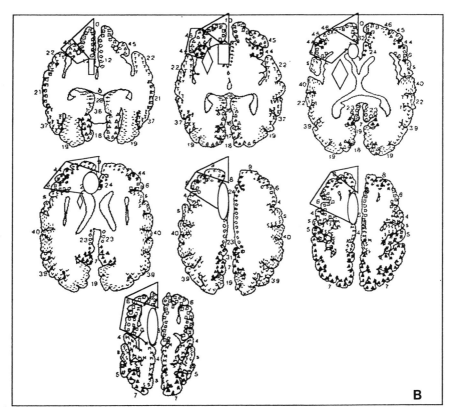

FIGURE 6. Templates for assignment of region of lesions. The cortical maps are divided by rough connectivity patterns (see text). The axial representations (**B**) from Damasio and Damasio[87] are typical CT plane templates. The relationship of cortical assignment (**A**) to subcortical white matter regions (**B**) is demonstrated. These divisions are topographically sensible but probably involve fibers of passage to frontal regions other than the one to which lesion is assigned. Note the intimate relationship of the deep extent of the dorsolateral frontal region to the head and body of the caudate nucleus.

TABLE 2. Anticipated Anatomical and Diagnostic Characteristics of Experimental Groups

Frontal Region	Laterality	Etiologies
Dorsolateral frontal cortical	Almost all unilateral	Single MCA infarctions, intracerebral hemorrhages, focal traumatic contusions
Dorsolateral caudate/ deep white matter	All unilateral	Single MCA infarctions, intracerebral hemorrhages
Posterior-inferior paramedian	Bilateral	ACoA aneurysms, cingulotomies
Superior paramedian/ cingulate	Bilateral/unilateral	ACoA aneurysms, focal contusions, meningioma resections, cingulotomies
	Unilateral	Single ACoA infarctions, intracerebral hemorrhages
Polar	Bilateral/unilateral	ACoA aneurysms, focal contusions, meningioma resections
	Unilateral	Intracerebral hemorrhages

Abbreviations: MCA, middle cerebral artery; ACoA, anterior communicating artery.

It is clear that several levels of theory are used in the approach. The overall Supervisory System model provides a framework that enables specific predictions concerning the individual attentional subprocesses to be made. Performance on each of the tasks examined requires yet more specific assumptions because, as the history of the investigation of the Stroop demonstrates (e.g., ref. 86), analyses of the component-structure of task performance are far from self-evident. Thus, any single method for testing specific predictions from the theoretical framework seems unlikely to be sufficiently powerful. If, however, each set of predictions can be reflected onto neurophysiological and anatomical dimensions as well as behavioral ones, and if each of these dimensions has its own internal constraints, the situation may become more tractable. We therefore propose that convergent evidence from neuropsychological, anatomical, and physiological techniques can provide sufficient support for a working theory of frontal lobe functions.

Our approach has certain theoretical implications. If we are correct that there is no central executive, neither can there be a dysexecutive syndrome. The frontal lobes (in anatomical terms) or the supervisory system (in cognitive terms) do not function (in physiological terms) as a simple (inexplicable) homunculus. Monitoring, energizing, inhibition, etc.—these are processes that exist at many levels of the brain, including those more posterior "automatic" processes. Because of their extensive reciprocal connections with virtually all other brain regions, the frontal lobes may be unique in the quality of the processes that have evolved, and perhaps in the level of processing which might be labeled "executive" or supervisory. The different regions of the frontal lobes provide multiple interacting processes. Because the level of processing allows the integration of information from other brain regions and because of the complexity of the frontal structures, the interacting processes can provide a sophisticated control of attention. The understanding of this, however, can be completed only at the level of processes and mechanisms, a concept that was a driving force in our approach.

We considered the functions of the frontal lobes using the example of attention. Although attentional control might be considered synonymous with the Supervisory System (or Supervisory Attentional System), we suggest that a more parsimonious approach might be to adapt our approach to other brain functions where the frontal lobe plays a major role, such as self-awareness and planning. These also might be explained in terms of multiple interacting simple processes.

ACKNOWLEDGMENTS

We thank Paula Mathews for typing the manuscript and Lisa Sayer and Dina Franchi for their help in the preparation of the manuscript.

REFERENCES

1. RADEMACHER, J., A. M. GALABURDA, D. N. KENNEDY, P. A. FILIPEK & V. S. CAVINESS, JR. 1992. Human cerebral cortex: Localization, parcellation, and morphometry with magnetic resonance imaging. J. Cognit. Neurosci. **4:** 352–374.
2. STUSS, D. T. & D. F. BENSON. 1986. The Frontal Lobes. Raven Press. New York.
3. FUSTER, J. M. 1989. The Prefrontal Cortex. Anatomy, Physiology, and Neuropsychology of the Frontal Lobe. 2nd edit. Raven Press. New York.
4. SCHACTER, D. L., A. W. KASZNIAK, J. F. KIHLSTROM & M. VALDISERRI. 1991. The relation between source memory and aging. Psychol. & Aging **6:** 559–568.
5. STUSS, D. T. 1991. Interference effects on memory functions in postleukotomy patients: An attentional perspective. *In* Frontal Lobe Function and Dysfunction. H. S. Levin, H. M. Eisenberg & A. L. Benton, Eds.: 157–172. Oxford University Press. New York.
6. BURGESS, P. & T. SHALLICE. Fractionnement du syndrome frontale. Rev. Neuropsychol. In press.
7. CUMMINGS, J. 1993. Frontal-subcortical circuits and human behavior. Arch. Neurol. **50:** 873–879.
8. REZAI, K., N. C. ANDREASEN, R. ALLIGER, G. COHEN, V. SWAYZE & D. S. O'LEARY. 1993. The neuropsychology of the prefrontal cortex. Arch. Neurol. **50:** 636–642.
9. SHALLICE, T. & P. W. BURGESS. 1991. Deficits in strategy application following frontal lobe damage in man. Brain **114:** 727–741.
10. STUSS, D. T., M. P. ALEXANDER, C. L. PALUMBO, L. BUCKLE, L. SAYER & J. POGUE. 1994. Organizational strategies of patients with unilateral or bilateral frontal lobe injury in word list learning tasks. Neuropsychology **8:** 355–373.
11. PICTON, T. W., O. G. LINS & M. SCHERG. 1995. The recording and analysis of event-related potentials. *In* Handbook of Neuropsychology. Event-Related Brain Potentials and Cognition. R. Johnson, Ed. Vol. 10: Elsevier. Amsterdam. In press.
12. NORMAN, D. A. & T. SHALLICE. 1986. Attention to action: Willed and automatic control of behaviour. *In* Consciousness and Self-Regulation: Advances in Research and Theory. R. J. Davidson, G. E. Schwartz & D. Shapiro, Eds. Vol. **4:** 1–18. Plenum. New York.
13. SHALLICE, T. 1982. Specific impairments of planning. Philos. Trans. R. Soc. Lond. B **298:** 199–209.
14. LURIA, A. R. 1973. The Working Brain: An Introduction to Neuropsychology. Basic Books. New York.
15. STUSS, D. T., J. POGUE, L. BUCKLE & J. BONDAR. 1994. Characterization of stability of performance in patients with traumatic brain injury: Variability and consistency on reaction time tests. Neuropsychology **8:** 316–324.

16. MESULAM, M-M. 1985. Patterns in behavioural neurology. In Principles of Behavioral Neurology. M-M. Mesulam, Ed.: 1–70. F. A. Davis. Philadelphia, PA.
17. POSNER, M. I. 1988. Structures and functions of selective attention. In Clinical Neuropsychology and Brain Function: Research, Measurement, and Practice. T. Boll & B. K. Bryant, Eds.: 173–202. American Psychological Association. Washington, DC.
18. POSNER, M. I. & S. E. PETERSEN. 1990. The attentional system of the human brain. Annu. Rev. Neurosci. 13: 25–42.
19. MARR, D. 1982. Vision. Freeman. San Francisco, CA.
20. SALMASO, D. & G. DENES. 1982. Role of the frontal lobes on an attention task: A signal detection analysis. Percept. Mot. Skills 54: 1147–1150.
21. WILKINS, A. J., T. SHALLICE & R. McCARTHY. 1987. Frontal lesions and sustained attention. Neuropsychologia 25: 359–365.
22. GLOSSER, G. & H. GOODGLASS. 1990. Disorders in executive control functions among aphasic and other brain damaged patients. J. Clin. Exp. Neuropsychol. 12: 485–501.
23. COHEN, R. M., W. E. SEMPLE, M. GROSS, H. H. HOLCOMB, M. S. DOWLING & T. E. NORDAHL. 1988. Functional localization of sustained attention: Comparison to sensory stimulation in the absence of instruction. Neuropsychiatry, Neuropsychol. Behav. Neurol. 1: 3–20.
24. PARDO, J. V., P. T. FOX & M. E. RAICHLE. 1991. Localization of a human system for sustained attention by positron emission tomography. Nature 349: 61–64.
25. DEUTSCH, G., A. C. PAPANICOLAOU, W. T. BOURBON & H. M. EISENBERG. 1987. Cerebral blood flow evidence of right frontal activation in attention demanding tasks. Int. J. Neurosci. 36: 23–28.
26. PETRIDES, M. 1991. Learning impairments following excisions of the primate frontal cortex. In Frontal Lobe Function and Dysfunction. H. S. Levin, H. M. Eisenberg & A. L. Benton, Eds.: 256–272. Oxford University Press. New York.
27. MILNER, B. 1982. Some cognitive effects of frontal lobe lesions in man. In The Neuropsychology of Cognitive Function. D. E. Broadbent & L. Weiskrantz, Eds.: 211–226. The Royal Society. London.
28. PETRIDES, M. & B. MILNER. 1982. Deficits on subject-ordered tasks after frontal- and temporal-lobe lesions in man. Neuropsychologia 20: 249–262.
29. PETRIDES, M., B. ALIVISATOS, A. C. EVANS & E. MEYER. 1993. Dissociation of human mid-dorsolateral from posterior dorsolateral frontal cortex in memory processing. Proc. Natl. Acad. Sci. USA 90: 873–877.
30. NÄÄTÄNEN, R. & T. W. PICTON. 1987. The N1 wave of the human electric and magnetic response to sound: A review and analysis of its component structure. Psychophysiology 24: 375–425.
31. ALCAINIM, M., M. H. GIARD, M. THÉVENET & J. PERNIER. 1994. Two separate frontal components in the N1 wave of the human auditory evoked response. Psychophysiology 31: 611–615.
32. GIARD, M. H., F. PERRIN, J. F. ECHALLIER, M. THÉVENET, C. FROMENT & J. PERNIER. 1994. Dissociation of temporal and frontal components in the human auditory N1 wave: A scalp current density and dipole model analysis. Electroencephalogr. Clin. Neurophysiol. 92: 238–252.
33. NÄÄTÄNEN, R. 1992. Attention and Brain Function. Lawrence Erlbaum. Hillsdale, NJ.
34. WOODS, D. L. & R. T. KNIGHT. 1986. Electrophysiologic evidence of increased distractibility after dorsolateral prefrontal lesions. Neurology 36: 212–216.
35. PANDYA, D. N., G. W. VAN HOESEN & M-M. MESULAM. 1981. Efferent connections of the cingulate gyrus in the rhesus monkey. Exp. Brain Res. 42: 319–330.
36. BENCH, C. J., C. D. FRITH, P. M. GRASBY, K. J. FRISTON, E. PAULESU, R. S. FRACKOWIAK & R. J. DOLAN. 1993. Investigations of the functional anatomy of attention using the Stroop test. Neuropsychologia 31: 907–922.
37. CORBETTA, M., F. M. MIEZIN, S. DOBMEYER, G. L. SHULMAN & S. E. PETERSEN. 1990. Attentional modulation of neural processing of shape, color, and velocity in humans. Science 248: 1556–1559.
38. FRITH, C. D., K. J. FRISTON, P. F. LIDDLE & R. S. J. FRACKOWIAK. 1991. Willed action

and the prefrontal cortex in man: A study with PET. Proc. R. Soc. Lond. B: Biol. Sci. **244:** 241–246.

39. GRASBY, P. M., C. D. FRITH, K. J. FRISTON, C. BENCH, R. S. J. FRACKOWIAK & R. J. DOLAN. 1993. Functional mapping of brain areas implicated in auditory-verbal memory function. Brain **116:** 1–20.

40. PARDO, J. V., P. S. PARDO, K. W. JANER & M. E. RAICHLE. 1990. The anterior cingulate cortex mediates processing selection in the Stroop attentional conflict paradigm. Proc. Natl. Acad. Sci. USA **87:** 256–259.

41. PETERSEN, S. E., P. T. FOX, M. I. POSNER, M. MINTUM & M. E. RAICHLE. 1988. Positron emission tomographic studies of the cortical anatomy of single-word processing. Nature **331:** 585–589.

42. ALEXANDER, M. P., D. F. BENSON & D. T. STUSS. 1989. Frontal lobes and language. Brain & Lang. **37:** 656–691.

43. GOODIN, D. S., M. J. AMINOFF & M. M. MANTLE. 1986. Subclasses of event-related potentials: Response-locked and stimulus-locked components. Ann. Neurol. **20:** 603–609.

44. PICTON, T. W. 1992. The P300 wave of the human event-related potential. J. Clin. Neurophysiol. **9:** 456–479.

45. PARKIN, A. J., N. R. C. LENG, N. STANHOPE & A. P. SMITH. 1988. Memory impairment following ruptured aneurysm of the anterior communicating artery. Brain & Cognition **7:** 231–243.

46. MOSCOVITCH, M. 1994. Cognitive resources and dual-task interference effects at retrieval in normal people: The role of the frontal lobes and medial temporal cortex. Neuropsychology **8:** 524–534.

47. FLETCHER, P. C., C. D. FRITH, P. M. GRASBY, T. SHALLICE, R. S. J. FRACKOWIAK & R. J. DOLAN. 1995. Brain systems for auditory-verbal memory: An in vivo study in humans. Brain **118:** 401–416.

48. HINK, R. F., S. T. VAN VOORHIS, S. A. HILLYARD & T. S. SMITH. 1977. The division of attention and the human auditory potential. Neuropsychologia **15:** 597–605.

49. DONCHIN, E., A. F. KRAMER & C. WICKENS. 1986. Applications of brain event-related potentials to problems in engineering psychology. *In* Psychophysiology, Systems, Processes, and Applications. G. H. Coles, E. Donchin & S. W. Porges, Eds. Guilford Press. New York.

50. WICKENS, C., A. KRAMER, L. VANASSE & E. DONCHIN. 1983. Performance of concurrent tasks: A psychophysiological analysis of the reciprocity of information-processing resources. Science **221:** 1080–1082.

51. SARAGA, E. & T. SHALLICE. 1973. Parallel processing of the attributes of single stimuli. Percept. & Psychophys. **13:** 261–274.

52. PERRET, E. 1974. The left frontal lobe of man and the suppression of habitual responses in verbal categorical behaviour. Neuropsychologia **12:** 323–330.

53. STUSS, D. T., D. F. BENSON, E. F. KAPLAN, W. S. WEIR & C. DELLA MALVA. 1981. Leucotomized and nonleucotomized schizophrenics: Comparison on tests of attention. Biol. Psychiatry **16:** 1085–1100.

54. RICHER, F., A. DÉCARY, M-P. LAPIERRE, I. ROULEAU, G. BOUVIER & J-M. SAINT-HILAIRE. 1993. Target detection deficits in frontal lobectomy. Brain & Cognition **21:** 203–211.

55. DE RENZI, E. & C. BARBIERI. 1992. The incidence of the grasp reflex following hemispheric lesion and its relation to frontal damage. Brain **115:** 293–313.

56. GUITTON, D., H. A. BUCHTEL & R. M. DOUGLAS. 1985. Frontal lobe lesions in man cause difficulties in suppressing reflexive glances and in generating goal-directed saccades. Exp. Brain Res. **58:** 455–472.

57. PAUS, T., M. KALINA, L. PATOCKOVA, Y. ANGEROVA, R. CERNY, P. MECIR, J. BAUER & P. KRABEC. 1991. Medial vs lateral frontal lobe lesions and differential impairment of central-gaze fixation maintenance in man. Brain **114:** 2051–2067.

58. GOLDBERG, G., N. H. MAYER & J. U. TOGLIA. 1981. Medial frontal cortex infarction and the alien hand sign. Arch. Neurol. **38:** 683–686.

59. SCHWARTZ, M. F., E. S. REED, M. MONTGOMERY, C. PALMER & N. H. MAYER. 1991.

The quantitative description of action disorganization after brain damage: A case study. Cogn. Neuropsychol. **8:** 381–414.

60. SHALLICE, T., P. W. BURGESS, F. SCHON & D. M. BAXTER. 1989. The origins of utilization behaviour. Brain **112:** 1587–1598.

61. DUNCAN-JOHNSON, C. C. & B. S. KOPELL. 1981. The Stroop effect: Brain potentials localize the source of interference. Science **214:** 938–940.

62. HILLYARD, S. A., E. COURCHESNE, H. I. KRAUSZ & T. W. PICTON. 1976. Scalp topography of the P3 wave in different auditory decision tasks. In The Responsive Brain. W. C. McCallum & J. R. Knott, Eds.: 81–87. John Wright and Sons. Bristol, UK.

63. ROBERTS, L. E., H. RAU, W. LUTZENBERGER & N. BIRBAUMER. 1994. Mapping P300 waves onto inhibition: Go/no-go discrimination. Electroencephalogr. Clin. Neurophysiol. **92:** 44–55.

64. MILNER, B. 1963. Effects of different brain lesions on card sorting. Arch. Neurol. **9:** 90–100.

65. STUSS, D. T., D. F. BENSON, E. F. KAPLAN, W. S. WEIR, M. A. NAESER, I. LIEBERMAN & D. FERRILL. 1983. The involvement of orbitofrontal cerebrum in cognitive tasks. Neuropsychologia **21:** 235–248.

66. OWEN, A. M., A. C. ROBERTS, J. R. HODGES, B. A. SUMMERS, C. E. POLKEY & T. W. ROBBINS. 1993. Contrasting mechanisms of impaired attentional set-shifting in patients with frontal lobe damage or Parkinson's disease. Brain **116:** 1159–1175.

67. ROGERS, R. & S. MONSELL. 1992. Task-set reconfiguration during a predictable task switch. Draft paper presented to the Experimental Psychology Society. Oxford, UK.

68. COURCHESNE, E., J. P. TOWNSEND, N. A. AKSHOOMOFF, R. YEUNG-COURCHESNE et al. 1993. A new finding: Impairment in shifting attention in autistic and cerebellar patients. In Atypical Cognitive Deficits in Developmental Disorders: Implications for Brain Function. S. H. Broman & J. Grafman, Eds.: 101–137. Lawrence Erlbaum. Hillsdale, NJ.

69. STUSS, D. T. & T. W. PICTON. 1978. Neurophysiological correlates of human concept formation. Behav. Biol. **23:** 135–162.

70. BLOXHAM, C. A., T. A. MINDEL & C. D. FRITH. 1984. Initiation and execution of predictable and unpredictable movements in Parkinson's disease. Brain **107:** 371–384.

71. GOODRICH, S., L. HENDERSON & C. KENNARD. 1989. On the existence of an attention-demanding process peculiar to simple reaction time: Converging evidence from Parkinson's disease. Cogn. Neuropsychol. **6:** 309–331.

72. PULLMAN, S. L., R. L. WATTS, J. L. JUNCOS & J. D. SANES. 1990. Movement amplitude choice reaction time performance in Parkinson's disease may be independent of dopaminergic status. J. Neurol. Neurosurg. Psychiatry **53:** 279–283.

73. SHERIDAN, M. R., K. A. FLOWER & J. HURRELL. 1987. Programming and execution of movement in Parkinson's disease. Brain **110:** 1247–1271.

74. DUBOIS, B., F. BOLLER, B. PILLON & Y. AGID. 1991. Cognitive deficits in Parkinson's disease. In Handbook of Neuropsychology. F. Boller & J. Grafman, Eds. Vol. **5:** 195–240. Elsevier. Amsterdam.

75. ALIVISATOS, B. & B. MILNER. 1989. Effects of frontal or temporal lobectomy on the use of advance information in a choice reaction time task. Neuropsychologia **27:** 495–503.

76. HARRISON, J. S., S. GOODRICH, C. KENNARD & L. HENDERSON. 1993. The consequence of "frontal" impairment for reaction time in Parkinson's disease. J. Neurol. Neurosurg. Psychiatry **56:** 726–727.

77. TECCE, J. J. 1977. Electrical brain activation (contingent negative variation) and related neuropsychological functions. Psychosurgery. U.S. Department of Health, Education and Welfare. DHEW Public. No. (OS) 77-0002. Washington DC 20402; II-44-II-64.

78. HILLYARD, S. A. & T. W. PICTON. 1987. Electrophysiology of cognition. In Handbook of Physiology. Sect. 1. The Nervous System Vol. 5. Higher Functions of the Nervous System. F. Plum, Ed.: 519–584. American Physiological Society. Bethesda, MD.

79. CHWILLA, D. J. & C. H. M. BRUNIA. 1991. Event-related potentials to different feedback stimuli. Psychophysiology **28:** 123–132.
80. STUSS, D. T., L. L. STETHEM, H. HUGENHOLTZ, T. W. PICTON, J. PIVIK & M. T. RICHARD. 1989. Reaction time after head injury: Fatigue, divided and focused attention and consistency of performance. J. Neurol. Neurosurg. Psychiatry **52:** 742–748.
81. STUSS, D. T., M. DELGADO & D. A. GUZMAN. 1987. Verbal regulation in the control of motor impersistence: A proposed rehabilitation procedure. J. Neurol. Rehabil. **1:** 19–24.
82. MESULAM, M-M. 1985. Attention, confusional states and neglect. *In* Principles of Behavioral Neurology. M-M. Mesulam, Ed.: 125–168. F. A. Davis. Philadelphia, PA.
83. MILNER, B. & M. PETRIDES. 1984. Behavioural effects of frontal-lobe lesions in man. Trends Neurosci. **7:** 403–407.
84. STUSS, D. T. & D. F. BENSON. 1983. Frontal lobe lesions and behavior. *In* Localization in Neuropsychology. A. Kertesz, Ed.: 429–454. Academic Press. New York.
85. ALEXANDER, G. E., M. R. DELONG & P. L. STRICK. 1986. Parallel organization of functionally segregated circuits linking basal ganglia and cortex. Annu. Rev. Neurosci. **9:** 357–381.
86. MACLEOD, C. M. 1991. Half a century of research on the Stroop effect: An integrative review. Psychol. Bull. **109:** 163–203.
87. DAMASIO, H. & A. R. DAMASIO. 1989. Lesion Analysis in Neuropsychology. Oxford University Press. New York.

Social and Emotional Self-Regulation[a]

DON M. TUCKER,[b,c] PHAN LUU,[b] AND KARL H. PRIBRAM[d,e]

bPsychology Department
University of Oregon
and
Electrical Geodesics, Inc.
Eugene, Oregon

dRadford University
Radford, Virginia

eStanford University
Stanford, California

The assumption of some form of frontal dysfunction in emotional disorder has long been important in psychiatry. In the United States during the 1940s and 1950s, this assumption led to many thousands of frontal lobotomies, leukotomies, and tractotomies for the treatment of affective and psychological dysfunctions.[1,2] Yet it was clear at the time that the scientific evidence relating these deliberate frontal lesions to psychiatric symptoms was thin at best.[3] The rationale was that psychosurgery treated the psychotic process by disrupting the "fixed" pathological ideation.[1,2] In fact, however, although orbital frontal and anterior cingulate lesions reliably decreased the symptoms of anxiety and depression, the clinical outcome studies of this era showed consistently that the psychotic disorder of schizophrenic patients was unchanged by the procedure.[4]

In Sweden, physicians evaluated the effects of lobotomy by talking with the patients' family members. The damage to personality was clear.

> The wife of patient 2 says, "Doctor, you have given me a new husband. He isn't the same man." The mother of patient 4 declares, "She is my daughter but yet a different person. She is with me in body but her soul is in some way lost. Those deep feelings, the tendernesses are gone. She is hard, somehow." The brother of patient 3, a clergyman, states that her personality is altered; her interests, her outlook on life, her behavior, are different. "I have lost my husband. I'm alone. I must take over all responsibilities now," says the wife of a schoolteacher. "I'm living with another person," says the friend of patient 7. "She is shallow in some way."[5] (p. 695)

With naturally occurring frontal lesions, such as from stroke or head injury, the psychosocial deficits are often unappreciated by clinicians until they have led to major failures in occupational and social adjustment.[6] For example, one patient appeared to have been a model citizen prior to sustaining a ventromedial frontal injury.[7] After the injury, although this patient scored well above average on standard tests of intelligence, he soon lost his job, his money, and his marriage.

[a] This work was supported by NIMH research grants MH42128 and MH42669 to the University of Oregon and small business innovation research grants MH50409 and MH51069 to Electrical Geodesics, Inc.
[c] Address correspondence to Don M. Tucker, Ph.D., Psychology Department, University of Oregon, Eugene, OR 97403.

213

An effective theory of human frontal lobe function must be able to explain the complex psychological and social skills that are impaired in such patients. The level of psychological description must go beyond the familiar concepts of cognitive neuroscience, such as spatial attention or working memory, and enter the domain of personality. On the other hand, the theoretical challenge at the neural level is to go beyond labeling the functions of the frontal lobe to formulate the key neurophysiological mechanisms. These mechanisms link the operations of frontal cortex to the multiple systems of the brain's control hierarchy, ranging from the control of arousal by brain-stem projection systems to the control of memory by reentrant corticolimbic interactions. When sufficiently understood, these mechanisms must be found to regulate not only the physiology of neural tissue, but the representation and maintenance of the self.

In this paper, we consider the social and emotional functions of the frontal lobe in terms of three anatomical dimensions. The first might be described as the "vertical" dimension because it emphasizes the integration of the lower functions—brain stem and limbic—with the highest operations—cognitive and motor planning—of the frontal neocortex. For this dimension, we provide a brief overview of theoretical approaches to vertical integration. Frontal lesions may disrupt self-regulation at the most elementary level by impairing the capacity to engage and maintain adequate levels of activation and arousal in service of long-range goals. At more complex levels, the adaptive control of frontal lobe contributions to attention and memory may be traced to the limbic networks that form the adaptive base for the operations of frontal neocortex.

The second dimension examines the functional differentiation between the dorsal and ventral anatomical pathways linking frontal cortex to the limbic structures, reflecting the dual origins of frontal cortex in the archicortical and paleocortical divisions of paralimbic cortex. We consider the differing clinical syndromes resulting from lesions to these pathways. Dorsomedial lesions may lead to apathy and a loss of initiative. Orbital (ventral) lesions may be more likely to lead to behavioral disinhibition. We interpret these syndromes in terms of a theory of differing motivational biases that shape the differential forms of motor control emerging in the dorsal and ventral pathways.

The third anatomical dimension is lateral, reflecting hemispheric specialization for emotion. We review the increasing evidence that the left and right frontal lobes contribute differently to emotional self-regulation. This evidence includes not only brain lesion studies, but brain function studies with both normal and psychiatric subjects using EEG, cerebral blood flow, and cerebral metabolism measures. The recent blood flow studies are particularly important in addressing the key theoretical issue of whether the emotional effect of a hemispheric lesion results from the disinhibition of the opposite hemisphere, or the disinhibition of the ipsilateral subcortical structures.

Although these three dimensions may seem to divide the frontal lobes along separate axes, they are not necessarily independent. The dorsal and ventral pathways may incorporate different forms of activation and arousal control, leading to different modes of vertical integration. Furthermore, lateral specialization for both cognition and emotion may involve differential elaboration of the dorsal and ventral corticolimbic pathways within each hemisphere, leading to different patterns of frontolimbic interaction on the two sides of the brain.

CONCEPTS OF VERTICAL INTEGRATION

To frame the problem of self-control in terms of the relevant neurophysiological systems is to face the theoretical problem of vertical integration. This is the problem of functionally coordinating the multiple levels of the vertebrate neural hierarchy, from brain stem through midbrain, striatal, and limbic to the extensive paralimbic and neocortical networks.[8] The frontal cortex appears able to recruit the multiple levels of the hierarchy in support of extended, goal-directed behavior. Whereas the perceptual systems of the posterior cortex are dedicated to *representational* operations, developing the internal model of the environmental context within each sensory modality, the networks of the frontal cortex are uniquely suited to achieve *regulatory* operations, linking the multiple levels of the neural hierarchy in service of effectively motivated actions.[9] In the human brain, the extensive frontal cortex also provides representational capacity—working memory—that is dedicated not just to the representation of the sensory context, but to a complex and flexible organization of the regulatory functions across the neural hierarchy. In this sense, the working memory of the frontal lobe could be described as the representation of the regulatory process. The most basic level of the regulatory process is the control of arousal.[10]

Self-Regulation through Activation and Arousal

Observations of frontal-lesioned patients have suggested that frontal cortex plays an integral role in the self-regulation of arousal in light of behavioral demands.[11] Mechanisms of this control may include both influences on brain-stem neuromodulator projection systems and frontal regulation of nonspecific thalamic projections.[12]

Psychological concepts of arousal have typically considered autonomic signs as the critical component.[13,14] The concept of the brain-stem reticular activating system was important in moving beyond the nineteenth century notion of arousal as a visceral mechanism, in order to consider neural mechanisms that regulate alertness as a function of both external and internal events.[15] However, even when framed within neurophysiological terms, a unidimensional construct of arousal has proven inadequate to account for the range of specific controls on the activity and attentional capacity of the brain. An important theoretical challenge has been to find concepts that bridge between the control of level of neural activity and the control of qualitative features of attention and memory.

Pribram and McGuinness[16] differentiated between an *arousal* system, centered on the amygdala, that responds in a phasic fashion to changes in stimulus input and an *activation* system, centered on the basal ganglia, that maintains the motor circuitry in preparation for action. In addition, an *effort* system regulated by the hippocampus was proposed to coordinate between arousal and activation.

Building upon this formulation, Tucker and Williamson[17] theorized how qualitative changes in attention could be produced by brain-stem neuromodulator systems regulating activation and arousal. Operating to apply a *redundancy bias* on working memory, the dopaminergic activation system routinizes actions and focuses attention. Operating under an opposite control system principle, a *habituation bias,* the noradrenergic arousal system allocates attention to a broad array of novel events, leading to an expansive, holistic perceptual mode.

Although these models remain controversial, they provide ways of understanding how elementary neurophysiological mechanisms could have fundamental psychological roles for the self-regulation not only of attention and cognition, but of personality. For example, a person who relies strongly on the phasic arousal system for self-control would be strongly regulated by external events. A child with this dominant mode of arousal control may be described as having an attention deficit.[18] An adult whose personality was dominated by this mode may be described as extraverted.[17]

The frontal lobe may fine-tune these qualitative controls on attention in accordance with ongoing adaptive demands. For example, lesions of the right frontal lobe may result in particularly severe cases of the neglect syndrome, in which the patient ignores objects, and even body parts, in the half of sensory space opposite to the lesion.[19] This syndrome appears to involve dysfunction of brain-stem, thalamic, and cortical alerting systems.[19] Positron emission tomography (PET) studies of attention have shown increased blood flow in right frontal cortex in a number of experiments that require orienting to targets.[20] The noradrenergic (NE) brainstem projection system courses through the frontal lobe before projecting caudally to posterior cortex, primarily of the dorsal (archicortical) pathway.[21] For human attention, Tucker and Williamson[17] proposed that the NE phasic arousal system is particularly important to the holistic attentional mode of the right hemisphere. Although many issues remain to be worked out, theoretical models that link frontal control to arousal regulation provide ways of understanding the deficits of motivation and initiative that may follow frontal lesions.[22] Further clarification of theoretical issues may help explain the normal role of frontal cortex in recruiting the appropriate state of arousal and alertness in service of effective behavior.

Corticolimbic Network Architecture

On the basis of both lesion and stimulation evidence and considering the connectivity of frontal cortex, Pribram and his associates have theorized that the frontal lobe is essential to integrating complex behavior because it represents the neocortical extension of the limbic system.[23-25] Recent research continues to confirm that areas of frontal cortex are closely connected to autonomic responses, as are areas of paralimbic cortex.[26] In addition, areas of frontal cortex appear to be important in integrating kinesthetic information with ongoing behavior, and impairment in kinesthetic processing may be a factor in the learning deficits of monkeys with frontal lesions.[27]

Any theory of the motivational basis of the function of the frontal lobe must consider the extensive frontal-limbic connectivity. For example, Nauta's formulation considered the limbic structures as providing interoceptive reference points to serve as adaptive guides for the frontal lobe's direction of behavior.[28] In a manner similar to Teuber's corollary discharge to perceptual systems,[29] an "efferent copy" of a frontal action plan could be evaluated in terms of the limbic reference points for desired outcomes.[28]

In the cognitive neuroscience model of today's research, the function of the frontal lobe is often considered in terms of working memory.[30] Corticolimbic connections are essential for memory as well as emotion. In monkeys, disruption of the cortical pathways linking perceptual systems to the hippocampus, amygdala, and associated paralimbic cortices results in severe memory impairments.[31,32] In humans, the amnesia syndromes can be traced to damage to limbic structures and paralimbic cortex.[33] Corticolimbic connections are often thought of in terms of the perceptual operations of the posterior brain, but they must also be important in guiding action on the basis of experience as well. The frontal neocortex shows a pattern of connectivity that links it to the archicortical and paleocortical paralimbic cortices, just as for the posterior brain.[34] However, the primary direction of information flow for the posterior brain appears to be from neocortical (sensory cortex) to limbic, whereas the primary flow for the anterior brain is from limbic to neocortical (primary motor).[35] An interesting theoretical question is whether the mechanisms of memory operate differently when the dominant direction of control reverses in the corticolimbic pathways.

Recognizing the dual functions of the limbic networks—memory and emotion—suggests important possibilities for theoretical insight into the adaptive base of frontal lobe function. To relate the anatomical and functional evidence to a theory of the cognition of the human frontal lobe, two theoretical questions arise. First, what does it mean that the networks that are most critical for consolidating memory (the paralimbic cortices) are also those that represent kinesthetic and visceral information? Second, how do these primitive regions of cortex shape the organization and control of actions?

For both these questions, psychological theory has provided an important perspective. Heinz Werner proposed that in the child's primitive, syncretic perception, motor attitudes, and bodily feelings form the elementary substrate for experience, the "postural-affective matrix." From this primitive experiential basis, specific thoughts and actions become articulated through a progressive developmental process.[36] Although the articulation becomes more differentiated in the adult's cognition, Werner believed that the adult's cognition still begins at a syncretic, primitive level of organization and becomes progressively articulated into each discrete act. This developmental process is said to be microgenetic, because it occurs within the milliseconds required for the formation of each thought and action.

Drawing from Werner's model, Brown[37] theorized that specific forms of apraxia (motor disorder) result from specific frontal lobe lesions because they represent the disruption of specific stages in the microgenetic process: frontal limbic lesions impair the initiation of actions; prefrontal lesions impair the direction and organization of actions once they are initiated; premotor and precentral lesions impair the final articulation of the action sequence. Each level of the reentrantly connected limbic-cortical progression thus serves to differentiate the action from the primitive motivational impetus.

In reviewing the theoretical issues in the research on frontal lobe anatomy and function, Pribam[27] proposed that Brown's microgenetic model provides a useful model for the development of motor plans across the linked limbic-neocortical networks of the frontal lobe. A microgenetic account might also explain the integration of visceral and kinesthetic representations within the organization of action programs. The frontal cortex may mediate between the interoceptive state represented within limbic networks and the external context as it is interfaced by primary sensory and motor cortices.[27,38]

Derryberry and Tucker[39] developed this line of reasoning by considering the computational architecture of the mammalian cortex. Within a connectionist or parallel-distributed model of information processing, the representational function of a network can be inferred in large part from its pattern of connectivity. The anatomical studies of Pandya and Yeterian[40] have shown that the interconnection among widespread cortical regions is sparse for neocortical networks (which therefore appear to process in a local fashion) and dense for paralimbic networks (which therefore appear to process in a more global fashion). This evidence shows that the most essential ''association'' cortex may not be that on the lateral convexity of the hemisphere, as traditionally thought. Rather, the greatest integration of sensory, motor, and evaluative information may occur in the primitive paralimbic cortex. In the cognitive domain, a central integrating role for paralimbic networks would be consistent with Brown's[37] observation that semantic language disorders involve damage to limbic cortex.

Thus the connectivity to limbic regions may help explain the cognitive as well as the motivational functions of the frontal lobe. Derryberry and Tucker[41] proposed that the representation of interoceptive information within paralimbic networks provides a reference for evaluating and motivating cognitive representations formed at this holistic level, before they are articulated as realized actions or fully conscious ideas. The limbic base for cognition may not be limited to thought and behavior that is obviously emotional. Tucker and Derryberry[42] theorized that the motivational substrate from limbic networks may be essential for guiding the higher executive functions of the frontal lobe. Thus anxiety, emerging from ventral limbic structures and becoming elaborated within orbital frontal cortex, may be an integral component of the focused attention and anticipation required for effective planning. Although pathologically high anxiety may disrupt frontal lobe function,[43] inadequate anxiety may contribute to the self-control deficits and personality disorder in the pseudopsychopathic syndrome that results from orbital frontal lesions.[44,45]

Although our purpose in this section has been to consider the vertical integration across limbic and neocortical networks in a general sense, the example of anxiety and the role of anticipation and planning pertains to a specific anatomical subdivision, the orbital frontal cortex emanating from the paleocortical limbic networks. The evolutionary parcellation of the cortex shown by the anatomical studies of Pandya and associates has given an important new perspective on the functional anatomy of the frontal lobe.[27] In the following section, we review the anatomy of the archicortical and paleocortical pathways, the interpretation of differing forms of motor control in each pathway by Goldberg,[46] and we propose that there are unique motivational biases for each pathway that are consistent with the different modes of motor control.

DORSAL AND VENTRAL CORTICOLIMBIC PATHWAYS

If the executive functions of the frontal lobe involve working memory,[27,30,47–52] these functions must be bound by the motivational constraints of limbic networks on one end of the processing stream and by the requirements of motor articulation on the other. The theoretical challenge is to characterize the progressive organization of behavior across frontal networks in a way that captures the integration of diverse motivational constraints, the recruitment of activation and arousal controls integral to the process, the extended working memory made possible by large networks, and the fine differentiation of motor programs that are suitably constrained by the extended representational process. In this section, we consider this process in reverse microgenetic order, beginning with a model of motor articulation, considering the role of working memory in planning action, and then theorizing on the emotional and motivational foundations from which the actions are organized. We argue that the theoretical challenge must be met twice, because different principles may be required to describe the dorsal and ventral limbic-cortical processing streams.

Clinical observations have long suggested that there may be differing motivational disorders resulting from damage to dorsal and ventral areas. Kleist noted in 1931 that patients with damage to the mediodorsal areas of the frontal lobes may show apathy and indifference, whereas patients with damage to orbital areas may show poor inhibition of impulses.[53] A number of recent findings have been consistent with Kleist's observations. A lack of initiative is often seen with bilateral dorsomedial frontal lesions. This condition may be confused with psychiatric depression, and has been called the "pseudodepression" syndrome.[44] An extreme form of apathy may be seen in the syndrome of akinetic mutism, in which the patient does not initiate action or speech even though capable of doing so. Although damage to basal ganglia or rostral brain stem may be required for a chronic form of this condition, it is not uncommon to see this syndrome in the period soon after cingulate and mediodorsal frontal lesions.[54] Thus, consistent with Kleist's formulation, an intact mediodorsal frontal lobe may be required for normal motivational initiative.

In contrast, lesions of the orbital frontal lobe may produce a deficit in controlling motivational impulses. Although the "disinhibition syndrome" has traditionally been related to frontal lesions generally, the classical neurological literature shows disinhibition of impulses, puerility, and euphoria to be associated with damage to the orbital surface specifically.[53] In the "pseudopsychopathic syndrome," damage to the orbital frontal region leads to the inability to maintain normal social constraints on behavior.[7,44] These deficits of inhibition form an interesting counterpoint to the overly restricted behavior of the anxious person, which may be associated with exaggerated activity of the orbital frontal lobe.[42,43]

We propose that understanding the role of the frontal lobe in human social and emotional behavior may require an appreciation of the differing modes of motivational control applied by the dorsal and ventral pathways that lead from limbic networks to the motor cortex. The anatomical differentiation of these pathways reflects the fact that the neocortex evolved from two points of origin: the dorsal, archicortical limbic cortex connected with the hippocampus and the ventral, paleocortical region associated with olfactory cortex.[55] This evolutionary perspective has provided new insights into the connectional architecture of the frontal lobe.[35]

In this section, we briefly outline the anatomical evidence for dual evolutionary origins of frontal cortex. We then propose that, just as the dorsal and ventral pathways display unique modes of motor control as they culminate in motor cortex,[46] these pathways may stem from unique modes of motivational control as each thought and action emerges from the archicortical and paleocortical substrate. Consistent with the principle of vertical integration, the unique motivational biases of the dorsal and ventral pathways may extend below the limbic networks, engaging differential modes of controlling activation and arousal by the brain-stem neuromodulator projection systems.

Dorsal and Ventral Cortical Moieties

The archicortical trend begins in the medial aspect of each hemisphere and projects to the mediodorsal surface of the frontal lobe.[34,56] The evolution of the archicortical moiety from the hippocampus gave rise to proisocortical areas (cingulate cortex, Brodmann areas 24, 25, and 32) and finally to the isocortical areas (9, 10, 46, and 8 on the dorsal surface). Within motor cortex, area 24 differentiated into premotor cortex,[6] which includes the supplementary motor area (SMA) and primary motor cortex (area 4). As it differentiated from primitive paralimbic cortex, the neocortex for both dorsal and ventral moieties accentuated the supragranular layers. Within the dorsal trend the architectonic differentiation emphasized the pyramidal cells. Within the ventral, paleocortical trend the differentiation emphasized the granular cells.

The paleocortical trend differentiated from the paleocortex on the ventral surface of the frontal lobe, into the proisocortex of the orbital and rostral insular regions, and finally into the isocortex on the ventrolateral surfaces of the prefrontal cortex, including Brodmann areas 10, 12, 46, 14, 8, and 11.[56] Paralleling the evolution of the dorsal trend, the paleocortical trend gave rise to the motor cortex on the ventral surface (area 6), which includes the face, head, and neck representations. Reflecting the shared paleocortical origin, researchers have noted the similarities between the insula and orbital cortex in terms of both architectonics and projections.[25,57]

Projectional and Responsive Modes of Motor Control

Luria and Homskaya[58] proposed that every frontal lesion may be understood as impairing the "psychological control of action" or the "synthesis of directed movements." Similarly, Pribram[27] proposed that the function of the frontal lobe may be discerned by understanding how internal experiences are translated into motor actions. An instructive theory of how motor control may be effected differentially by the archicortical and paleocortical limbic-cortical pathways was proposed by Goldberg.[46]

Goldberg suggested that the mediodorsal frontal pathway, derived from archicortex, is concerned with projecting actions based on probabilistic models of the future. Within this network, motor behavior is organized according to the organism's internal model of the world that is based on experience in similar contexts.[59] In this pathway, the control of action is achieved through a projectional or "feedforward" mode, in that the motor plan is directed by a preexisting model of the action rather than ongoing feedback about the course of the action in the environmental situation.[46] The entire action sequence is organized and launched as a holistic unit.

The ventrolateral motor system, in contrast, appears to link motor sequences to perceptual objects in a responsive manner.[46] This system must be able to identify objects and their motivational significance, and then a "feedback" guidance of motor action causes the motor plan to be articulated with specific reference to the ongoing perceptual input. The ventral motor plan seems to be more differentiated in time than that in the dorsal stream, in that each segment can be linked to perceptual data about its progress.

Observing the separation of these systems of motor control in the frontal lobe suggests that evolution has encountered the same dilemma faced by artificial intelligence researchers in designing intelligent machines (Hendler, this volume). A deliberate system, one that projects actions in future scenarios, is poorly suited to reacting to unforeseen events. A reactive system, on the other hand, is geared for feedback control, and this architecture may not support control by plans.

Could the dorsal and ventral modes of motor control be dependent on differing motivational biases? Are these biases unmasked by the personality deficits resulting from dorsal versus orbital frontal lesions? If the patient with a dorsomedial lesion is apathetic and lacks behavioral initiative, this may suggest that the projectional mode of action in the dorsal pathway has a characteristic motivational basis—a bias toward initiation of action that results in holistic motor plans being projected into the environmental context. If the patient with ventrolateral lesions is impulsive and inappropriate, this may reflect an unbalanced exaggeration of the impulsiveness of the dorsal stream. If so, the normal contribution of the ventral pathway would be to restrict and monitor motivational impulses, perhaps in a manner analogous to the feedback guidance of the action plan by perceptual data on Goldberg's model of the ventral trend.

Learning Mechanisms and Working Memory

If there are inherent relations between the motivational biases suggested by clinical observations and the modes of motor control in Goldberg's analysis, we should expect to find these biases of motivational control integral to the cognitive operations of dorsal and ventral regions of frontal cortex. In a general sense, goal-directed behavior must be organized over time, and therefore it must be guided by the working memory capacities of frontal networks. Given the essential role of corticolimbic interaction in memory consolidation,[60] we can assume that frontal connections with limbic networks will be necessary to consolidate the cognitive representations that support extended motor planning. Although there is substantial evidence that limbic networks are integral to memory and that there are unique memory capacities for dorsal and ventral pathways in the frontal lobe, it is an unanswered question how these memory capacities relate specifically to differing methods of motor control.

Several lines of evidence suggest that the archicortical and paleocortical moieties support functionally as well as anatomically differentiated memory circuits. The ventral memory system appears to be dependent upon rhinal sulcus, the mediodorsal thalamus, and the orbital cortex.[32,61] In contrast, the dorsal circuit appears to be centered on the hippocampus, anterior nucleus of the thalamus, and the cingulate lobe.[61] Lesions to both the orbitoventral and cingulate cortices result in memory deficits,[62] and similar memory impairments are observed after lesions to the mediodorsal and anterior thalamic nuclei.[63]

Although the functional differentiation of these two memory circuits remains to be clarified, a strong hypothesis is that they are differentially involved in object and spatial memory. The dorsal memory circuit centered on the hippocampus may be involved in spatial memory.[64] One speculation is that the dorsal pathway is important to contextual memory, which may be analogous to spatial relations.[42] The ventral trend, on the other hand, may be especially involved in object memory and the fine-tuning of the neocortical representation of objects, whether the objects are conceptual or perceptual.[42]

A similar framework for cognition was suggested by Kleist in 1934 in a remarkable anticipation of today's cognitive neuroscience model of dorsal and ventral memory systems.[65] The studies of perceptual memory by Ungerleider and Mishkin[31] have led to the realization that objects, the "what" of perception, are represented in the ventral processing stream, whereas spatial relations, the "where" of perception, are represented in the dorsal processing stream. Kleist proposed that "what" is represented in orbital frontal cortex, whereas the "how" of organizing actions is organized in dorsal regions of frontal cortex.[65]

Although generalizations to complex cognitive processes remain speculative, there is substantial experimental evidence with monkeys to differentiate between object and spatial memory capacities of ventral and dorsal frontal regions. In the monkey, the principal sulcus is the boundary dividing the two cortical trends.[56] It has long been known that lesions to the dorsal areas above the principal sulcus result in poor performance on spatial delay tasks, and that lesions to areas ventral to the principal sulcus result in poor performance on object alternation tasks.[27] Current work with single-cell recording in monkeys has provided support for these observations.[30,49]

Studies by Goldman-Rakic and associates have provided convincing evidence that the dorsal and ventral pathways of the posterior cortex, with their respective archicortical and paleocortical targets, are continuous with the dorsal and ventral pathways of the frontal lobe. Neurons below the principal sulcus are responsive to foveal visual stimulation and to recognition of objects in the perceptual field.

Both of these functions are linked to the posterior ventral pathway of the visual system proceeding from occipital to inferior temporal areas.[51] Neurons above the principal sulcus are responsive to peripheral visual stimulation and to spatial aspects of the perceptual task, consistent with the posterior dorsal visual pathway through parietal lobe to cingulate cortex.[51] The working memory operations of frontal cortex appear to maintain the functional continuity with the dorsal and ventral processing streams of posterior cortex.[30]

Fuster[49,66] proposes that the memory capacities of the frontal lobe provide the primate brain with an extended time frame within which more complex patterns of behavior may be organized. Many human cognitive processes can be said to be motor plans that are rehearsed, and evaluated for their adaptive significance, covertly. The most complex forms of cognition require the capacity to evaluate events after they have occurred and to anticipate action before it is required. These are skills that draw explicitly on the temporal span of experience that Fuster describes.

If the dorsal and ventral pathways represent integrated networks for higher cognitive functions, we might expect there would be general principles that could relate the specialized forms of spatial and object working memory to the projectional and reactive modes of motor control, respectively. Do peripheral vision and spatial memory provide a holistic context to support the ballistic, projectional mode of action in the dorsal pathway? Do foveal vision and object identification provide a parsing of the sensory stream in a way that supports a differentiated feedback-monitoring of sequential actions?

If there are coherent systems of working memory that are integral to dorsal and ventral motor control pathways, these may provide clues to the initiative versus inhibitory motivational biases suggested for the dorsal and ventral pathways by clinical neurology. Substantial evidence indicates that the memory operations of the limbic circuitry are closely linked with motivational mechanisms. Clues to the unique adaptive controls inherent to the archicortical and paleocortical substrates of the neocortex may be present in this evidence.

Motivational Bias of the Ventral Pathway

The ventrolateral motor system, with its limbic cortical base in the orbital frontal lobe, may derive its affective influences through extensive connections with the amygdala, insular, and temporal pole cortices.[25,57] The temporal and insula regions provide the ventrolateral system with data from the auditory, visual, and somesthetic modalities for evaluation. In addition, the interconnections of the ventral trend with the insula may be important for linking visceroautonomic associations to perceptual events and to the organization of action plans.[25,39] Based upon their review of the literature, Buchanan and Powell[67] emphasized the importance of sympathetic autonomic responses to ventral limbic cortex. By integrating sensory information with autonomic responses, the ventral limbic complex is well suited to evaluate stimuli for their motivational significance in relation to internal states. Given the evidence linking the ventral trend to the flight/fight response,[42] sympathetic regulation may be particularly important for dealing with threat.

The amygdala appears important to integrating the sensory data that lead to fear responses in rats.[68] In primates, Pribram and his associates have observed effects of amygdala lesions that may suggest ways that memory consolidation in the ventral trend is associated with a specific motivational bias. This bias may be consistent with a role of the ventral limbic networks in anxiety[42] and in the inhibition of impulses suggested by classical and by more recent[69] clinical observations.

Pribram[70] suggests that the amygdala integrates visceroautonomic information with ongoing perception in a process of memory consolidation—familiarization—that marks an episode in time. This parsing of an episode from the flow of experience may be relevant for the learning deficits of amygdalectomized monkeys. In addition, the behavioral abnormalities of these monkeys are consistent with the classical Kluver-Bucy syndrome:[71] they show inappropriate approach behavior to previously feared objects, and they appear hypersexual and hyperoral. These examples of disinhibited behavior may be consistent with the loss of the normal inhibition of hedonic impulses that would stem from the anxiety and threat-monitoring operations of the ventral trend. This tight, inhibitory control in the affective domain may represent the motivational counterpart to the reactive, feedback mode of control of the ventrolateral system in the motor domain.[46]

Motivational Bias of the Dorsal Pathway

In considering the control of learning by the hippocampus, Pribram[70] has suggested that it may support a representation of the context in which behavior occurs. The mechanism for doing this is an interesting one. Several findings suggest the hippocampus may code information about nonreinforced stimuli. This form of discrimination may be important to the extinction of ineffective attention and behavior, and it may be important in relegating nonreinforced stimuli to the background or context of the current behavior.

This framing of the context may be related to the emergence of spatial attention and memory skills of the archicortical pathway[31,72] and perhaps to the notion that the dorsal cortical regions represent contextual information in more general semantic cognition in humans.[42] There is also the suggestion that the learning and memory mechanisms of the hippocampus are associated with a particular motivational bias. Monkeys with hippocampectomy become more conservative and take fewer risks in task performance.[73] This appears to be an opposite bias to the fearless impulsivity of the amygdalectomized monkeys.[70] These differential effects of amygdala versus hippocampal lesions may provide clues to the limbic substrate of the apathy and loss of initiative with dorsal frontal lesions versus the disinhibition of impulses observed with ventral frontal lesions.[5,44,53,74]

Some researchers have argued that the motivational and emotional processes of the limbic circuitry are centered on the amygdala and that the hippocampus and associated dorsal limbic cortex are more relevant to cognition than emotion.[75] However, this view ignores the substantial evidence of the importance of the cingulate cortex to emotion in both animals and humans.[76] The cingulate cortex runs along the superior surface of the corpus callosum and is separated from it by the callosal sulcus. Recent studies suggest the cingulate is a highly heterogeneous structure. In addition to being divided in the rostral/caudal dimension, it is also differentiated in the dorsal/ventral dimension.[77] The anterior cingulate (areas 24, 25, and 32) can be differentiated from the posterior cingulate based upon cytoarchitecture and patterns of projections, as well as function.[78] Most notably, the anterior cingulate receives afferents from the amygdala, whereas the posterior cingulate does not.[79] The posterior cingulate does not have direct projections to the premotor areas of the frontal lobe, whereas the anterior cingulate does.[80] Consistent with a general rostral/caudal motor/sensory distinction, the anterior cingulate is characterized as "executive" in function, whereas the posterior is characterized as "evaluative."[78]

One way of interpreting the apathy and loss of initiative resulting from dorsomedial frontal lesions would be to attribute these effects to impairment of the dorsal limbic contribution to integrating hedonic value with potential action plans. Patients with cingulate lesions are found to lose interest in formerly important activities, such as hobbies.[81] This evidence is consistent with the view that the cingulate cortex contributes to attention by monitoring the motivational significance of stimuli.[82]

MacLean has emphasized that the dorsal limbic structures have become enlarged in mammalian evolution in parallel with the appearance of complex social and emotional behavior, including care for the young, emotional vocalization, and play.[76,83] Research examining this hypothesis for emotional vocalization has supported the importance of cingulate cortex. Ploog and associates[54,84] have used a combination of lesion and stimulation studies to show the control hierarchy for emotional vocalization in the monkey, with fragmentary motor features represented in brain-stem motor nuclei, patterned species-specific calls represented in the midbrain, emotional coloration of calls deriving from limbic influences, and voluntary call initiation being controlled by cingulate cortex.[54,84] In contrast, lateral motor cortex appears to control "voluntary call formation" through articulated actions mediated by direct pyramidal pathways from motor cortex to brain-stem motor nuclei.

The motivated initiation of holistic patterns of vocalization by the cingulate region bears interesting similarities to both the motivational initiative[44] and the projectional mode of motor control[46] ascribed to dorsomedial frontal cortex. In humans, there are suggestions that the cingulate region may be important in attaching motivational significance, and self-relevance, to the organization of actions in the dorsal limbic-frontal pathway. The decrease in agitation following cingulate lesions for chronic anxiety or for intractable pain[4] may be interpreted as a loss of caring about the condition. The fact that patients lose interest in formerly valued activities[81] suggests that the cingulate contribution to motivational significance is not limited to aversive initiation of action, but that it may involve hedonic value as well. The incorporation of motivational significance, visceral tone, and kinesthetic sensation within the organization of an action may be integral to perceiving the action as part of the self. Goldberg[46] describes the "alien hand" syndrome resulting from dorsomedial frontal lesions, in which an action of the hand contralateral to the lesion, apparently arising within the ventrolateral motor system, is perceived as belonging to someone else.

Redundancy and Habituation Biases as Adaptive Attentional Modes

In theorizing about the motivational basis of the orbital frontal lobe's contribution to the executive functions, Tucker and Derryberry[42] proposed that anxiety may be the affective characteristic of the preparation for fight/flight within the extended amygdala and ventral limbic-frontal pathway. This interpretation would be consistent with the decreases in anxiety with psychosurgery of the orbital region[4] and with the increases in blood flow in ventral frontal cortex seen in clinical anxiety states.[43] This view would not be consistent with Jeffrey Gray's view that anxiety is regulated by the hippocampus. Gray, however, emphasized behavioral inhibition as the key feature of anxiety, whereas Tucker and Derryberry emphasized vigilance and attentional focusing. Although anxiety is often considered to be a pathological state, it may have an integral role in optimal brain function, focusing attention on adaptively important objects.

Tucker and Derryberry[42] argued that the redundancy bias of the dopaminergic tonic activation system[17] may mediate the attentional focusing associated with anxiety. This elementary mode of controlling working memory may have both primitive and sophisticated influences on behavior. In the primitive form, a redundancy bias would facilitate routinized actions, such as in habit formation or in the stereotyped motor sequences of fight/flight responses. In the more sophisticated form, the redundancy bias may focus the representation of plans in working memory on motivationally significant issues, allowing an extended representation that supports the continuity of goal-directed behavior over time. Tucker and Derryberry suggest that the focused attention of the dopaminergic redundancy bias may be especially important to the analytic cognition of the left hemisphere.[42]

In both primitive and sophisticated forms, the redundancy bias may be integral to the feedback modulation of discrete motor sequences in the ventrolateral motor system. The pathological symptoms of exaggerated redundancy in working memory, such as the ruminations and compulsions of the chronically anxious person, may represent the distortion of a neurocybernetic mode that is essential to the normal maintenance of motivated attention.[42]

We speculate that the dorsal motor system may also be regulated by a qualitatively-specific activity control system, the habituation bias of the noradrenergic phasic arousal system. The noradrenergic projections from the brain stem densely innervate cingulate cortex, ascend to the frontal pole, then proceed caudally to innervate the dorsal regions of the neocortex preferentially.[21] Tucker and Williamson[17] theorized that, by decrementing attention to constant features of the environment, a habituation bias would create the positive control of a selection for novelty. They proposed that this novelty selection is integral to the orienting response and that in humans the resulting expansive allocation of working memory is important to the holistic spatial cognitive skills of the right hemisphere. Whereas right hemisphere specialization is an integral aspect of spatial attention in humans, this must be an elaboration of the more fundamental organization of spatial attention and memory within the primate dorsal corticolimbic pathway.[85]

At the limbic root of the archicortical pathway, the hippocampus may regulate learning and memory through mechanisms that are consistent with a habituation bias. The extinction of activity in relation to nonreinforced stimuli theorized by Pribram[70] may be the key limbic mechanism of the habituation bias. The representation of the context for behavioral activity created by this mechanism may be consistent with the holistic attentional mode attributed to the noradrenergic phasic arousal system by Tucker and Williamson.[17] A critical link in this theorizing, unknown to us at this time, would be between the hippocampus and its associated cortices and the brain-stem noradrenergic and serotonergic projection systems theorized to mediate the habituation bias.

Connections between the parietal lobe (dorsal pathway of the posterior brain) and the brain-stem noradrenergic and serotonergic nuclei have been proposed by Mesulam to be integral to the neglect syndrome.[82] In this disorder, the patient fails to orient to stimuli contralateral to the lesion.[19] Heilman and associates have pointed out that frontal lesions may also produce neglect, and they proposed that the frontal cortex regulates brain-stem reticular and thalamic arousal mechanisms.[86] In rats, right but not left frontal lesions deplete norepinephrine in the locus coeruleus and cortex bilaterally.[87] In humans, the fact that the neglect syndrome is more severe with right-hemisphere lesions suggests that the right hemisphere is particularly important to the higher-order elaboration of the orienting response in attention and working memory.

The neural mechanisms of phasic arousal and the habituation bias appear to have inherent affective qualities, reflecting the depression of mood at low levels of function and mania at high levels.[17] A critical role of the phasic arousal system in the dorsomedial frontal lobe may be relevant to the pseudodepression seen with dorsomedial frontal lesions.[44,88] In some patients, treatment of depression with tricyclics reverses both spatial memory deficits and left neglect.[89,90] In normal subjects, a depressed mood produces a mild attentional neglect that is lateralized to the left visual field.[91] The psychomotor retardation of severe psychiatric depression may be seen as a form of motor initiative deficit that is not unlike the akinetic mutism seen with dorsomedial frontal lesions.

If this line of reasoning is correct, a specific motivational bias may be integral to the cognition and motor organization in the dorsomedial frontal lobe. Closely linked to the individual's mood state, the projectional motor system would be highly charged by motivational directives in manic or euphoric mood states, leading to an impulsive mode of behavior. Although the pathological extreme is instructive, the motivational control of the habituation bias may be integral to the optimal function of the dorsal frontal lobe as well, leading to a bias toward initiating hedonically charged thoughts and actions in the mild elation associated with successful coping, and a specific attenuation of cognitive and behavioral hedonic initiative under conditions of failure.

HEMISPHERIC SPECIALIZATION FOR EMOTION

In addition to the inherent asymmetries of arousal, attention, and memory systems, it has become apparent over the last two decades that important aspects of emotional experience and behavior are asymmetrically distributed in the human brain.[92] The majority of the evidence pertains to emotional communication, the understanding and expression of emotion that is accomplished largely through nonverbal means. In right-handers, the right hemisphere plays the major role for both the comprehension and the expression of emotion. Understanding facial expressions of emotion, for example, is particularly impaired by right-hemisphere damage.[92] Normal subjects show greater expressivity of emotion on the left side of the face,[93] and they show greater attention to the speaker's emotional tone of voice when passages are presented to the left ear.[94]

This evidence of the importance of the right hemisphere to emotion may be consistent with certain clinical observations suggesting that right frontal lobe lesions are particularly likely to produce the personality disinhibition of the frontal lobe syndrome.[10] However, other evidence has suggested that the left hemisphere also plays an important role in emotional experience and behavior, and a number of recent findings point to the importance of left–frontal lobe function in particular. For both right and left frontal lobes, a key question is how the frontal cortex relates to the emotional processes mediated by subcortical circuits.

Lateralization of Positive and Negative Emotions

Altered emotional and personality processes with right-hemisphere lesions had been recognized since Babinski's observation that anosognosia, denial of illness, was most common with left hemiplegia. However, the "depressive-catastrophic response" to stroke or other brain damage was recognized by Goldstein[95] to occur more frequently with left-hemisphere lesions. The obvious interpretation of this association was that the loss of language is more devastating than loss of nonverbal intelligence. However, a number of studies have failed to correlate the degree of depressive response with the degree of language or cognitive impairment,[96] suggesting that a more fundamental relation may exist between hemispheric specialization and the balance between positive and negative emotional orientations.

An important milestone in this literature was Gainotti's confirmation that catastrophic responses are more likely with left-hemisphere lesions, whereas indifference denial of problems may be more likely with right-hemisphere lesions.[97] Assuming that these findings provide an insight into human emotional balance, the interpretive question became whether damage to a hemisphere results in a release of the contralateral hemisphere's normal emotional orientation,[98] or a release of the damaged hemisphere's subcortical circuits.[99]

In support of the contralateral release interpretation, Sackeim et al.[98] reviewed several forms of evidence from the neurological literature. A strong association between the laterality of the lesion and emotional valence was found for cases of pathological laughing (more common with right-hemisphere lesions) and crying (more common with left-hemisphere lesions). The classical interpretation of such cases of "pseudobulbar palsy" is a release of brain-stem emotional mechanisms.[100–102] Rinn points out that whereas corticobulbar projections to brain-stem motor nuclei are contralateral, the pathways disrupted in pseudobulbar palsy involve the reticular formation and, therefore, are bilateral.

In their review, Sackeim et al.[98] also observed that outbursts of laughter were frequently associated with left-hemisphere seizures. Reasoning that seizures represent an exaggeration of hemispheric function, Sackeim et al. concluded that this evidence implicates a positive emotional bias for the left hemisphere. This conclusion would fit with a contralateral release view of the effects of lesions, assuming that the left hemisphere normally tends toward positive emotion and the right hemisphere toward negative emotion. Particularly important to this issue was the evidence on chronic changes in emotional outlook in temporal lobe epilepsy.[103] In this research, patients with left-hemisphere pathology showed a negative, critical orientation in self-report measures, whereas those with right-hemisphere pathology showed an inappropriately positive approach to self-evaluation. A form of ipsilateral release was suggested by the cognitive styles of these patient groups. The patients with a left focus were highly intellectualized as well as self-critical, suggesting exaggerated if degraded left-hemisphere cognitive function. The patients with a right focus were emotionally expressive as well as inappropriately positive, suggesting exaggerated right-hemisphere function.

Asymmetric Frontal Lobe Contributions

Although temporal lobe mechanisms are obviously critical to this controversy, the frontal lobe has been found to have an integral role as well. Some of the initial evidence came from EEG studies with normal emotion, which have found asymmetries in frontal lobe alpha activity in a number of paradigms. The initial report[104] observed greater EEG activation (alpha suppression) over the right frontal lobe in response to negative emotional material, in contrast to EEG activation over the left frontal lobe in response to positive emotional material. Independently, Tucker *et al.* found a consistent pattern of results: normal subjects in an induced depressed mood showed alpha suppression (EEG activation) over the right frontal lobe.[105]

Although the findings of frontal lobe EEG asymmetry were consistent in these initial studies, the functional interpretations were not. In line with Sackeim *et al.*'s reasoning, Davidson and associates proposed that the left hemisphere contributes to positive emotion and to approach behavior generally,[106] whereas the right hemisphere is responsible for negative emotion and behavioral withdrawal. In contrast, Tucker *et al.*[105] interpreted their frontal EEG results in line with the ipsilateral release interpretation of the neurological evidence, proposing that the frontal activity may be inhibitory in nature. In their mood induction study, Tucker *et al.* had observed that the depressed mood was associated not only with right frontal EEG activation, but impaired visuospatial performance suggestive of decreased right-hemisphere cognitive functioning.

The evidence of poor visuospatial perception in depression is now quite substantial, and a number of findings implicate impaired right-hemisphere function specifically.[91] In addition to replicating and extending their findings of frontal-lobe alpha asymmetries in a number of experiments, Davidson and associates have also observed poor right-hemisphere cognitive function in depression.[107] The interpretation that the role of the frontal lobe could be inhibitory is consistent with the many findings of disinhibition with frontal lesions. Knight and associates,[108] for example, observed increased auditory ERP responses over the ipsilateral hemisphere in frontal-lesioned patients, suggesting the normal attentional control of frontal cortex may be inhibitory.

An important recent addition to this line of evidence has been the finding that, in normal subjects, left-frontal alpha suppression is related less to the subject's current emotional state than it is to the tendency to deny negative characteristics.[109] In this research it was repressors, subjects who present themselves in a favorable light, who showed the greatest left-frontal alpha suppression in the normal sample of university students. This finding, coupled with an inverse relation between left-frontal blood flow and bilateral amygdala activity in depressed patients, has led Davidson[110] to propose that an important role of left-frontal activity may be the inhibition of negative affect.

Frontal lobe function has been found to be critical to the interpretation of hemispheric contributions to emotion in lesioned patients as well as in normal subjects. In studies of acute depression in stroke patients, Robinson and associates confirmed the previous reports of greater depression with left-hemisphere lesions, and they found a striking trend for greater depression with lesions of more anterior regions of the left hemisphere.[96] Tucker and Frederick[111] interpreted these observations in line with an inhibitory role for the left-frontal region, specifically inhibiting the left-hemisphere limbic and subcortical contributions to anxiety and negative affect. However, at least for striatal contributions to emotional responsivity, this reasoning does not seem to hold. Starkstein et al.[112] examined emotional responses in patients with lesions of the caudate nucleus as well as frontal cortex; depression was common in patients with left-caudate lesions as well as left frontal cortex.

If the left frontal lobe is important in inhibiting negative affect, the subcortical structures that are inhibited may be the limbic structures of the left hemisphere. Recent PET blood flow findings have suggested that increased functioning of the amygdala of the left hemisphere may accompany negative affect in both normal subjects and depressed patients. Coupled with previous reports of increased activity of left frontal cortex in negative emotion, these findings raise interesting questions about hemispheric frontal-limbic interactions in emotional self-regulation.

A number of studies have observed increased blood flow and metabolism of regions of left frontal cortex in negative affect. With the Xenon surface rCBF (regional cerebral blood flow) method, Johanson and associates examined anxiety disorder patients as they considered the source of their anxiety. Increased blood flow was observed in inferior regions of the left hemisphere.[113] Using positron emission tomography (PET) measures of rCBF with normal volunteers, Pardo et al.[114] found increased orbitofrontal blood flow bilaterally for women in their sample, but only on the left for the men.

An important question for mood induction research is the uncontrolled cognition, such as self-verbalization, that may be induced by the instructions in addition to the affect. Extending their study of anxious patients with a high-resolution rCBF scanner, Johanson et al. also included a control condition of a neutral mood induction that served to equate the possible demands for self-verbalization.[43] They again found high flow over inferior (orbital) left-frontal areas in anxiety. Given the chronic high anxiety of most obsessive-compulsive patients, a consistent finding may be that of Baxter *et al.*, who found increased metabolism in both caudate nuclei and the left orbital frontal cortex in a PET study of obsessive-compulsives.[115]

The improved anatomical precision of PET rCBF, particularly with registration with magnetic resonance anatomical images, has allowed estimates of activity in the amygdala. Examining unipolar depressed patients, Drevets and associates found increased blood flow in the left amygdala and in left frontal cortex.[116] Converging findings with normal emotion have come from the PET rCBF study of Schneider, Gur and associates,[117] who used viewing of emotional faces as a mood induction procedure. In the negative-emotion condition of this experiment, the subjects showed increased flow of the left amygdala. In the positive-emotion condition, they showed increased blood flow in the right amygdala. Interestingly, in a manner similar to that described by Davidson,[110] several measures of frontal cortical flow were found to be inversely correlated with amygdala blood flow.

These several findings may be consistent with the unilateral release interpretation of the effect of hemispheric lesions on emotional orientation.[99] The inherent negative affect (anxiety and hostility) of the left hemisphere may be seen to be modulated by cortical control in the normal brain, such that the depressive catastrophic response to left frontal damage reflects a release of the ipsilateral limbic emotionality. Similarly, the inherently positive emotional tone of right limbic regions may be normally modulated by the right frontal lobe, such that right frontal damage leads to personality disinhibition and denial of problems. Within this framework, the exaggerated corticolimbic interconnection in temporal lobe epilepsy[103] reflects the inherent relations between a self-critical emotional tone and the intellectual ideation of the left hemisphere, compared to the optimistic, self-aggrandizing emotional tone and emotional expressivity of the right hemisphere. These inherent relations between hemispheric cognitive styles and hemispheric affective styles are important clues to the structure of both normal personality and the personality disorders that include avoidant, schizoid, and anxious personalities on the one hand, and histrionic, antisocial, and narcissistic personalities on the other.[118]

The implications of this line of reasoning for frontal lobe function in emotional self-regulation are interesting and somewhat complex. The frontal lobe has been described as inhibitory for hemispheric emotionality;[105] this would be consistent with a release (disinhibition) of emotional behavior following a frontal lesion. Yet, at least for orbitofrontal regions, the rCBF findings suggest that the emotional state is associated with increased frontal activity. The interesting question is whether that increased activity during the emotional state reflects frontal inhibitory modulation of the limbic emotional response, or whether it reflects an elaboration of the emotional process itself.

ASYMMETRIES OF CORTICOLIMBIC ARCHITECTURE

Very likely, the frontal lobe contribution to emotional experience and behavior involves both excitatory and inhibitory influences from both left and right frontal regions. As neuroimaging methods provide increasingly detailed views of human brain activity, they should provide new answers to the major empirical question of how asymmetric frontal activity relates to positive and negative emotional states. The theoretical question, however, will remain: why are these differing emotional orientations asymmetric in the human brain?

We propose that hemispheric specialization, for both emotion and cognition, has evolved in humans by elaborating upon the more fundamental dorsal/ventral dimension of neocortical organization. Specifically, the right hemisphere's skills in emotional communication, and its integral relation to the depression-elation dimension, may have evolved in close correspondence with the motivational bias toward hedonic initiation of behavior of the dorsal limbic pathways. Similarly, the left hemisphere's motivational links to anxiety and hostility may reflect its close interdependence with the self-preservation, fight/flight mechanisms of the ventral limbic pathways.

The initial speculation that hemispheric specialization involves differential elaboration of dorsal and ventral pathways was offered by Bear.[85] In considering the importance of the right hemisphere to emotional processes, he pointed out that its specialization for both emotion and spatial cognition may be consistent with a strong reliance on the dorsal pathway, which he suggested may support "emotional surveillance." Other recent theories of hemispheric asymmetries in emotional processes have emphasized that the left hemisphere has a unique motivational and emotional basis as well, and that this basis may emerge from the ventral limbic pathways that are integral to anxiety and hostility.[38,42] Liotti and Tucker[119] reviewed several lines of evidence that suggest that hemispheric cognitive skills may be differentially linked to the archicortical and paleocortical moieties. Several findings have suggested left-hemispheric specialization for object perception; in the more general sense, the left hemisphere's competence in analytic processing may emerge from the focal attention and object-formation capacities of the ventral corticolimbic pathway.[119] Similarly, the right hemisphere's spatial skills, and its competence in holistic conceptual as well as perceptual organization, may be dependent on the unique cybernetics of the dorsal corticolimbic pathway.

This line of theorizing may offer new ways of considering the evidence on hemispheric specialization for emotion, particularly the issues of frontal-limbic control that are emerging in both the blood flow and frontal lesion studies. Each hemisphere includes both archicortical and paleocortical divisions, of course, so that a theory that describes an emphasis on one "dominant" division in that hemisphere would need to explain the specialized role of the "nondominant" corticolimbic division.

An adequate explanation of hemispheric specialization for emotion will be essential for a general theory of the motivational control of human cognition. However, it is important to keep in mind the general implication of corticolimbic architecture that occurs for both dorsal and ventral pathways in both hemispheres: the most global integration of cognition must occur in the most densely interconnected networks, and these are the paralimbic networks.[38] Brown[120] points out from his aphasia studies that semantic deficits are most common with lesions of paralimbic cortex. Because the anatomy of cortical connections has been inadequate, we have assumed for many years that sensory information is projected to "association" cortex, which represents "higher" cognitive representations. Although this view is not necessarily wrong, it is incomplete. The higher "association" areas of posterior and frontal cortex represent intermediate networks between sensory and motor isocortex and the densely interconnected paralimbic networks.[34] For the posterior brain, memory consolidation seems to involve recruitment and organization of the processing in neocortical networks under motivational control from paralimbic networks. For the frontal lobes, the process is reversed, with the organization of action emerging from paralimbic cortices—where the representation is inextricably bound with its motivational significance—and then progressively articulated into discrete actions in the multilevel network recursion culminating in motor cortex.[37]

This general limbic-frontal progression in behavioral organization appears to take different forms in the dorsal and ventral corticolimbic pathways. For the dorsal pathway, the "projectional" or feedforward mode of motor control appears to be based on a motivational mode that readily spawns behavioral impulses. The exaggerated case may be the hypomanic or sociopathic personality whose actions are readily generated by hedonic impulses with inadequate feedback from critical self-monitoring. For the ventral pathway, the tight sensorimotor links suggest a high degree of monitoring feedback in the generation of each action from the initial global paralimbic representation. Dominated by this control mode, the chronically anxious or obsessive-compulsive personality may show highly constrained, articulated actions that are seldom tainted by the hedonic impulse. These exaggerated personality styles may be understood in terms of exaggerated neurophysiological mechanisms, providing clues to the motivational biases that must be integrated to balance effective frontal lobe contributions to social and emotional self-regulation.

SUMMARY

In humans, frontal lesions result in deficits of social and emotional behavior that are often surprising in the presence of intact language and other cognitive skills. The connections between the motivation and memory functions of limbic cortex and the motor planning functions of frontal neocortex must be fundamental to meeting the daily challenges of self-regulation. The connectional architecture of limbic and neocortical networks suggests a model of function. The densely interconnected paralimbic cortices may serve to maintain a global motivational context within which specific actions are articulated and sequenced within frontal neocortical networks. The paralimbic networks represent the visceral and kinesthetic information that is integral to the representation of the bodily self. In a general sense, the implicit self-representation within paralimbic networks may shape the significance of perceptions and the motivational context for developing actions. The network architecture of the frontal lobe reflects the dual limbic origins of frontal cortex, in the dorsal archicortical and ventral paleocortical structures. In this paper, we speculated that these two limbic-cortical pathways apply different motivational biases to direct the frontal lobe representation of working memory. The dorsal limbic mechanisms projecting through the cingulate gyrus may be influenced by hedonic evaluations, social attachments, and they may initiate a mode of motor control that is holistic and impulsive. In contrast, the ventral limbic pathway from the amygdala to orbital frontal cortex may implement a tight, restricted mode of motor control that reflects adaptive constraints of self-preservation. In the human brain, hemispheric specialization appears to have led to asymmetric elaborations of the dorsal and ventral pathways. Understanding the inherent asymmetries of corticolimbic architecture may be important in interpreting the increasing evidence that the left and right frontal lobes contribute differently to normal and pathological forms of self-regulation.

REFERENCES

1. VALENSTEIN, E. S. 1992. Therapeutic exuberance: A double-edged sword. *In* So Human a Brain: Knowledge and Values in the Neurosciences. A. Harrington, Ed. Birkhausen. Boston, MA.
2. VALENSTEIN, E. S. 1990. The prefrontal area and psychosurgery. Prog. Brain Res. **85:** 539–554.
3. PRIBRAM, K. H. 1950. Psychosurgery in midcentury. Surg. Gynecol. Obstet. **91:** 364–367.
4. FLOR-HENRY, P. 1977. Progress and problems in psychosurgery. *In* Current Psychiatric Therapies. J. H. Masserman, Ed.: 283–298. Grune and Stratton. New York.
5. RYLANDER, G. 1948. Personality analysis before and after frontal lobotomy. *In* The Frontal Lobes: Proceedings of the Association for Research in Nervous and Mental Disease, Vol. 27. J. F. Fulton, C. D. Aring & S. B. Wortis, Ed. Williams & Wilkins. Baltimore, MD.
6. LEZAK, M. D. 1976. Neuropsychological Assessment. Oxford University Press. New York.
7. DAMASIO, A. R., D. TRANEL & H. DAMASIO. 1990. Individuals with sociopathic behavior caused by frontal damage fail to respond autonomically to social stimuli. Behav. Brain Res. **41:** 81–94.
8. TUCKER, D. M. 1993. Emotional experience and the problem of vertical integration. Neuropsychology 7: 500–509.
9. PRIBRAM, K. H. 1981. Emotions. *In* Handbook of Clinical Neuropsychology. S. K. Filskov & T. J. Boll, Eds. Wiley-Interscience. New York.
10. LURIA, A. R. 1973. The working brain; an introduction to neuropsychology. Basic Books. New York.
11. LURIA, A. R. & E. D. HOMSKAYA. 1970. Frontal lobe and the regulation of arousal processes. *In* Attention: Contemporary Theory and Research. D. Mostofsky, Ed. Appleton-Century-Crofts. New York.
12. YNGLING, C. D. & J. E. SKINNER. 1977. Gating of thalamic input to cerebral cortex by nucleus reticularis thalami. *In* Attention Voluntary Contraction and Event-related Cerebral Potentials; Progress in Clinical Neurophysiology. Vol. 1. J. E. Desmedt, Ed.: 70–96. Karger. Basel.
13. JAMES, W. 1884. What is emotion? Mind **4:** 118–204.
14. SCHACHTER, S. & J. E. SINGER. 1962. Cognitive, social, and physiological determinants of emotional state. Psychol. Rev. **69(5):** 379–399.
15. MORUZZI, G. & H. W. MAGOUN. 1949. Brain stem reticular formation and activation of the EEG. Electroencephalogr. Clin. Neurophysiol. **1:** 455–473.
16. PRIBRAM, K. H. & D. McGUINNESS. 1975. Arousal, activation, and effort in the control of attention. Psychol. Rev. **82:** 116–149.
17. TUCKER, D. M. & P. A. WILLIAMSON. 1984. Asymmetric neural control systems in human self-regulation. Psychol. Rev. **91(2):** 185–215.
18. MALONE, M. A., J. R. KERSHNER, L. SIEGEL & J. SWANSON. Hemispheric processing and methylphenidate effects in ADHD. J. Child Neurol. In press.
19. HEILMAN, K. M. 1979. Neglect and related disorders. *In* Clinical Neuropsychology. K. M. Heilman & E. Valenstein, Eds. Oxford University Press. New York.

20. PARDO, J. V., P. J. PARDO, K. W. JANER & M. E. RAICHLE. 1990. The anterior cingulate cortex mediates processing selection in the Stroop attentional conflict paradigm. Proc. Natl. Acad. Sci. USA **87**: 256–259.
21. FOOTE, S. L. & J. H. MORRISON. 1987. Extrathalamic modulation of cortical function. Annu. Rev. Neurosci. **10**: 67–95.
22. HECAEN, H. & M. L. ALBERT. 1978. Human neuropsychology. Wiley. New York.
23. BUCY, P. C. & K. H. PRIBRAM. 1943. Localized sweating as part of a localized convulsive seizure. Arch. Neurol. Psychiatry **50**: 456–461.
24. KAADA, B. R., K. H. PRIBRAM & J. A. EPSTEIN. 1949. Respiratory and vascular responses in monkeys from temporal pole, insula, orbital surface, and cingulate gyrus. J. Neurophysiol. **12**: 347–356.
25. PRIBRAM, K. H. & P. D. MACLEAN. 1953. Neuronographic analysis of medial and basal cerebral cortex. II. Monkey. J. Neurophysiology **16**: 324–340.
26. NEAFSEY, E. J. 1990. Prefrontal cortical control of the autonomic nervous system: Anatomical and physiological observations. *In* The Prefrontal Cortex: Its Structure, Function and Pathology. H. B. M. Uylings *et al.*, Eds.: 147–166. Elsevier. New York.
27. PRIBRAM, K. H. 1987. The subdivision of the frontal cortex revisited. *In* The Frontal Lobes Revisited. E. Perecman, Ed.: 11–39. IRBN Press. New York.
28. NAUTA, W. J. H. 1971. The problem of the frontal lobe: A reinterpretation. J. Psychiatr. Res. **8**: 167–187.
29. TEUBER, H. L. 1964. The riddle of the frontal lobe function in man. *In* The Frontal Granular Cortex and Behavior. J. M. Warren & K. Akert, Eds.: 410–444. McGraw Hill. New York.
30. GOLDMAN-RAKIC, P. 1995. Ann. N.Y. Acad. Sci. This volume.
31. UNGERLEIDER, L. G. & M. MISHKIN. 1982. Two cortical visual systems. *In* The analysis of visual behavior. D. J. Ingle, R. J. W. Mansfield & M. A. Goodale, Eds.: 549–586. MIT Press. Cambridge, MA.
32. MISHKIN, M. 1982. A memory system in the monkey. Philos. Trans. R. Soc. Lond. B **298**: 85–95.
33. SQUIRE, L. R. 1986. Mechanisms of memory. Science **232**: 1612–1619.
34. PANDYA, D. N., B. SELTZER & H. BARBAS. 1988. Input-output organization of the primate cerebral cortex. *In* Comparative Primate Biology, Vol. 4: Neurosciences.: 39–80. Allen Ardlis, Inc. New York.
35. PANDYA, D. N. & C. L. BARNES. 1987. Architecture and connections of the frontal lobe. *In* The Frontal Lobes Revisited. E. Perecman, Ed.: 41–72. IRBN Press. New York.
36. WERNER, H. 1957. The comparative psychology of mental development. Harper. New York.
37. BROWN, J. 1987. The microstructure of action. *In* The Frontal Lobes Revisited. E. Perecman, Ed. IRBN Press. New York.
38. TUCKER, D. M. 1992. Development of emotion and cortical networks. *In* Minnesota Symposium on Child Development: Developmental Neuroscience. M. Gunnar & C. Nelson, Eds. Oxford University Press. New York.
39. DERRYBERRY, D. & D. M. TUCKER. 1991. The adaptive base of the neural hierarchy: Elementary motivational controls on network function. *In* Nebraska Symposium on Motivation. R. Dienstbier, Ed. University of Nebraska Press. Lincoln, NE.
40. PANDYA, D. N. & E. H. YETERIAN. 1985. Architecture and connections of cortical association areas. *In* Cerebral Cortex. Vol. 4. Association and auditory cortices. A. Peters & E. G. Jones, Eds.: 3–61. Plenum Press. New York.
41. DERRYBERRY, D. & D. M. TUCKER. 1991. The adaptive base of the neural hierarchy: Elementary motivational controls of network function. *In* Nebraska Symposium on Motivation. A. Dienstbier, Ed.: 289–342. University of Nebraska Press. Lincoln, NE.
42. TUCKER, D. M. & D. DERRYBERRY. 1992. Motivated attention: Anxiety and the frontal executive functions. Neuropsychiatry Neuropsychol. Behav. Neurol. **5**: 233–252.

43. JOHANSON, A., G. SMITH, J. RISBERG, P. SILFVERSKIOLD & D. TUCKER 1992. Left orbital frontal activation in pathological anxiety. Anxiety Stress Coping **5:** 313–328.
44. BLUMER, D. & D. F. BENSON. 1975. Personality changes with frontal and temporal lobe lesions. *In* Psychiatric Aspects of Neurologic Disease. D. F. Benson & D. Blumer, Eds.: 151–170. Grune and Stratton. New York.
45. DAMASIO, A. 1995. Ann. N.Y. Acad. Sci. This volume.
46. GOLDBERG, G. 1985. Supplementary motor area structure and function: Review and hypotheses. Behav. Brain Sci. **8:** 567–616.
47. FUSTER, J. M. 1980. The Prefrontal Cortex: Anatomy, Physiology, and Neuropsychology of the Frontal Lobe. Raven Press. New York.
48. FUSTER, J. M. 1985. The prefrontal cortex, mediator of cross-temporal contingencies. Hum. Neurobiol. **4:** 169–179.
49. FUSTER, J. M. 1995. Ann. N.Y. Acad. Sci. This volume.
50. GOLDMAN-RAKIC, P. S. 1987. Circuitry of the primate prefrontal cortex and regulation of behavior by representational memory. *In* Handbook of Physiology. Sect. 1. The nervous system. Vol. 5. Higher functions of the brain, Part 1. F. Plum, Ed.: 373–417. Am. Physiol. Soc. Bethesda, MD.
51. WILSON, F. A. W., S. P. O. SCALAIDHE & P. S. GOLDMAN-RAKIC. 1993. Dissociation of object and spatial processing domains in primate prefrontal cortex. Science **260:** 1955–1958.
52. PRIBRAM, K. H. & W. E. TUBBS. 1967. Short-term memory, parsing and the primate frontal cortex. Science **156:** 1765–1767.
53. STARKSTEIN, S. E., J. D. BOSTON & R. G. ROBINSON. 1988. Mechanisms of mania after brain injury: 12 case reports and review of the literature. J. Nerv. Ment. Dis. **176:** 87–100.
54. PLOOG, D. W. 1992. Neuroethological perspectives on the human brain: From the expression of emotions to intentional signing and speech. *In* So Human a Brain: Knowledge and Values in the Neurosciences. A. Harrington, Ed.: 3–13. Birkhauser. Boston, MA.
55. SANIDES, F. 1970. Functional architecture of motor and sensory cortices in primates in the light of a new concept of neocortex evolution. *In* The Primate Brain: Advances in Primatology, Vol. 1. C. R. Noback & W. Montagna, Eds.: 137–201. Appleton-Century-Crofts. New York.
56. PANDYA, D. N. & E. H. YETERIAN. 1990. Prefrontal cortex in relation to other cortical areas in rhesus monkey: Architecture and connections. *In* The Prefrontal Cortex: Its Structure, Function and Pathology. H. B. M. Uylings *et al.*, Eds.: 63–94. Elsevier. New York.
57. MESULAM, M. M. & E. J. MUFSON. 1982. Insula of the old world monkey. III. Efferent cortical output and comments on function. J. Comp. Neurol. **212:** 38–52.
58. LURIA, A. R. & E. D. HOMSKAYA. 1964. Disturbance in the regulative role of speech with frontal lobe lesions. *In* The Frontal Granular Cortex and Behavior. J. M. Warren & K. Akert, Eds.: 353–371. McGraw Hill. New York.
59. GOLDBERG, G. 1987. From intent to action: Evolution and function of the premotor systems of the frontal lobe. *In* The Frontal Lobes Revisited. E. Perecman, Ed.: 273–306. IRBN Press. New York.
60. SQUIRE, L. R. 1987. Memory and Brain. Oxford University Press. New York.
61. MISHKIN, M. & E. A. MURRAY. 1994. Stimulus recognition. Curr. Opin. Neurobiol. **4:** 200–206.
62. BACHEVALIER, J. & M. MISHKIN. 1986. Visual recognition impairment follows ventromedial but not dorsolateral prefrontal lesions in monkeys. Behav. Brain Res. **20:** 249–261.
63. AGGLETON, J. P. & M. MISHKIN. 1986. The amydala: Sensory gateway to the emotions. *In* Emotion: Theory, Research and Experience. R. Plutchik & H. Kellerman, Eds.: 281–299. Academic Press. New York.
64. NADEL, L. 1992. Multiple memory systems: What and why. J. Cognit. Neurosci. **4(3):** 179–188.
65. DEECKE, L., H. H. KORNHUBER, W. LANG & H. SCHREIBER. 1985. Timing function

of the frontal cortex in sequential motor and learning tasks. Hum. Neurobiol. **4:** 143–154.

66. FUSTER, J. M. 1985. The prefrontal cortex and temporal integration. *In* Cerebral Cortex, Vol. 4. Association and Auditory Cortices. A. Peters & E. G. Jones, Eds.: 151–177. Plenum Press. New York.

67. BUCHANAN, S. L. & D. POWELL. 1993. Cingulothlamic and prefrontal control of autonomic function. *In* Neurobiology of the Cingulate Cortex and Limbic Thalamus. B. A. Vogt & M. Gabriel, Eds.: 381–414. Birkhauser. Boston, MA.

68. LEDOUX, J. E. 1991. Information flow from sensation to emotion: Plasticity in neural computation of stimulus value. *In* Learning and Computational Neuroscience: Foundations of Adaptive Networks. M. Gabriel & J. Moore, Eds.: 3–51. MIT Press. Cambridge, MA.

69. LEHRMITTE, F., B. PILLON & M. SERDARU. 1986. Human autonomy and the frontal lobes. Part I. Imitation and utilization behavior: A neuropsychological study of 75 patients. Ann. Neurol. **19:** 326–334.

70. PRIBRAM, K. H. 1991. Brain and Perception: Holonomy and Structure in Figural Processing. Erlbaum. Hillsdale, NJ.

71. KLUVER, H. & P. C. BUCY. 1939. Preliminary analysis of functions of the temporal lobes in monkeys. Arch. Neurol. Psychiatry **42:** 979–1000.

72. PANDYA, D. N. & E. H. YETERIAN. 1984. Proposed neural circuitry for spatial memory in the primate brain. Neuropsychologia **22:** 109–122.

73. SPEVACK, A. & K. H. PRIBRAM. 1973. A decisional analysis of the effects of limbic lesions in monkeys. J. Comp. Physiol. Psychol. **82:** 211–226.

74. DAMASIO, A. R., G. W. VAN HOESEN & J. VILENSKY. 1981. Limbic-motor pathways in the primate: A means for emotion to influence motor behavior. Neurology **31:** 60–84.

75. LEDOUX, J. E. 1987. Emotion. *In* Handbook of Physiology. Sect. 1: The Nervous System. Vol. 5. Higher Functions of the Brain, Part 1., F. Plum, Ed.: 419–459. American Physiological Society. Bethesda, MD.

76. MACLEAN, P. D. 1993. Introduction: Perspectives on cingulate cortex in the limbic system. *In* Neurobiology of the Cingulate Cortex and Limbic Thalamus. B. A. Vogt & M. Gabriel, Eds.: 1–15. Birkhauser. Boston, MA.

77. VOGT, B. A., D. N. PANDYA & D. L. ROSENE. 1987. Cingulate cortex of the rhesus monkey. I. Cyto architecture and thalamic afferents. J. Comp. Neurol. **262:** 256–270.

78. VOGT, B. A., D. M. FINCH & C. R. OLSON. 1993. Functional heterogeneity in the cingulate cortex: The anterior executive and posterior evaluative regions. Cereb. Cortex **2:** 435–443.

79. VOGT, B. A. & D. N. PANDYA. 1987. Cingulate cortex of the rhesus monkey. II. Cortical afferents. J. Comp. Neurol. **262:** 271–289.

80. PANDYA, D. N., G. W. VAN HOESEN & M.-M. MESULAM. 1981. Efferent connections of the cingulate gyrus in the rhesus monkey. Exp. Brain Res. **42:** 319–330.

81. DEVINSKY, O. & D. LUCIANO. 1993. The contributions of cingulate cortex to human behavior. *In* Neurobiology of the Cingulate Cortex and Limbic Thalamus. B. A. Vogt & M. Gabriel, Eds.: 427–556. Birkhauser. Boston, MA.

82. MESULAM, M. 1981. A cortical network for directed attention and unilateral neglect. Ann. Neurol. **10(4):** 309–325.

83. MACLEAN, P. D. 1990. The Triune Brain in Evolution: Role in Paleocerebral Functions. Plenum Press. New York.

84. PLOOG, D. 1981. Neurobiology of primate audio-vocal behavior. Brain Res. Rev. **3:** 35–61.

85. BEAR, D. M. 1983. Hemispheric specialization and the neurology of emotion. Arch. Neurol. **40:** 195–202.

86. HEILMAN, K. M. & T. VAN DEN ABLE. 1980. Right hemisphere dominance for attention: The mechanism underlying hemisphere asymmetry of inattention (neglect). Neurology **30:** 327–330.

87. PEARLSON, G. D. & R. G. ROBINSON. 1981. Suction lesions of the frontal cerebral

cortex in the rat induce asymmetrical behavioral and catecholaminergic responses. Brain Res. **218:** 233–242.

88. FLOR-HENRY, P. 1979. On certain aspects of the localization of cerebral systems regulating and determining emotion. Biol. Psychiatry **14:** 677–698.

89. FOGEL, B. S. & F. R. SPARADEO. 1985. Focal cognitive deficits accentuated by depression. J. Nerv. Ment. Dis. **173(1):** 120–124.

90. BRUMBACK, R. A., R. D. STATON & H. WILSON. 1980. Neuropsychological study of children during and after remission of endogenous depressive episodes. Percept. Mot. Skills **50(0):** 1163–1167.

91. LIOTTI, M. & D. M. TUCKER. 1992. Right hemisphere sensitivity to arousal and depression. Brain & Cognition **18:** 138–151.

92. BOROD, J. C. 1992. Interhemispheric and intrahemispheric control of emotion: A focus on unilateral brain damage. J. Consult. Clin. Psychol. **60:** 339–348.

93. SACKEIM, H. A., R. C. GUR & M. C. SAUCY. 1978. Emotions are expressed more intensely on the left side of the face. Science **202:** 434–436.

94. SAFER, M. A. & H. LEVENTHAL. 1977. Ear differences in evaluating emotional tones of voice and verbal content. J. Exp. Psychol. Hum. Percept. Perform. **3(1):** 75–82.

95. GOLDSTEIN, K. 1952. The effect of brain damage on the personality. Psychiatry **15:** 245–260.

96. ROBINSON, R. G., K. L. KUBOS, K. RAO & T. R. PRICE. 1984. Mood disorders in stroke patients: Importance of location of lesion. Brain **107:** 81–93.

97. GAINOTTI, G. 1972. Emotional behavior and hemispheric side of the lesion. Cortex **8:** 41–55.

98. SACKEIM, H. A., M. S. GREENBERG, A. L. WEIMAN et al. 1982. Hemispheric asymmetry in the expression of positive and negative emotions: Neurologic evidence. Arch. Neurol. **39:** 210–218.

99. TUCKER, D. M. 1981. Lateral brain function, emotion, and conceptualization. Psychol. Bull. **89:** 19–46.

100. BRODAL, A. 1969. Neurological Anatomy in Relation to Clinical Medicine. Oxford University Press. New York.

101. RINN, W. E. 1984. The neuropsychology of facial expression: A review of the neurological and psychological mechanisms for producing facial expressions. Psychol. Bull. **95:** 52–77.

102. MONRAD-KROHN, G. H. 1924. On the dissociation of voluntary and emotional innervation in facial paresis of central origin. Brain **47:** 22–35.

103. BEAR, D. M. & P. FEDIO. 1977. Quantitative analysis of interictal behavior in temporal lobe epilepsy. Arch. Neurol. **34:** 454–467.

104. DAVIDSON, R. J., G. E. SCHWARTZ, C. SARON et al. 1979. Frontal versus parietal EEG asymmetry during positive and negative affect. Psychophysiology **16:** 202–203.

105. TUCKER, D. M., C. E. STENSLIE, R. S. ROTH & S. SHEARER. 1981. Right frontal lobe activation and right hemisphere performance decrement during a depressed mood. Arch. Gen. Psychiatry **38:** 169–174.

106. DAVIDSON, R. J. 1984. Affect, cognition and hemispheric specialization. In Emotion, Cognition and Behavior. C. E. Izard, J. Kagan & R. Zajonc, Eds. Cambridge University Press. New York.

107. HENRIQUES, J. B. & R. J. DAVIDSON. 1990. Regional brain electrical asymmetries discriminate between previously depressed and healthy control subjects. J. Abnorm. Psychol. **99:** 22–31.

108. KNIGHT, R. T., S. A. HILLYARD, D. L. WOODS & H. J. NEVILLE. 1981. The effects of frontal cortex lesions on event-related potentials during auditory selective attention. Electroencephalogr. Clin. Neurophysiol. **52:** 571–582.

109. TOMARKEN, A. J. & R. J. DAVIDSON. Brain activation in repressors and non-repressors: Implications for affective regulation. J. Abnorm. Psychol. In press.

110. DAVIDSON, R. J. 1994. Role of prefrontal activation in the inhibition of negative affect. Psychophysiology **31:** S7 (Abstr.).

111. TUCKER, D. M. & S. L. FREDERICK. 1989. Emotion and brain lateralization. In Hand-

book of Psychophysiology: Emotion and Social Behaviour. H. Wagner & T. Manstead, Eds. John Wiley. New York.

112. STARKSTEIN, S. E., R. G. ROBINSON & T. R. PRICE. 1987. Comparison of cortical and subcortical lesions in the production of poststroke mood disorders. Brain **110:** 1045–1059.

113. JOHANSON, A. M., J. RISBERG, P. SILFVERSKIOLD & G. SMITH. 1986. Regional changes of cerebral blood flow during increased anxiety in patients with anxiety neurosis. *In* The Roots of Perception. U. Hentschel, G. Smith & J. G. Draguns, Eds. North-Holland. Amsterdam.

114. PARDO, J. V., P. J. PARDO & M. E. RAICHLE. 1993. Neural correlates of self-induced dysphoria. Am. J. Psychiatry **150:** 713–719.

115. BAXTER, L. R., M. E. PHELPS, J. C. MAZZIOTTA & B. H. GAZE. 1987. Local cerebral glucose metabolic rates in obsessive-compulsive disorder. Arch. Gen. Psychiatry **44:** 211–218.

116. DREVETS, W. C., T. O. VIDEEN, J. L. PRICE, S. K. PRESKORN *et al.* 1992. A functional anatomical study of unipolar depression. J. Neurosci. **12:** 3628–3641.

117. GUR, R. C. 1994. Personal communication.

118. AMERICAN PSYCHIATRIC ASSOCIATION. 1994. Diagnostic and Statistical Manual of Mental Disorders, 4th edit. American Psychiatric Press. Washington, DC.

119. LIOTTI, M. & D. M. TUCKER. 1994. Emotion in asymmetric corticolimbic networks. *In* Human Brain Laterality. R. J. Davidson & K. Hugdahl, Eds. Oxford University Press. New York.

120. BROWN, J. W. 1989. The nature of voluntary action. Brain & Cognition **10:** 105–120.

On Some Functions of the Human Prefrontal Cortex[a]

ANTONIO R. DAMASIO[b]

Department of Neurology
Division of Behavioral Neurology and Cognitive Neuroscience
University of Iowa College of Medicine
Iowa City, Iowa

INTRODUCTION

In one way or another structures in the frontal lobe participate in several functions that are primarily associated with other brain regions. This is true of visual and auditory perception, of motor function, of memory, and of language, and it should constitute no surprise given the vastness of the frontal lobe and its varied connections to other brain regions. In addition, however, the frontal lobe is also presumed to be the primary source of functions such as reasoning, decision making, and creativity—those functions that, together with language, best distinguish humanity in the full sense of the term. This paper is focused on this latter set of frontal lobe functions, specifically, on the kind of reasoning and decision-making processes we usually describe as rationality. I will suggest that, here too, those complex functions do not arise from the frontal lobe alone but rather from large-scale systems that include, along with critical frontal lobe structures, other cortical and subcortical components; and that those functions depend critically on neural structures that regulate homeostasis and partly express their operations in the processes of emotion and feeling.

AN ACQUIRED DISTURBANCE OF PERSONAL AND SOCIAL BEHAVIOR

For many years, my colleagues and I have reported that patients with damage to the prefrontal region, especially when the damage is centered in ventral and medial aspects of this region, develop severe impairments in personal and social decision making, in spite of otherwise largely preserved intellectual abilities (see refs. 1 and 2 for a description of standard examples of such patients).

This class of patients can be described as intelligent, creative, and successful until a specific form of brain damage occurs, after which a pattern of abnormal decision making in personal and social space ensues. Such patients have difficulty planning their work day; difficulty planning their future at immediate, medium,

[a] This work was supported in part by National Institutes of Health NINDS Grant No. PO1 NS19632.

[b] Address correspondence to Antonio R. Damasio, MD, PhD, Department of Neurology, University of Iowa Hospitals & Clinics, Iowa City, Iowa 52242.

and long ranges; and have difficulty choosing suitable friends, partners, and activities. The plans they organize, the persons they elect to join with, or the activities they undertake, often lead to financial losses, losses in social standing, and losses to family and friends. Clearly, the choices these patients make are no longer personally advantageous, are socially inadequate, and are remarkably different from the kind of choices the patients were known to make in the premorbid period.

Yet these patients' intellect remains normal, as measured by conventional IQ tests, and so do the learning and the retention of factual knowledge at both unique and nonunique levels, and the learning and retention of skills. The ability to use logic in the solution of problems commonly posed in neuropsychological testing is also normal, and so is language. Of no lesser importance, basic attention and working memory are not affected, nor are the abilities to make estimates, to judge recency and frequency of events, and to perform normally in the Wisconsin Card Sorting Test. Given that impairment in the latter set of abilities and test performances have traditionally been seen as a hallmark of frontal lobe dysfunction, it is noteworthy indeed that they are not compromised. Finally, there is the fact that these patients' repertoire of social knowledge is still retained, and can be accessed, in a laboratory situation.[3] In brief, this particular class of patients presents a puzzling disturbance that cannot be easily accounted for in terms of a defect in the pertinent knowledge, intellectual ability, language, or basic working memory and attention. The patients pose, in fact, a double challenge: although the impairment is obvious in its ecological niche, there has been neither a laboratory probe to detect it or measure it, nor a satisfactory account of the neural and cognitive mechanisms underlying it. In this paper, I report some progress on both fronts. First I will outline the somatic marker hypothesis, which is part of a framework to account for the condition. Then I will describe new laboratory probes designed to detect and measure aspects of the condition. The reader should note that I will not address, in this text, the condition of other patients with frontal lobe damage whose lesions are located in other anatomical sectors and who, although they too may have defects in reasoning or decision making, also have measurable defects in many of the abilities that are preserved in patients with ventromedial lesions. Patients with other lesion patterns are also important as an object of study, and my group is studying them too, but they do not offer the same window into the process of reasoning and decision making. Moreover, the conditions with which they present may or may not be accountable by the somatic marker hypothesis.

THE SOMATIC MARKER HYPOTHESIS

The idea for the somatic marker hypothesis came from the realization that, although the ventromedial patients were intact in every neuropsychological laboratory test we tried, the patients did have a compromised ability to express emotion and to experience feelings in situations in which emotions would normally have been expected and would presumably have been present during the premorbid period. In other words, along with normal intellect and abnormal decision making, there were abnormalities in emotion and feeling. In the absence of other cognitive impairments that might effectively account for the salient aspects of the condition,

I then assumed that the defect in emotion and feeling, along with its underlying neurobiological components, would constitute a plausible cause. I proposed the following:

1. Some structures in prefrontal cortex are required to learn the association between certain classes of complex situation, on the one hand, and the type of emotional state usually associated with that class of situation in prior individual experience. Because I see emotion as expressing itself most importantly (though not solely) through changes in body state, and because I believe that the results of emotion are primarily represented in the brain in the form of transient changes in the activity pattern of somatosensory structures, I designated the emotional changes under the umbrella term "somatic state." Note that by somatic I refer to musculoskeletal, visceral, and internal milieu components of the soma and not just to the musculoskeletal aspect (see refs. 2 and 4 for details).

2. When a situation of a given class recurs, the system in the prefrontal cortex which has previously acquired the link between the class of situation and the class of somatic state, that is, the cortices in the ventromedial region, can now trigger the reactivation of the somatosensory pattern that describes the appropriate somatic state. This reactivation can be carried out via a "body loop," in which the soma actually changes in response to the activation, and the ensuing changes are relayed to somatosensory cortices; or via an "as if" loop, in which the reactivation signals are conveyed to the somatosensory cortices which then adopt the appropriate pattern. The body is bypassed. The results of either mechanism may be overt (conscious) or covert (nonconscious).

3. The establishment of a somatosensory pattern appropriate to the situation (again, via the "body loop" or the "as if" loop and either overt or covert), together with factual evocations pertinent to the situation, operate to constrain the process of reasoning over multiple options and multiple future outcomes. The constraint operates by a mechanism of qualification. Specifically, when the image that results from the somatosensory pattern is juxtaposed to the images that triggered the somatic state and which describe a scenario of future outcome, the somatosensory pattern *marks* the scenario as good or bad. If the process is overt, the somatic state can thus operate as an alarm signal or an incentive signal. When it operates covertly the somatic state constitutes a biasing signal.

4. Certain somatosensory patterns also act as boosters to attention and working memory.

5. The operation of logical reasoning is facilitated by steps 3 and 4.

In other words, the hypothesis suggests that somatic markers normally help constrain the decision-making space by making that space manageable for logic-based, cost-benefit analyses. In situations in which there is remarkable uncertainty about the future and in which the decision can be influenced by previous individual experience, such constraints permit the organism to decide efficiently within short time intervals.

In the absence of a somatic marker, all options and outcomes become equalized and logic must then operate over too many option-outcome pairs and necessarily more slowly. This is the pattern of behavior we often see in ventromedial frontal lobe patients. Other possibly related patterns include that of random and impulsive decision making.

A NEURAL NETWORK FOR SOMATIC MARKERS

We do not know yet if lesions located elsewhere in the frontal lobe can cause the condition we described above, although we are certain that damage to several other sites in the frontal lobe does *not* cause this pattern, and we are also certain that the relation between this pattern of behavior and ventromedial damage is not spurious.

The finding of this relation, however, raises a question: Why is it that ventral and medial prefrontal cortices are critical to the type of personal and social reasoning and decision-making defects noted in our patients? These cortices, judging from what is known of nonhuman primate neuroanatomy, receive projections from all sensory modalities, directly or indirectly.[5-8] In turn, they are the only known source of projections from frontal regions toward central autonomic control structures,[9] and such projections have a demonstrated physiological influence on visceral control.[10] The ventromedial cortices have extensive bidirectional connections with the hippocampus and amygdala.[11-15]

This anatomical design is quite compatible with the role we propose for the ventromedial cortices. We believe these cortices contain convergence zones, which hold a record of temporal conjunctions of activity in varied neural units (e.g., sensory cortices, limbic structures) hailing from both external *and* internal stimuli (see refs. 16–18 for details of convergence zones). This would be a record of signals from regions that were active simultaneously and which, as a set, defined a given situation. A critical output of the ventromedial convergence zones would be to autonomic effectors. The system would operate as follows: When parts of certain exteroceptive-interoceptive conjunctions are reprocessed, consciously or not, their activation is signaled to ventromedial cortices, which in turn activate somatic effectors in amygdala, hypothalamus, and brain-stem nuclei. One might describe this process as an attempt to reconstitute the kind of somatic state that belonged to the conjunction. The reenacted somatic state can then be signaled to cortical and subcortical somatosensory processing structures, and can either be consciously perceived or trigger a covert process modifying appetitive or aversive behaviors. Ventromedial frontal damage would preclude this chain of events.

In other words, ventral and medial prefrontal cortices are the natural recipients of signals concerning the multiple-site representation of scenarios of complex situations, in several early sensory cortices. Moreover, ventromedial cortices are also recipients of signals from somatosensory structures and bioregulatory structures. Finally, ventromedial frontal structures can originate signals to bioregulatory structures such as the amygdala, hypothalamus, and brain stem (see ref. 2 for details).

The systems network necessary for somatic markers to operate thus includes the following structures: (1) Ventromedial frontal cortices which contain convergence zones that record links between (a) the dispositions that represent categorizations of certain complex situations and (b) the dispositions that represent the somatic states that have been prevalently associated with the situations referred above; (2) central autonomic effectors, for example, the amygdala, which can activate somatic responses in viscera, vascular bed, endocrine system, and nonspecific neurotransmitter systems; and (3) somatosensory cortices and their interlocking projections (especially in the nondominant hemisphere).

It is important to note that the evocation of a somatic marker for stimuli that are unconditioned and basic—for instance, a startling noise or a flash of light—requires a different and simpler network, that is, a network that can cope with behaviorally relevant stimuli that do not need the complex informational processing that social configurations do. The alternate network would bypass the cerebral cortex altogether and activate autonomic centers (e.g., amygdala and others) directly from thalamus.[19,20] My formulation in this regard predicts a dissociation between responses to complex stimuli which require cortical processing and to basic stimuli which do not.

OVERT AND COVERT SOMATIC MARKERS

The somatic marker itself has more than one avenue, specifically, it has one through consciousness (overt) and another outside consciousness (covert). Whether body states are real or vicarious (what I term "as if"), the corresponding neural pattern can be made conscious and constitutes a feeling. However, although many important choices involve feelings, a number of our daily decisions undoubtedly proceed without feelings. That does not mean that the evaluation that normally leads to a body state has not taken place, or that the body state or its surrogate has not been engaged, or that the dispositional machinery underlying the process has not been activated. It simply means that the body state or its surrogate has not been attended. Without attention, neither will be part of consciousness, although either can be part of a covert action on the mechanisms that govern, without willful control, our appetitive (approach) or aversive (withdrawal) attitudes toward the world. Although the hidden machinery underneath has been activated, our consciousness will never know it. Moreover, triggering of activity from neurotransmitter nuclei, which is part of an "emotional response," can bias cognitive processes in a covert manner, thus influencing the reasoning and decision-making mode (see also ref. 21).

THE ROLE OF EMOTION

One may ask why some signals are so critical to the process of reasoning and decision making. My answer is that certain classes of situation, namely those that concern personal and social matters, are frequently linked to punishment and reward, and thus to pain, pleasure, and the regulation of homeostatic states, including the part of the regulation that is expressed by emotion and feeling. It is not possible to represent neurally any of these aspects of cognition and biology without involving the somatosensory system.

A more general question is why a signal is needed at all, external to the representations over which one reasons. The answer I have already suggested above has to do with the uncertainty of outcomes, the dimension of the logical operations required by deciding under uncertainty, and the advantage of a signal which helps constrain the decision-making space.

Assuming that the brain has available a means to select good responses from bad ones in social situations, I suspect it is likely that the mechanism has been co-opted for behavioral guidance that is outside the realm of social cognition. The argument here is that nature would have evolved a highly successful mechanism of guidance to cope with problems whose answers might maximize survival or lead to danger. Although a large range of those problems pertains to the social realm directly, it is apparent that many other problems, albeit not social, are indirectly linked to precisely the same framework of survival versus danger, of ultimate advantage versus disadvantage, of ultimate gain and balance versus loss and disequilibrium. It is therefore plausible that a system geared to produce markers and signposts to guide "social" responses would have been adapted to assist with "intellectual" decision making. Naturally, the somatic markers would not necessarily be perceived in the form of "feelings." But they would still act covertly to highlight, in the form of an attentional mechanism, certain components over others, and to direct, in effect, the go, stop, and turn signals necessary for much decision making and planning on even the most abstract of topics. (Shallice[22] has also proposed that some form of marker is needed in decision making, although he has not specified the neurobiological nature of his marker, and it may be different from mine).

In conclusion, in normal individuals, certain situations require high-order composite memories formed by "facts" and by the "body states" that usually accompany those facts in an individual's experience. The "fact" memories are held in dispositional form in the appropriate association cortices. The "body state" memories do not need to be held permanently, because body states can be re-enacted on demand. Only the memory of the *linkage* between certain classes of situation and certain body states must be held permanently, and I believe the requisite system is in ventral and medial prefrontal cortices.

Patients with ventromedial frontal lobe damage fail to evoke part of the composite memory for a class of situation—the part that describes the association between the class of situation and the somatosensory state linked to the situation. The factual knowledge component of the composite memory can still be evoked, but somatic states cannot be re-enacted, overtly or covertly, relative to those facts. This limitation poses no problem for situations that have minimal somatic state associations in previous experience, but is catastrophic for situations that do.

TESTING THE SOMATIC MARKER HYPOTHESIS

We began a series of experiments aimed at providing a possible physiopathological explanation for the defect. The salient results are described below.

Somatic Responses to Emotionally Charged Stimuli

In these experiments we tested the hypothesis that patients with bilateral damage in the ventromedial prefrontal cortices would not generate somatic states in response to emotionally charged stimuli. The basic idea was that the processing of stimuli with emotional significance would be affected by the previous experiences the subjects had had with those stimuli, and that the ventromedial prefrontal cortex would be pivotal to reactivate the somatic states that had been usually engendered when those stimuli were experienced.

In order to assess the presence or absence of a change in somatic state we decided to measure a standard autonomic index, the skin conduction response (SCR). We studied three groups of subjects. The first was composed of normal controls, without neurological or psychiatric illness. The second comprised subjects with lesions located outside the frontal cortices. The third comprised subjects with lesions in the ventromedial frontal cortex. All subjects in the third group had both bilateral damage in the target region and the index condition, that is, acquired defects in decision making in their real-life real-time behavior.

The experimental condition called for the subjects to view two types of visual images. One type was emotionally neutral, such as landscapes or abstract patterns. The other was emotionally charged, such as scenes of social catastrophe or body mutilation.

The state of responsivity of the autonomic nervous system was assessed in all three groups of subjects by their SCRs to startling stimuli such as loud noises, or to the behaviors that reliably elicit SCRs, for example, deep breath. All three groups had normal SCRs in that condition. In the experimental condition, however, although both normal controls and nonfrontal brain-damaged groups exhibited standard SCR responses to the emotionally charged stimuli and little or no response to the neutral stimuli, the subjects with ventromedial frontal damage failed to react to the emotionally charged stimuli.[23-26] The findings suggest that indeed patients with bilateral ventromedial frontal damage and decision-making defects in the personal and social domain, no longer have a normal ability to generate somatic responses to stimuli with an emotional component.

The Gambling Experiments

Another approach to the testing of the somatic marker hypothesis relied on a novel card-gambling task.[27] The task is an attempt to create in the laboratory a realistic situation in which subjects gradually learn how to play a card game, to their best advantage, in situations of limited knowledge about the rules and under the control of rewards and penalties. As described in our original publication, the task operates as follows: The subjects sit in front of four decks of cards equal in appearance and size, and are given a $2000 loan of play money (facsimile U.S. bills). They are told that the game requires a series of card selections, one card at a time, from any of the four decks, until they are told to stop. The subjects are also told that (1) the goal of the task is to maximize profit on the loan of play money; (2) they are free to switch from any deck to another, at any time, and as often as wished; but (3) they are not told ahead of time how many card selections must be made. The task is stopped after 100 card selections. After *each* card turning, the subjects receive some money. The amount is announced after the turning and varies with the deck. Turning any card from deck A or deck B yields $100; turning any card from deck C or deck D yields $50. After turning *some* cards of any deck, however, the subjects are *both* given money *and* asked to pay a penalty. Again the amount is announced after the card is turned and varies with the deck and the position in the deck according to a schedule unknown to the subjects. The ultimate yield of each deck varies because the penalty amounts are higher in the high-paying decks (A and B), and lower in the low-paying decks (C and D). For example, after turning 10 cards from deck A, the subjects earned $1000, but they have also encountered five unexpected punishments, bringing their total cost to $1250 and incurring a net loss of $250. They encounter the same problem with deck B. On the other hand, after turning 10 cards from decks C or D, the subjects earned $500, but their unpredicted punishments only amounted to $250—that is, the subject netted $250. In short, decks A and B are equivalent in terms of overall net loss over the trials. The difference is that with deck A, the punishment is more frequent, but of smaller magnitude, whereas with deck B, the punishment is less frequent but of higher magnitude. Decks C and D are also equivalent in terms of overall net loss. With deck C, the punishment is more frequent and of smaller magnitude, although with deck D the punishment is less frequent but of higher magnitude. Decks A and B are "disadvantageous" because they cost the most in the long run, whereas decks C and D are "advantageous" because they result in an overall gain in the long run.

The performances of a group of normal control subjects (21 women and 23 men) in this task were compared to those of ventromedial prefrontal subjects (4 men and 2 women). The age range of normal controls was from 20 to 79 years; for ventromedial subjects, from 43 to 84 years. About half the number of subjects in each group had a high-school education, and the other half had a college education.

The results were strikingly clear cut. Normal controls and patients without frontal damage sample from all decks for a while and gradually begin playing more frequently from the good deck than from the bad. About half way through the game they finally adopt this strategy and never abandon it. As a result they come out ahead. Ventromedial frontal lobe patients, on the contrary, continue to play predominantly from the bad decks, in spite of repeated losses. As a result they lose all of their loan and need to borrow money.

Although the gambling task involves a long series of gains and losses, it is not possible for subjects to perform an exact calculation of the net gains or losses generated from each deck as they play. (A group of normal control subjects with superior memory and IQ, whom we asked to think aloud while performing the task and keep track of the magnitudes and frequencies of the various punishments, could not provide figures for the net gains or losses from each deck). The subjects must rely on their ability "to sense," overtly or not, which decks are risky and which are profitable. The performance profile of ventromedial patients is comparable to their real-life inability to decide advantageously, especially in personal and social matters—a domain for which in life, as in the task, an exact calculation of the future outcomes is not possible and where choices must be based on approximations. We believe this task offers, for the first time, the possibility of detecting and measuring in the laboratory, these patients' elusive impairment.

We considered three possibilities for why the target patients make choices that have high immediate reward but severe delayed punishment. The first is that patients are so *sensitive to reward* that the prospect of future (delayed) punishment is outweighed by that of immediate gain. The second is that they are *insensitive to punishment,* and thus the prospect of reward always prevails, even if they are not abnormally sensitive to reward. The third is that they are generally *insensitive to future consequences,* positive or negative, and thus their behavior is mostly guided by immediate prospects. Subsequent work with variants of these tasks (to be published) suggests that neither insensitivity to punishment nor hypersensitivity to reward accounts for the defect. Rather, the subjects seem unresponsive to future consequences, whatever they are.

Evidence from other studies indicate that these patients retain and access the knowledge necessary to conjure up options of actions and scenarios of future outcomes.[3] What they fail to do is act on such knowledge. Elsewhere we have proposed several possible mechanisms of defect.[2,27] For instance, it is possible that the representations of future outcomes that these patients evoke are unstable—that is, they are not held in working memory long enough for attention to enhance them and for reasoning strategies to operate on them. This mechanism invokes a defect along the lines proposed for behavioral domains dependent on dorsolateral prefrontal cortex networks.[28] Defects in temporal integration and attention would be related to this account.[29,30] Another possibility is that the representations of future outcomes might be stable but would not be *marked* with a negative or positive value; the *value mark* for a cognitive scenario would be missing.[2,24]

Psychophysiological Dimension of the Gambling Experiments

In a further test to the somatic marker test hypothesis we undertook a continuous monitoring of SCR, while normal subjects and patients were engaged in the gambling task.[31] The most salient result of this study was the finding that, in normal subjects, during the time window that precedes the selection of a card from a given deck—an interval of about 4 seconds—normal subjects begin to respond with high-amplitude SCRs whenever they are about to make a selection from a bad deck. They show no comparable responses when they are about to make a selection from a good deck. As the task unfolds, the SCRs to the bad decks continue to appear systematically and they rise in amplitude. This does not happen for the responses associated with the good decks. Quite remarkably, *no such anticipatory responses are seen at all in the patients with ventromedial frontal damage*.

One possible interpretation is that the SCR is part of a very early and automated alarm signal, which is triggered, as proposed in the somatic marker hypothesis, from the ventromedial region. The signal affects further processing of the factual knowledge connected with the situation by marking a particular option-outcome pair with a negative bias. Incidentally, this interpretation holds whether the signal is overt and fully appreciated in consciousness, or covert and entirely operated at an unconscious level.

An alternative interpretation is that normal subjects reason, early on, that certain decks are bad and certain decks are good, and that, on the basis of their cognition of "badness" and "goodness," they generate a somatic response which is indexed by the SCR. I find the latter interpretation less plausible for reasons that have to do with my perspective on the evolutionary biology and adaptive value of an automated somatic marker device. Moreover, recent studies in our laboratory suggest that normal subjects begin producing their SCRs to bad decks long before they have, according to their testimony, any notion whatsoever of the good or bad nature of each deck and of the diabolical design of the game they are playing.

CONCLUDING REMARKS

Rationality, the process of reasoning and decision making in a personal and social domain, does seem to depend on prefrontal cortices and, quite critically, on the ventromedial sector of those cortices. I outlined a system network which, together with the ventromedial region, would be essential for the maintenance of rational decision making. The network relies importantly on structures that regulate homeostasis, namely, those whose operations are normally expressed by emotion and feeling. I called the hypothesis that subsumes my idea of the process the "somatic marker hypothesis" because I view somatic changes, enacted in the body or just neurally signaled, as the essential aspect of the process of emotion, albeit not the only one. I note, however, that rationality depends on systems other than the ones I outlined as required for somatic markers to operate—namely, those that depend on knowledge concerning past situations as well as the basic intellectual manipulation of such knowledge. Regarding the latter, recent studies by Grafman and colleagues on the management of "scripts" are especially relevant.[32]

REFERENCES

1. DAMASIO, A. R. 1979. The frontal lobes. *In* Clinical Neuropsychology. K. M. Heilman & E. Valenstein, Eds.: 360–412. Oxford University Press. New York.
2. DAMASIO, A. R. 1994. Descartes' Error: Emotion, Reason, and the Human Brain. Grosset/Putnam. New York.
3. SAVER, J. L. & A. R. DAMASIO. 1991. Preserved access and processing of social knowledge in a patient with acquired sociopathy due to ventromedial frontal damage. Neuropsychologia 29: 1241–1249.
4. DAMASIO, A. R. 1995. Toward a neurobiology of emotion and feeling: Operational concepts and hypotheses. Neuroscientist 1: 19–25.
5. CHAVIS, D. A. & D. N. PANDYA 1976. Further observations on corticofrontal connections in the rhesus monkey. Brain Res. 117: 369–386.
6. JONES, E. G. & T. P. S. POWELL. 1970. An anatomical study of converging sensory pathways within the cerebral cortex of the monkey. Brain 93: 793–820.
7. PANDYA, D. N. & H. G. J. M. KUYPERS. 1969. Cortico-cortical connections in the rhesus monkey. Brain Res. 13: 13–36.
8. POTTER, H. & W. J. H. NAUTA. 1979. A note on the problem of olfactory associations of the orbitofrontal cortex in the money. Neuroscience 4: 316–367.
9. NAUTA, W. J. H. 1971. The problem of the frontal lobe: A reinterpretation. J. Psychiatr. Res. 8: 167–187.
10. HALL, R. E., R. B. LIVINGSTON & C. M. BLOOR. 1977. Orbital cortical influences on cardiovascular dynamics and myocardial structure in conscious monkeys. J. Neurosur. 46: 638–647.

11. AMARAL, D. G. & J. L. PRICE. 1984. Amygdalo-cortical projections in the monkey (*Macaca fascicularis*). J. Comp. Neurol. **230:** 465–496.
12. GOLDMAN-RAKIC, P. S., L. D. SELEMON & M. L. SCHWARTZ. 1984. Dual pathways connecting the dorsolateral prefrontal cortex with the hippocampal formation and parahippocampal cortex in the rhesus monkey. Neuroscience **12:** 719–743.
13. PORRINO, L. J., A. M. CRANE & P. S. GOLDMAN-RAKIC. 1981. Direct and indirect pathways from the amygdala to the frontal lobe in rhesus monkeys. J. Comp. Neurol. **198:** 121–136.
14. VAN HOESEN, G. W., D. N. PANDYA & N. BUTTERS. 1972. Cortical afferents to the entorhinal cortex of the rhesus monkey. Science **175:** 1471–1473.
15. VAN HOESEN, G. W., D. N. PANDYA & N. BUTTERS. 1975. Some connections of the entorhinal (area 28) and perirhinal (area 35) cortices of the rhesus monkey: II. Frontal lobe afferents. Brain Res. **95:** 25–38.
16. DAMASIO, A. R. 1989. The brain binds entities and events by multiregional activation from convergence zones. Neural Computation **1:** 123–132.
17. DAMASIO, A. R. 1989. Time-locked multiregional retroactivation: A systems level proposal for the neural substrates of recall and recognition. Cognition **33:** 25–62.
18. DAMASIO A. R. & H. DAMASIO. 1994. Cortical systems for retrieval of concrete knowledge: The convergence zone framework. *In* Large-Scale Neuronal Theories of the Brain. C. Koch, Ed.: 61–74. MIT Press. Cambridge, MA.
19. CLUGNET, C., J. E. LeDOUX, S. F. MORRISON & D. J. REIS. 1988. Soc. Neurosci. Abstr. **14:** 1227.
20. FARB, C. F., D. A. RUGGIERO & J. E. LeDOUX. 1988. Soc. Neurosci. Abstr. **14:** 1227.
21. TRANEL, D. & A. R. DAMASIO. 1993. The covert learning of affective valence does not require structures in hippocampal system or amygdala. J. Cognit. Neurosci. **5:** 79–88.
22. SHALLICE, T. & P. W. BURGESS. 1993. Supervisory control of action and thought selection. *In* Attention: Selection, Awareness, and Control. A Tribute to Donald Broadbent. A. Baddeley & L. Weiskrantz, Eds.: 171–187. Clarendon Press. Oxford, UK.
23. DAMASIO, A. R., D. TRANEL & H. DAMASIO. 1990. Individuals with sociopathic behavior caused by frontal damage fail to respond autonomically to social stimuli. Behav. Brain Res. **41:** 81–94.
24. DAMASIO, A. R., D. TRANEL & H. DAMASIO. 1991. Somatic markers and the guidance of behavior: Theory and preliminary testing. *In* Frontal Lobe Function and Dysfunction. H. S. Levin, H. M. Eisenberg & A. L. Benton, Eds.: 217–229. Oxford University Press. New York.
25. TRANEL, D. 1994. "Acquired sociopathy": The development of sociopathic behavior following focal brain damage. *In* Progress in Experimental Personality and Psychopathology Research. D. C. Fowles, P. Sutker & S. H. Goodman, Eds. Vol. 17: 285–311. Springer. New York.
26. TRANEL, D., H. DAMASIO & A. R. DAMASIO. 1995. Double dissociation between overt and covert face recognition. J. Cognit. Neurosci. In press.
27. BECHARA, A., A. R. DAMASIO, H. DAMASIO & S. W. ANDERSON. 1994. Insensitivity to future consequences following damage to human prefrontal cortex. Cognition **50:** 7–12.
28. GOLDMAN-RAKIC, P. 1987. Circuitry of primate prefrontal cortex and regulation of behavior by representational memory. *In* Handbook of Physiology: The Nervous System. F. Plum & V. Mountcastle, Eds. Vol. 5: 373–401. The American Physiological Society. Bethesda, MD.
29. FUSTER, J. M. 1989. The Prefrontal Cortex: Anatomy, Physiology, and Neuropsychology of the Frontal Lobe (2nd edit.) Raven Press. New York.
30. POSNER, M. I. & S. E. PETERSEN. 1990. The attention system of the human brain. Annu. Rev. Neurosci. **13:** 25–42.
31. BECHARA, A., D. TRANEL, H. DAMASIO & A. R. DAMASIO. Failure to respond autonomically to anticipated future outcomes following damage to prefrontal cortex. Cereb. Cortex. In Press.
32. GRAFMAN, J., A. SIRIGU, L. SPECTOR & H. HENDLER. 1993. Damage to the prefrontal cortex leads to decomposition of structured event complexes. J. Head Trauma Rehabil. **8:** 73–87.

Forms of Reasoning: Insight into Prefrontal Functions?[a]

KEITH J. HOLYOAK AND JAMES K. KROGER

Department of Psychology and Brain Research Institute
University of California, Los Angeles
Los Angeles, California 90095

INTRODUCTION

The faculties that have historically been attributed to the prefrontal cortex on the basis of clinical and neuropsychological studies parallel the mental abilities traditionally called "higher cognitive functions" by cognitive psychologists. The frontal lobes appear to be directly involved in such important cognitive tasks as planning, problem solving, and determination of social behavior.[1-7] At the same time, patients with frontal damage often remain capable of performing within normal limits on standard intelligence tests. Frontal deficits appear to be both broad in scope and yet selective in important ways, suggesting that models of frontal function could provide important constraints on theories of human cognition.

Nonetheless, only a loose correspondence exists between the recent work of cognitive psychologists on reasoning and brain research, including both clinical studies of the effects of brain damage and neurophysiological studies. Although connectionist models inspired by brain structure have been proposed as models of mechanisms underlying high-level cognition, cognitive theories of reasoning have typically not been based on data from brain research. Conversely, neuro-psychological investigations of brain damage seek to specify the contributions of different neural regions to complex human cognition, but their conceptions of high-level cognition are often very general and fail to reflect the intricacies of the cognitive mechanisms involved. This gap is likely attributable to the difficulty neuroscientists have had in formulating detailed descriptions of neural operations in association areas.

Clinical researchers as well as cognitive psychologists have been concerned with such varieties of thinking as deductive and inductive inference, categorization, judgment and decision making, and problem solving. Thinking, unlike vision and language, has generally been viewed as nonmodular and hence unlikely to be tightly localized in the brain. Human reasoning appears to be in many respects more complex and variegated than the types of conditional responding typically investigated in primate work on frontal functions. Many of the major theoretical constructs that have been influential in cognitive models of thinking—for example, schemas, mental models, and condition-action rules—have not been defined in a way that can be readily related to brain mechanisms. In this paper we sketch some possible links between models of human thinking and models of frontal functions.

[a] This work was supported by National Science Foundation grant SBR-9310614.

Are there particular varieties of thinking and reasoning that selectively depend on brain mechanisms realized in prefrontal cortex? Are there characteristics of the reasoning process that correlate with the emerging picture of neural operation in the frontal lobes? Our aim is limited to exploring how these questions might be developed, rather than proposing any firm answers.

FUNCTIONS OF PREFRONTAL CORTEX

Different models of prefrontal cortex have emphasized a number of major cognitive functions it may subserve, including executive control, various forms of behavioral inhibition, temporal ordering, and working memory. Perhaps the most general description of the overall function of the frontal system is that it serves to mediate behavioral responses to complex environmental contingencies in the absence of control by direct and immediate perceptual cues.[8,9] This function may involve maintaining an association across time to permit successful matching of a proper response to a stimulus,[8,10] or the monitoring of a condition so that an appropriate response may be made.[11] Meditation of contingencies involves the frontal lobes when behavior must be directed in the absence of guiding environmental cues.[9,12] In particular, the dorsolateral area (Brodmann's area 46) appears to be responsible for maintaining a representation needed to mediate contingencies across time, after the stimulus being responded to has been withdrawn. It has been shown that subareas within this region are differentially responsible for maintaining representations of identity[13] and spatial position.[14] Other tasks that are frontal-dependent do not require stimulus representations to be actively maintained in working memory; rather, stimuli are monitored and conditional rules must be retrieved from long-term memory and applied so that behavior is determined by internal mediation and application of contingencies.[11]

It is clear that many high-level cognitive tasks performed by humans depend on behavioral responses controlled by contingencies remote from immediate perceptual cues. Indeed, the most distinctively human cognitive activities include hypothetical reasoning, long-term planning, manipulation of abstract concepts, and internal reorganization of knowledge—activities that require systematic application of internally controlled knowledge. How can performance on such tasks be related to frontal functions? One general approach to delineating the neural substrate of a particular kind of higher cognition is to analyze complex tasks in terms of the simpler cognitive components that comprise it. Working memory is a prime example of a basic cognitive function that has been convincingly associated with a particular brain region and characteristic activity of that region.[3,8,10,13] Reasoning tasks inevitably require the maintenance of a representation of that which is reasoned about; it is likely that this function depends on working memory and the neural substrates that have been shown to underlie it.[15] We would therefore expect reasoning tasks to evoke activation in the dorsolateral region.[2,3,12] Further, based on evidence of topographical distribution of working memory function for different kinds of content (serial order, spatial, and object identity) across subareas of dorsolateral cortex,[16] we might expect to find neurological correlates that are selective for specific types of reasoning content. It is certainly the case that content can have dramatic effects on reasoning and problem solving.[17]

Similarly, attention is almost certainly required for focusing on the various items reasoned about; some of the neural structures associated with attention have been identified.[18–20] Carefully designed reasoning experiments should produce activation of some or all of the brain regions responsible for such basic cognitive functions as working memory and attention. By systematically varying the task, it may be possible to learn the role each component plays in reasoning, and how the ability to reason results from the cooperative operation of the components.

Nonetheless, the details of how component mechanisms yield complex thought remain to be specified. Understanding the interaction of systems of specialized brain regions is an essential step, but ultimately we need to know not only that a particular brain region is responsible for a certain cognitive component, but also *how* it performs its specialization in concert with other regions. At the present time we have only a sketchy understanding of either the system level of brain organization or the neurophysiological underpinnings of component mechanisms.

Thinking is an adaptive evolutionary response to the challenges of survival, incorporating the ability to apprehend the environment and to mediate representations of it in an organized and purposeful manner. At the more abstract level of cognitive theories, work has focused on describing such representations and on revealing the mechanisms of their manipulation. In the remainder of this paper we will consider some general properties of human thinking and how they might be connected to frontal functioning.

SOME COGNITIVE COMPONENTS OF HUMAN THINKING

Symbols and Variables

Robin and Holyoak[21] argued that the diverse tasks that reveal impairment after frontal damage, including planning, sequencing of actions, using context to modulate social behavior, learning contingencies between spatiotemporally separate stimuli and responses, and forming flexible categories, all share a common requirement: the need to bind independently varying elements to specific roles with respect to relations. This point of view suggests that the frontal cortex plays an important role in the development of explicit representations of knowledge, which allow systematic manipulation of symbols. The acquisition of explicit knowledge appears to be based on slow, effortful, and conscious processing that is directly dependent on working memory, and contrasts with implicit knowledge based on relatively rapid, effortless, and unconscious processing.

One of the key contributions of modern connectionism has been demonstrations that many varieties of intelligent behavior do not necessarily depend on either symbols or rules.[22] However, these demonstrations have led to refined arguments that a subset of human (and possibly other primate) knowledge is indeed symbolic. The most fundamental argument for the necessity of symbolic representations in human cognition was presented by Fodor and Pylyshyn,[23] who pointed out that knowledge is *systematic* in the sense that the ability to think particular thoughts seems to imply the ability to think certain related thoughts. For example, if a person understands the meaning of the concepts "love," "boy," and "girl," and can understand the proposition "The boy loves the girl," then it would seem extremely bizarre if the person were nonetheless unable to understand the proposition "The girl loves the boy." Such systematic reasoning with composable constituents requires symbols. A "symbol," fundamentally, is a locally available code that can provide access to distal information relevant to a task. In a symbol system, information acquired in one task context has the potential to be made available in a different task context. Knowledge is symbolic, in this sense, when it can be decoupled from a particular context. In our example above, we can understand both "the boy loves the girl" and "the girl loves the boy" because the concepts "girl" and "boy" are represented in a manner that keeps each distinct from both the "lover" and "beloved" contexts, and therefore potentially available for use in either context. This notion of a symbol being separate from, yet composable with, a given context may be related to evidence that frontal damage can impair both modulation of performance by the context[24] and memory for the spatiotemporal context of events.[25]

Systematicity is related to the use of rules of inference, such as "If X sells Y to Z, then Z owns Y." Smith et al.[26] argue that several empirical criteria can be used to demonstrate that some knowledge used in human reasoning is coded as abstract rules. One criterion is that it seems just as easy to draw inferences about unfamiliar instantiations—including nonsense ones—as about familiar ones. Thus if we are told that "Henry sold the floogle to Sam," we conclude that Sam now owns the floogle (whatever that might be). The inference follows directly from the role that "floogle" plays in the argument structure of the rule, without any requirement that floogles somehow resemble familiar objects that have been sold and then owned by someone else.

Perhaps, then, the human frontal cortex is selectively involved in encoding and manipulating explicit symbolic knowledge, which is based on a predicate-argument (or slot-filler) structure. A key requirement for representing a proposition with a systematic slot-filler structure is that its constituents must be kept distinct, yet interrelated, by creating a set of bindings between the arguments of the proposition and the case roles they fill. Although controversial, there is some neurophysiological evidence that some aspects of perception, as well as the representation and manipulation of information in the frontal lobes, may be accomplished via synchronized neural oscillations.[27–31] Particular components of the total representation may consist of groups of distributed neurons with phase-locked firing oscillations. A representation held in working memory involves not only dorsolateral prefrontal cortex, but also the modality-specific sensory areas and association areas that enable perception of such objects.[2,12] One may envision a distributed network of frontal and sensory brain regions, the activation of which is controlled by area 46, such that their collective activity would constitute the construction and maintenance of propositional representations.

Hummel and colleagues[32,33] have used a synchrony-based computational model to represent abstract propositions. Their model allows units representing roles to be temporarily bound to units representing the arguments of those roles by synchrony relations. The essential idea is that two or more units can indicate a binding of the properties they represent (i.e., that the properties belong to the same entity or otherwise stand in correspondence) by firing in synchrony with one another. For example, *love (boy, girl)* could be represented by units for "boy" firing in synchrony with units for the agent role of "love," with units for "girl" firing in synchrony with units for the patent role. The agent/boy units must fire out of synchrony with the patient/girl set. This simple mechanism provides a way to distinguish the representation of *love (boy, girl)* from the representation of *love (girl, boy)* without requiring separate units to represent the meaning of *boy-as-agent-of-love* and *boy-as-patient-of-love*.

Relational Complexity and Analogical Mapping

It remains to be seen whether neural synchrony involving the frontal cortex plays a role in forming and manipulating propositions. However, regardless of the specific neural mechanisms, good grounds exist for supposing that the human brain is capable of distinguishing roles from their fillers. Robin and Holyoak,[21] adapting a taxonomy proposed by Halford,[34] argued that the human frontal cortex has evolved to cope with role-filler relationships at increasing levels of complexity. Similar complexity analyses have been proposed both in work on primate intelligence[35] and human analogical reasoning.[36] One version of the complexity hierarchy distinguishes *holistic* representations, which do not involve representations of variables and presumably do not depend on frontal functions, from a series of levels of complexity based on predicate-argument structure. An *attribute* requires abstraction of a single dimension of variation, the minimal requirement for differentiating a role from its filler, as in

brown (dog).

A *relation* connects two fillers to each other, as in

chase (dog, cat).

A *higher-order relation* takes a lower-order proposition as a filler, which makes it possible to define a relation between relations, as in

cause [chase (dog, cat), run-away (cat)].

Holyoak and Thagard[37] have argued that these levels of relational complexity are related to progressive increases in the abstraction of analogical mapping, both in evolution and in human cognitive development. Evidence from variations of the match-to-sample task suggests that language-trained chimpanzees can solve analogies on the basis of correspondences at the relational level, but probably not on the basis of higher-order relations.[35] Adult humans can readily find mappings based on higher-order relations.[38] Mappings at this level are primarily constrained by consistency of role correspondences. For example, Aesop's "sour grapes" fable ("A fox wanted some grapes, but couldn't reach them, so announced to his friends that the grapes were sour anyway") can be compared to the tale of a disgruntled job-seeker ("Harry hoped to get the new position of marketing manager, but was passed over, so he told his wife the job would have been boring"). The resulting correspondences are: fox ⟨--⟩ Harry, grapes ⟨--⟩ job, friends ⟨--⟩ wife. It is noteworthy that comprehension of fables at an abstract level appears to depend on brain regions that include part of the right prefrontal cortex.[39]

Systematic relational correspondences also play a role in judgments of perceptual similarity.[40–42] For example, suppose people are shown three pairs of geometric shapes, with each pair arranged vertically. One pair consists of two identical triangles, one of identical squares, and one of identical circles. People tend to evaluate the pair of triangles as more similar to the pair of squares than to the pair of circles. But if a square is now added as a third form below the two items in each of the pairs, the relative similarity reverses: two triangles and a square are viewed as less similar to three squares than to two circles and a square. This similarity reversal reflects differences in relational correspondences: both the first and the third triad can readily be represented as "two same forms plus a square," whereas the middle triad is most naturally represented as "three squares." Thus, the first and third triads have a better match in terms of relational correspondences.

The evidence for relational influences on human analogical mapping and similarity judgments thus spans very different content and tasks, suggesting the possibility that the brain may support a "relational mapping module" based on explicit, structured representations. Although the possibility remains speculative, the prefrontal cortex may play an important role in the neural substrate for such a mechanism.

Human Conditional and Social Reasoning

Many forms of human reasoning appear to involve the representation and manipulation of contingencies (see ref. 17 for a review). In the area of deductive reasoning, the Wason[43] selection task has been employed for almost three decades to investigate the factors affecting subjects' success at solving a problem requiring manipulation of a conditional rule (e.g., refs. 43–45). In the standard "arbitrary" version of this task, subjects view four cards. They are also given a rule, such as, "If there is a vowel on one side of the card, then there must be an even number on the other side." This rule has the logical form "If p then q." Only the fronts of the cards are showing; in this example, either a number or a letter is on the face of each card. Subjects must choose, based on the rule and what is showing on each card, which cards need to be turned over in order to determine if the rule is violated. Only two of the cards need to be turned over: the cases corresponding to vowel (p) and odd number (not q). However, only around 15% of subjects are successful in choosing these two cards; most select either the p case only, or the p and q cases.[43]

The Wason task is of particular interest for models of prefrontal functions because performance is greatly enhanced when the content taps into types of knowledge closely related to everyday social interactions, a type of knowledge that appears to depend on the integrity of ventromedial cortex, the medial portion of Brodmann's area 11.[46,47] People are much more likely to select the "correct" alternatives for conditional rules that tap into knowledge about social regulations based on permission or obligation.[44,48–51] Cheng and Holyoak[44] attributed the facilitation due to social-regulation content to the application of pragmatic reasoning schemas, which are generalized sets of rules for assessing violation of and conformity with social regulations. The application of such schemas may be expected to be mediated by the frontal lobes, because making correct responses depends on fitting the correct rule from the schema to each card. The rules that comprise the schemas are in the form of contingencies; each card must be turned over only when what shows on its front indicates that it may match one of the relevant contingency rules. Successful performance depends on subjects' correctly using these contingencies in relation to unobserved aspects of the environment (i.e., the hidden sides of the cards). It is possible that social regulations tap into portions of the frontal cortex specialized for making social inferences.

Is there a relation between the cognitive ability to perform relational mapping and the improvement of problem-solving efficacy when a logic problem is recast in terms of social rules of conduct for goal satisfaction? At one level, it is useful to ask how the components of a representation are bound together physically. At another level, it is useful to ask how the components of a representation are bound together functionally, because any representation that an organism bothers to maintain or manipulate likely has some functional significance. The structure of a representation can be guided by the goals or needs of the reasoner. A number of investigators have demonstrated that subjects will represent a problem differently depending on the perspective they are encouraged to take when reading the problem.[52–54] For example, Holyoak and Cheng[51] administered a Wason selection task based on the rule, "If an employee works on the weekend, then that person gets a day off during the week." The cards indicated people who had or had not worked on the weekend, and had or had not taken the day off. Subjects were to select cards representing people who might have violated the rule. The rule was presented in a context that encouraged the subject to view the problem from the perspective of either the employer or the employee. This particular rule is ambiguous with respect to which kind of deontic schema it corresponds: a permission or an obligation. The correct solution when the rule is viewed as an obligation is different from the solution when the problem is viewed as a permission. When the context favored viewing the problem from the employer's point of view, the rule was interpreted as a conditional permission (if the employee worked on the weekend, the employee was permitted a day off); when viewed from the employee's point of view, the same rule was best interpreted as a conditional obligation (if the employee worked on the weekend, the employer was obliged to provide a day off). These different perspectives are correlated with different goals of the two actors. The employer's goal is for his employees to work; the employee's goal is to obtain time off. In both cases, the goals are defined by potential losses or benefits to one's self. In this and similar experiments, the pattern of subjects' card selections was reversed across the two perspective conditions.

Humans have a variety of needs that motivate their behavior. In acting to satisfy them, they must operate within a social milieu in which interactions are governed by rules of behavior. As mentioned, evidence suggests that damage to the basal forebrain interferes with patients' ability to interact effectively in the social environment.[46–47] It is possible that this inability arises from difficulties in mapping one's needs to a set of actions that would constitute an effective solution in conformance with rules of social interaction. We might expect patients with this type of damage to be deficient in the kind of reasoning that leads to the correct solution when a Wason selection task is presented in the form of a deontic obligation or permission. The deficiency may lie in the failure to produce a relational mapping between the goal in the social context and the appropriate action-governing schema. Such a deficiency might be caused by an absence of a well-formulated goal, a lack of access to the action-governing schema, or a breakdown in the mapping process itself.

When a Wason selection task is presented that is not phrased in terms of a deontic permission or obligation, subjects' poor performance may result from having no appropriate schemas in long-term memory to which the problem can be mapped. Conversely, clear social content may encourage binding the constituents of the rule to a relevant schema. It has been proposed that the frontal cortex and especially the basal forebrain give form to one's needs and reactions to the environment, which are communicated from the limbic system.[46,55] To the degree that we are social animals, it is sensible that reasoning about social interaction would be especially likely to bring these brain regions to bear on the problem. Not only might such activation make available schemas that permit problem solution, but it may also activate brain areas that support the binding process (e.g., dorsolateral prefrontal cortex). Emotional influences on cognition,[46,55] processing of social interaction,[47] and inhibition of incorrect responses[12] have all been attributed to the basal forebrain. Perhaps these influences are functions of discrete cortical units within the larger area of inferior frontal cortex; however, it may be that different experimental paradigms have produced differing perspectives of what is a single contribution to higher cognitive function—the signifying of components of representations relevant to our goals. The resulting representation of a situation will constrain the solution which is mapped to it. However, the neurophysiological relation between the formulation of a problem representation and the mapping of its solution remains to be resolved.

CONCLUSION

Clearly, much remains to be learned about the neural underpinnings of complex human thought. We have pointed to a few aspects of human thinking—symbols and variables, relations and analogical mapping, and the content specificity of conditional reasoning—that may provide candidates for closer scrutiny of the role played by the prefrontal cortex. The promise of cognitive neuroscience is an understanding of how multiple cortical mechanisms act in concert to permit human behavior. Evidence from both behavioral and neural research will constrain future descriptions of higher cognitive function, so that our expanding ability to observe the brain in action will ultimately shape our understanding of human cognition.

ACKNOWLEDGMENT

We thank François Boller for helpful comments on an earlier draft.

REFERENCES

1. DAMASIO, A. R., D. TRANEL & H. DAMASIO. 1990. Individuals with sociopathic behavior caused by frontal damage fail to respond autonomically to social stimuli. Behav. Brain Res. **41:** 81–94.
2. FUSTER, J. M. 1989. The Prefrontal Cortex. Raven Press. New York.
3. GOLDMAN-RAKIC, P. S. 1992. Working memory and the mind. Sci. Am. **267:** 110–117.
4. MILNER, B., M. PETRIDES & M. L. SMITH. 1985. Frontal lobes and the temporal organization of memory. Hum. Neuropsychol. **4:** 137–142.
5. PETRIDES, M. 1994. Frontal lobes and behavior. Curr. Opin. Neurobiol. **4:** 207–211.
6. SHALLICE, T. 1982. Specific impairments of planning. Phil. Trans. R. Soc. Lond. **B298:** 199–209.
7. STUSS, D. T. & D. F. BENSON. 1986. The Frontal Lobes. Raven Press. New York.
8. FUSTER, J. M. 1990. Prefrontal cortex and the bridging of temporal gaps in the perception-action cycle. Ann. N. Y. Acad. Sci. **608:** 318–329; 330–336 (discussion).
9. GOLDMAN-RAKIC, P. S., J. F. BATES & M. V. CHAFEE. 1992. The prefrontal cortex and internally generated motor acts. Curr. Opin. Neurobiol. **2:** 830–836.
10. QUINTANA, J. & J. M. FUSTER. 1993. Spatial and temporal factors in the role of prefrontal and parietal cortex in visuomotor integration. Cereb. Cortex **3:** 122–132.
11. PETRIDES, M., B. ALIVISATOS, A. C. EVANS & E. MEYER. 1993. Dissociation of human mid-dorsolateral from posterior dorsolateral frontal cortex in memory processing. Proc. Natl. Acad. Sci. USA **90:** 873–877.
12. FUSTER, J. M. 1993. Frontal lobes. Curr. Opin. Neurobiol. **3:** 160–165.
13. DiMATTIA, B. V., K. A. POSLEY & J. M. FUSTER. 1990. Crossmodal short-term memory of haptic and visual information. Neuropsychologia **28:** 17–33.
14. WILSON, F. A., S. P. SCALAIDHE & P. S. GOLDMAN-RAKIC. 1993. Dissociation of object and spatial processing domains in primate prefrontal cortex. Science **260:** 1955–1958.
15. KIMBERG, D. Y. & M. J. FARAH. 1993. A unified account of cognitive impairments following frontal lobe damage: The role of working memory in complex, organized behavior. J. Exp. Psychol. Gen. **122:** 411–428.
16. COHEN, J. D., S. D. FORMAN, T. S. BRAVER, B. J. CASEY, D. SERVAN-SCHREIBER & D. C. NOLL. 1994. Activation of the prefrontal cortex in a nonspatial working memory task with functional MRI. Hum. Brain Mapping **1:** 293–304.
17. HOLYOAK, K. J. & B. A. SPELLMAN. 1993. Thinking. Annu. Rev. Psychol. **44:** 265–213.
18. POSNER, M. 1994. Attention: The mechanisms of consciousness. Proc. Natl. Acad. Sci. USA **91:** 7398–7403.
19. POSNER, M. & S. DEHAENE. 1994. Attentional networks. Trends Neurosci. **17:** 75–79.
20. VENTRIGLIA, F. 1990. Activity in cortical-like neural systems: Short-range effects and attention phenomena. Bull. Math. Biol. **52:** 397–429.
21. ROBIN, N. & K. J. HOLYOAK. 1994. Relational complexity and the functions of prefrontal cortex. *In* The Cognitive Neurosciences. M. S. Gazzaniga, Ed.: 987–997. MIT Press. Cambridge, MA.
22. RUMELHART, D. E. & J. L. McCLELLAND. 1986. PDP models and general issues in cognitive science. *In* Parallel Distributed Processing: Explorations in the Microstructure of Cognition, Vol. 1. D. E. Rumelhart, J. L. McClelland & the PDP Research Group, Eds.: 110–146. MIT Press. Cambridge, MA.
23. FODOR, J. A. & Z. W. PYLYSHYN. 1988. Connectionism and cognitive architecture: A critical analysis. *In* Connections and Symbols. S. Pinker & J. Mehler, Eds.: 3–71. MIT Press. Cambridge, MA.
24. COHEN, J. D. & D. SERVAN-SCHREIBER. 1992. Context, cortex, and dopamine: A connectionist approach to behavior and biology in schizophrenia. Psychol. Rev. **99:** 45–77.
25. JANOWSKY, J. S., A. P. SHIMAMURA & L. R. SQUIRE. 1989. Source memory impairment in patients with frontal lobe lesions. Neuropsychologia **27:** 1043–1056.
26. SMITH, E. E., C. LANGSTON & R. E. NISBETT. 1992. The case for rules in reasoning. Cognit. Sci. **13:** 145–182.
27. BRESSLER, S., R. COPPOLA & R. NAKAMURA. 1993. Episodic multiregional cortical

coherence at multiple frequencies during visual task performance. Nature **366:** 153–156.

28. DESMEDT, J. & C. TOMBERG. 1994. Transient phase-locking of 40 Hz electrical oscillations in prefrontal and parietal human cortex reflects the process of conscious somatic perception. Neurosci. Lett. **168:** 126–129.

29. NEUENSCHWANDER, S. & F. VARELA. 1993. Visually triggered neuronal oscillations in the pigeon: An autocorrelation study of tectal activity. Eur. J. Neurosci. **5:** 870–881.

30. TOVEE, M. & E. ROLLS. 1992. Oscillatory activity is not evident in the primate temporal visual cortex with static stimuli. Neuroreport **3:** 369–372.

31. VAADIA, E., I. HAALMAN, M. ABELES, H. BERGMAN, Y. PRUT, H. SLOVIN & A. AERTSEN. 1995. Dynamics of neuronal interactions in monkey cortex in relation to behavioural events. Nature **373:** 515–518.

32. HUMMEL, J. E. & K. J. HOLYOAK. 1992. Indirect analogical mapping. *In* Proceedings of the Fourteenth Annual Conference of the Cognitive Science Society.: 516–521. Erlbaum. Hillsdale, NJ.

33. HUMMEL, J. E., E. R. MELZ, J. THOMPSON & K. J. HOLYOAK. 1994. Mapping hierarchical structures with synchrony for binding: Preliminary investigations. *In* Proceedings of the Sixteenth Annual Conference of the Cognitive Science Society. A. Ram & K. Eiselt, Eds.: 433–438. Erlbaum. Hillsdale, NJ.

34. HALFORD, G. S. 1993. Children's Understanding: The Development of Mental Models. Erlbaum. Hillsdale, NJ.

35. PREMACK, D. 1983. The codes of man and beasts. Behav. Brain Sci. **6:** 125–167.

36. GENTNER, D. 1983. Structure-mapping: A theoretical framework for analogy. Cognit. Sci. **7:** 155–170.

37. HOLYOAK, K. J. & P. THAGARD. 1995. Mental Leaps: Analogy in Creative Thought. MIT Press. Cambridge, MA.

38. GICK, M. L. & K. J. HOLYOAK. 1980. Analogical problem solving. Cogn. Psychol. **12:** 306–355.

39. NICHELLI, P., J. GRAFMAN, P. PIETRINI, K. CLARK, K. Y. LEE & R. MILETICH. 1995. Where the brain appreciates the moral of a story. In preparation.

40. GOLDSTONE, R. L., D. L. MEDIN & D. GENTNER. 1991. Relational similarity and the nonindependence of features in similarity judgments. Cogn. Psychol. **23:** 222–262.

41. MARKMAN, A. B. & D. GENTNER. 1993. Structural alignment during similarity comparisons. Cogn. Psychol. **23:** 431–467.

42. MEDIN, D. L., R. L. GOLDSTONE & D. GENTNER. 1993. Respects for similarity. Psychol. Rev. **100:** 254–278.

43. WASON, P. C. 1966. Reasoning. *In* New Horizons in Psychology. B. M. Foss, Ed. Vol. 1. Penguin. Harmondsworth, UK.

44. CHENG, P. W. & K. J. HOLYOAK. 1985. Pragmatic reasoning schemas. Cogn. Psychol. **17:** 391–416.

45. JOHNSON-LAIRD, P. N., P. LEGRENZI & S. M. LEGRENZI. 1972. Reasoning and a sense of reality. Br. J. Psychol. **63:** 395–400.

46. DAMASIO, A. R. 1995. Toward a neurobiology of emotion and feeling: Operational concepts and hypotheses. Neuroscientist **1:** 19–25.

47. SAVER, J. L. & A. R. DAMASIO. 1991. Preserved access and processing of social knowledge in a patient with acquired sociopathy due to ventromedial frontal damage. Neuropsychologia **29:** 1241–1249.

48. CHENG, P. W., K. J. HOLYOAK, R. E. NISBETT & L. M. OLIVER. 1986. Pragmatic versus syntactic approaches to training deductive reasoning. Cogn. Psychol. **18:** 293–328.

49. COSMIDES, L. 1989. The logic of social exchange: Has natural selection shaped how humans reason? Studies with the Wason selection task. Cognition **31:** 187–276.

50. KROGER, J. K., P. W. CHENG & K. J. HOLYOAK. 1993. Evoking the permission schema: The impact of explicit negation and a violation-checking context. Q. J. Exp. Psychol. **46A:** 615–635.

51. HOLYOAK, K. J. & P. W. CHENG. Pragmatic reasoning with a point of view. Thinking & Reasoning. In press.

52. MANKTELOW, K. I. & D. E. OVER. 1991. Social roles and utilities in reasoning with deontic conditionals. Cognition **39:** 85–105.
53. GIGERENZER, G. & K. HUG. 1992. Domain-specific reasoning: Social contracts, cheating, and perspective change. Cognition **43:** 127–171.
54. POLITZER, G. & A. NGUYEN-XUAN. 1992. Reasoning about promises and warnings: Darwinian algorithms, mental models, relevance judgments or pragmatic schemas? Q. J. Exp. Psychol. **44A:** 402–421.
55. DERRYBERRY, D. & D. M. TUCKER. 1990. The adaptive base of the neural hierarchy: Elementary motivational controls on network function. Nebr. Symp. Motiv. **38:** 289–342.

Types of Planning: Can Artificial Intelligence Yield Insights into Prefrontal Function?[a]

JAMES A. HENDLER

Department of Computer Science
University of Maryland
College Park, Maryland 20742

INTRODUCTION

The prefrontal cortex of the brain is a relatively recent evolutionary development, and well-developed frontal lobes are only observed in species high on the phylogenetic ladder—particularly in humans. In addition, in humans, the frontal lobes do not mature until well into the teenage years. Thus, there is reason to believe that the frontal lobes are an important center of human social and abstract thought. This has given rise to a very active neurobehavioral interest in studying the cognitive deficits and mood disorders that emerge subsequent to frontal lobe lesions.

Early research into frontal lobe disorders resulted primarily from anecdotal studies of patients suffering acute trauma, and from patients with psychiatric disorders resulting in neurosurgery—notably lobotomy and leukotomy. The brain damage resulting from such traumatic injuries or psychosurgery typically involved significant-sized lesions that destroyed large segments of the frontal lobes or, particularly in the case of psychosurgery, disconnected the frontal cortex from other brain regions. Nevertheless, the most striking observation was that many patients, following injury or psychosurgery, were able to continue to function in society although often with a noticeable amount of impairment, particularly mood dysregulation.[1]

More recent research has focused on more carefully controlled experimentation and comparison between patients with frontal lobe lesions and other population samples. Some of the important results show that frontal lesions result in:

- A pattern of impaired processing of temporal relations and order[2-4]
- A tendency towards inattention[5,6]
- Impairments in planning and problem solving[7-12]
- Trouble remembering the spatiotemporal contexts of episodic information[13]
- Only minor effects on standard memory tests, although some impairment of memory span and spatial location memory have been noted.[14,15]

[a] This research was supported in part by grants from NSF (IRI-9306580), ONR (N00014-J-91-1451), AFOSR (F49620-93-1-0065), the ARPA/Rome Laboratory Planning Initiative (F30602-93-C-0039), and the ARPA I3 Initiative (N00014-94-10907). J.A.H. is also affiliated with the University of Maryland Institute for Systems Research (NSF EEC 94-02384).

Perhaps the most important conclusion of these studies is that despite specific deficits, patients with frontal lobe lesions typically do quite well on conventional psychological tests. In addition, the effects seen under controlled experimentation were not intended to account for the social-behavioral disorders most often reported anecdotally by those living or working with the lesioned subjects. Based on these reports, it appears that patients with frontal lesions tend to appear abnormal primarily when required to maintain a behavioral or cognitive set. Of particular note in light of the problems with temporal and planning behaviors that have been observed in these subjects is a difficulty in the ability to proceed smoothly through an overlearned event (such as going shopping or eating in a restaurant).

Despite this large body of anecdotal and experimental evidence, no testable model of cognition has yet emerged that addresses the specific symptomology observed in patients with frontal lobe lesions. One important piece of work toward the development of such a model is that of Norman and Shallice[16–17] who proposed a cognitive model aimed at accounting for the neuropsychological data on human frontal lobe processing. Their model focused on the role of attention in retrieving information stored in the frontal lobes.

The Norman and Shallice model focused on the selection of memory schemata based on a contention scheduler that was supervised by an attentional system. Their model assumed that two different methods were used for selecting memory schemata to govern behavior: lower-level schemata were selected automatically via activation from specific environmental triggers whereas high-level schemata required a specific centralized supervisory system. It was assumed that information managed by the supervisory system included the knowledge needed to perform and monitor long-term planning.

Although this work provided an important starting point in explaining some of the deficits seen in patients with frontal lobe lesions, it did not actually present a testable model. In particular, the model of knowledge embodied in the schemata assumed by their model was only weakly determined. Although they opined that a knowledge structure such as the memory organization packages representation of Schank[18] could be used, no commitment was made. Thus, though perhaps viable as a model of explaining aspects of frontal function, their model didn't present a specific enough "planning" module to allow testing or a detailed enough account to explain neuropsychological effects.

Other neuropsychologists have attempted to develop models that would help to fill in some of the details in the Norman and Shallice model, or that functioned as competing theories. Grafman,[19,20] for example, has developed a model of knowledge representation known as Managerial Knowledge Units (MKUs) to account for the knowledge representation deficits of patients with frontal damage. In his model, he attempts to account for various aspects of human planning behavior that must be present in any explanation of frontal processing. In particular, he argues that a representation of planning knowledge that could be used by a supervisory (or managerial) "executive" must have the following features:

- A memory of complex planning information that is used in guiding long-term behavior
- Hierarchically ordered schemata that are used to represent this information

- Activation effects that occur both in the choice of the memory schemata to use and in monitoring the processing during the execution of those schemata
- Schemata processing that is activated and/or effected by environmental stimuli
- A model in which multiple schemata with differing temporal extents can be active in parallel.

Interestingly, at a very different end of the research spectrum—that of artificial intelligence research—models of problem solving that met Grafman's criteria were being explored. Researchers in this field, often unmotivated by cognitive issues, were rejecting earlier, more formal models of planning, arguing that more complex systems were needed to get robots (simulated or real) to display useful competences in complex, natural environments. This emerging part of the field of artificial intelligence (AI) is focused on trying to explain the processing requirements that are encumbent upon "agents" that are trying to function while embedded in a dynamic (changing) environment. Although these models are not at the point where they directly address neuropsychology, they may provide a fruitful starting place for researchers interested in exploring more detailed models of frontal functioning.

In the remainder of this paper, background on the AI considerations in the field of planning that led to these new models and discussion of one such model—a planning model developed at the University of Maryland in the thesis of Lee Spector are provided. This model is presented as a "point of departure" for interested neuropsychologists, and my motivation in presenting this paper is the hope that a synergism between such AI models and the prescriptive models of neuropsychology could lead to a new understanding and deeper modeling of human frontal processing. Indeed, several promising starts have been made along these lines.[21,22]

ARTIFICIAL INTELLIGENCE PLANNING—A BRIEF HISTORICAL RETROSPECTIVE

In AI terminology, *planning* is simply defined as designing the behavior of some entity that acts—either an individual, a group, or an organization. The output is some kind of blueprint for behavior, which we call a *plan*. People make a lot of plans, sometimes for themselves, sometimes for other people, sometimes for machines. The question that defines the topic for AI people is, How can we automate planning? Although for some the motivation is that automating planning might shed light on how people and other animals design their behaviors, for more of the AI community the focus has been on helping humans to solve complex planning problems with the aid of computers.

When planning research started in the late 1950s, it was formulated as the process of producing an ordered sequence of actions that would, starting in some particular state of the world, produce some desired "goal" state. This led to a formalization of planning which (1) assumes plans are sequences of actions, (2) assumes the purpose of a plan is solely to bring about a situation satisfying a particular description, and (3) treats the outcome of every action as perfectly predictable. These assumptions essentially define what is now called *classical planning*.

Classical planning is largely derived from work in the area of theorem proving. As early as 1960, John McCarthy proposed the use of predicate-calculus reasoning to guide intelligent behavior, and the first big realization of this idea was Green's[23] program QA3, which solved a variety of simple problems expressed in predicate calculus. Among them was a set of planning problems, expressed in terms of McCarthy's *situation calculus* in which axioms about what actions led to what situations were used to deduce action sequences. These axioms embodied assumptions equivalent to those above. Unfortunately, just turning a theorem prover loose on the axioms led to a search problem that was hard to solve. Theorem provers look for chains of inferences that lead to conclusions, and these chains are only indirectly related to the chains of action we are interested in.

In 1969, the AI group at Stanford Research Institute in Palo Alto, California, found a way to get the best of this approach while avoiding many of the weaknesses. This group devised a system worked directly from action definitions stated in a form similar to that of the situation calculus.[24] Each action was defined in terms of its *preconditions* and *effects,* stated as predicate-calculus atomic formulas. The action definition was used to *edit* situation descriptions instead of *deducing* them as required. This problem solver was called STRIPS (STanford Research Institute Problem Solver). It was able to solve bigger problems than previous approaches and was used as the planner for a robot named Shakey.[25]

Starting in the mid-1970s, the field of planning shifted away from some of the main commitments in STRIPS, initially for the purpose of improving search control and later to allow for the solution of nonclassical planning problems. The new approach was seen in two influential programs: NOAH[26] and NONLIN[27] These programs explored a search space of *partial plans,* collections of plan steps that achieved some of the goals in the problem statement. In these planners, the plan steps did not have to be kept in a linear order, and thus they have often been referred to as "nonlinear."

By coincidence, systems based on the approach used in STRIPS were attacked with more theoretical rigor than the "nonlinear" systems. In fact, as often happens in AI, theoretical rigor seemed inversely proportional to practical applicability. Descendants of NONLIN and NOAH, especially Wilkins's SIPE system,[28] were attempts to build software systems that could be applied to real problems. So they included a lot of tools for handling user interaction, knowledge representation, inference, and so on. Thus, although the work in STRIPS-style planning produced a series of theorems about search techniques, these theorems did not seem to have much bearing on the behavior of practical systems.

The disillusionment with the gap between theory and practice led to the exploration of a wide variety of new approaches that were aimed at extending the classical framework. In addition, an influential paper by Chapman[29] was published that attempted to synthesize a number of existing approaches, and to show that classical planning problems could be undecidable in many situations. These factors led to the exploration of a number of new approaches that attempted to go beyond the classical framework. Techniques included the use of memory-based approaches,[30,31] activation spreading,[32] temporal reasoning,[33] simulation and debugging,[34] and plan reuse.[35] Other work attempted to repudiate the classical approach and to work without explicit goal-based planning. People in the field talked about the "death of the classical planning framework," and the planning community flourished as exciting new approaches were debated.

In fact, classical planning refused to die, and it continues as the primary thrust in the traditional AI literature. New algorithms have been developed that prove to be "sound" and "complete" under the classical assumptions, and these have been made both more efficient and more expressive. Thus, the neuropsychological researcher approaching today's planning literature is likely to find it full of complex mathematics and many Greek symbols, with little discussion of the use of memory or dynamic effects. However, the strands that grew out of this tradition in the mid- and late 1980s are also active today, and we argue that they can be the basis of a potentially fruitful cooperation between the AI scientist and the neuropsychologist.

ARTIFICIAL INTELLIGENCE INTRODUCES "INTELLIGENT AGENTS"

As stated above, in the mid-1980s, many researchers were becoming dissatisfied with the classical assumptions about planning. One often-cited argument was that the field had originated in attempts to find plans for robots, but, in fact, robots do not satisfy the classical assumptions at all well. As robots must survive in environments that are changing and imperfectly known, they must constantly sense their surroundings and react to what they perceive. In these conditions, it does not seem reasonable to model behavior as a predictable sequence of actions. In fact, a whole new breed of robots that repudiated the notion of symbolic planning was being developed at the Massachusetts Institute of Technology (MIT).[36] In the mid-1980s, a number of approaches to planning in dynamically changing worlds were explored, and papers by Agre and Chapman,[37] Georgeff and Lansky,[38] Kaelbling and Rosenschein,[39] Sanborn and Hendler,[40] Firby,[41] and others developed models of planning agents that could function in dynamically changing environments. Oversimplifying somewhat, one can look at all these approaches as attempting to create agents that could react by direct coupling of sensing (stimulus) to effecting (response). In most of this work the design was carried out by humans. The more complex the behaviors got, the harder it became to design them automatically.

In addition to the design problems, a second issue became clear. Although these new models had the ability to deal with changing worlds, they were unable to demonstrate the sorts of "intelligent" behavior that the researchers desired. The low-level actions tended to function without the guidance of longer-term goals, and at the risk of anthropomorphizing, the programs tended to reproduce the functions of lower animals. Thus, instead of "intelligent agents" the field seemed to be building "robotic cockroaches," an interesting pursuit in its own right, but not the one AI planners largely wished to follow. This work was also a major contributor to the burgeoning field of "artificial life," and many approaches such as genetic algorithms and neural networks have been tested and refined in the area of agents that react to environmental change.

The failing of these approaches has led to a trend which tries to couple the strengths of classical planning (the ability to project into the future) with those of reacting (the ability to handle dynamicity and unexpected events). This has led to a variety of "multilevel" planning approaches, several of which have been shown to be useful with simulated and/or real robots. To present a general overview of this field would be well beyond the limits of this paper. Instead, we will present one such system, which we believe emphasizes many of the potentially interesting features of "multilevel" planning approaches. (Overviews and discussion of related work can be found in works by Gat[42] and Spector.[43])

The Abstraction-Partitioned Evaluator

One system which demonstrates the integration of reaction and deliberation via a multilevel approach is work performed in the ParalleL Understanding Systems (PLUS) Laboratory at the University of Maryland. In particular, the thesis of Dr. Lee Spector, now at Hampshire College, involved the implementation of a planning system (called APE, for Abstraction-Partitioned Evaluator) which can merge reaction and deliberation in a number of tasks, particularly the control of a simulated robot operating in a complex household task domain.

APE was based on some important computational considerations. For example, it has long been recognized that an AI system can profit from the division of its computational components into relatively independent modules and from the decomposition of its knowledge into relatively disjoint areas of expertise. Systems partitioned in this manner exhibit several desirable characteristics, including parallelizability, improved program comprehensibility, and significant reductions in the size of problem-solving search spaces. Although these and other virtues of such "abstraction-based" modularization were well known, little work had been done on providing such a strong partitioning in the planning domain.

We felt that the need for an abstraction-based model became clear as one examined issues related to planning in complex and changing domains. Because many of the reasoning processes used in early AI systems have exponential complexity, they quickly become impractical as domains become more realistic (and hence larger). Additionally, as mentioned previously, events in the world continue to occur while an agent is thinking and acting, and the agent's reasoning processes must be capable of accommodating a changing, usually only semipredictable world. It was clear to us that multilevel architectures, if employed properly, could help handle such problems. The modularity of partitioned systems mitigates against combinatorial complexity, and hierarchical organization is a powerful tool for obtaining real-time behavior particularly in low-level robotics control.[44] To realize this partitioning, our system was based on an advanced blackboard system architecture to provide a mechanism for integrating knowledge about multiple facets of the world in a computationally viable way.

The multilevel architecture used in APE provided for the direct coupling of sensation to action only at the lowest level of the system. Thus, the lowest levels could provide basic "competencies" without the intervention of higher, more complex levels. On the other hand, the architecture allowed for the higher levels to receive their knowledge of the world via the lower levels of the system, and also permitted higher levels to pass commands for action through to the lower levels. An abstract architecture was designed to allow any combination of levels to be hooked up in certain ways, but one particular model proved extremely useful and I will focus on that for the remainder of this paper. In particular, the levels for APE were chosen on the basis of an analysis of the general structure of event-related knowledge, as exposed in the philosophical and psychological literature. (A detailed discussion of the motivations for this choice of levels can be found in Spector's thesis[43]).

The levels used in APE, from lowest to highest, are: perceptual/manual, spatial, temporal, causal, and conventional. A linear order is imposed on the levels, but representations must sometimes be passed through intervening levels. The perceptual/manual level represents events as simple sensory reports and as operators for effector manipulation. Perceptual/manual representations might be rendered in English as "I see a sock at position 12, 17, 26, at time 3:45 P.M." or "To move forward, I should gain control of the main body motor, run it forward, and check to see that I've moved." The only "reasoning" at this level is the composition of such sequences of perceptual and manual tasks. The coupling of perception to action that results is in some ways analogous to simple "reflex arcs" in animals. Note that although spatial and temporal data is *present* at this level, reasoning *about* space and time occurs elsewhere.

The spatial level contains structures that organize perceptual data with respect to spatial relations. Synthetic spatial relations such as *on, above, near,* etc., arise at this level, and hence representations such as "The cat is on the mat" become expressible. At the perceptual/manual level this would be represented only as the conjunction of two sensory reports: one describing the position of the cat and one describing the position of the mat. Representations about events and actions that *change* the status of spatial relations (for example, "I put the banana peel into the trash can at 12:15 P.M.") are expressible here, but the temporal and causal dimensions of such changes are not the subjects of spatial level reasoning. Operators for complex spatial reasoning (for example, path planning) *do* reside here.

The temporal level augments spatial representations with temporal relations, allowing for reasoning about deadlines and temporal projection. New concepts at this level include synthetic temporal relations such as *before, during,* and *after,* and other concepts specific to temporal reasoning such as *expect, delay,* and *late.* Although every level represents time in some manner (and certainly every level acts *in* time), only at the temporal level do representations such as "The chicken has been in the oil too long" arise. Lower levels simply tag representations with temporal information and perform actions as quickly as they can. It is at the temporal level that the system can reason *about* time, scheduling actions to meet deadlines.

The causal level contains representations that embody the agent's conception of the causal structure of the world. This may include causal rules and causally deduced facts such as "I prevented the human from falling." At this level concepts that are defined on the basis of causal models of the world are introduced; for example, *cause, effect, boil,* and *melt.* Although the representation of a melting of an ice cube might be represented at the temporal level as a conjunction of observations or predictions about the relative sizes of the cube and of the resulting puddle over time, at the causal level there may be a *melt* concept that is integrated into a theory of temperatures, state changes, etc. (representing, for example, the fact that heat causes the melting to occur).

The conventional level contains knowledge about facts that are true by convention; for example, that a certain hand gesture is a signal for a turn, or that a dirty sock "belongs" in the dirty clothes hamper. Procedures at this level should embody some theory of social rules and interaction. For example, the knowledge that it is *impolite* to leave the room when being addressed might be encoded here.

These levels partition the system's knowledge (both declarative and procedural) into a set of connected, communicating systems, each of which exhibits expertise at a particular level of "abstraction" from the world. Note that this is *not* to say that the representations characteristic of one level are entirely absent from all other levels. As mentioned earlier, for example, temporal representations exist at all levels of the system, even though explicit reasoning *about* time occurs only at the temporal level. Similar statements can be made for the other levels as well.

To see the need for all of this mechanism, consider the following problem which is referred to as the "Ice Cube Problem." We imagine a household-cleaning robot in the midst of a routine household chore (putting a dirty sock into the laundry). An ice cube is on the floor in the middle of a room, and at some point it is seen by the robot. The assumption of a built-in "ice cube reaction rule" is problematic; ice cubes do not always present problems, and any reaction rule that checks all contextual circumstances to determine if there *is* a problem upon each sighting of an ice cube would be computationally complex if constructible at all. We therefore assume that no such rule exists, and hence we can expect no immediate response to the sighting of the cube. Assuming that the robot has sufficient causal knowledge to infer that the ice cube will melt over time, however, and assuming that it can also infer that puddles may be dangerous (since people tend to slip in them), it would be appropriate for the robot to *eventually* make such inferences and to alter its behavior accordingly. The robot should then suspend work on its current task, take care of the potential safety hazard, and then resume the original task with as little replanning as possible.

The details of how the robot would handle such problems are myriad, and there is insufficient space for them in this paper. Complete details of the ice cube problem, as well as several others, can be found in the work of Spector and Hendler,[45] as can details of the computational apparatus used to implement such as system. For now, what I wish to point out is that we proposed a model in which many kinds of knowledge must function together in solving problems. Higher knowledge about the world (for example, where dirty socks go) and expectations of behavior (it is good to clean up hazards) interact with perceptual clues (I see an ice cube), temporal reasoning (I must clean up the ice cube before it melts), and low-level competences (move forward to approach where the ice cube is). The multiple levels, functioning in parallel, allow the integration of these capabilities and provide a model that can solve "knowledge-rich" problems without giving up the reactive (low-level) competences.

CAN APE MEET MAN? ONWARD TO A SYNERGY OF NEUROPSYCHOLOGY AND ARTIFICIAL INTELLIGENCE PLANNING

As should be clear from the above discussion, the APE planning system was not primarily motivated by neuropsychological issues. The need for multiple levels was based on computational requirements; the choice of levels, although somewhat influenced by cognitive concerns, was mainly derived from the literature of artificial intelligence; and the architecture of the system was based on the needs of solving certain problem classes with no regard for neuroscience and brain structure. Why then can I argue that this work should be of interest to neuropsychologists?

First, it should be noted that the multilevel systems, such as APE, seem to have certain resemblances to the Norman and Shallice model discussed in the INTRODUCTION. As I pointed out there, their model assumed that a range of memory schemata existed that were, essentially, competing for supervision by an attentional system. Two methods were used for selecting among these schemata: lower-level schemata were selected automatically via activation from specific environmental triggers whereas higher-level schemata required a specific centralized supervisory system. It was assumed that information managed by the supervisory system included the knowledge needed to perform and monitor long-term planning.

This can also be said of AI models like APE. Notice that in our program, stimulus from the environment (sight of the ice cube) feeds only to the lowest level (perceptual/manual competences). However, a higher-level "planner" is used to manage the top-level goals of the system, residing in the so-called conventional level. The lower-level behaviors are effected by the higher-level control, but they are also effected by information flowing up from the lower levels; reflexive actions can occur, but their results are propagated up. Thus, the control systems explored by neuropsychologists may have a dual in the control regime prescribed by the AI scientists. Many differences are found in the details of these levels (APE could not be directly plugged into the neuropsychological model without much work), but there are also striking similarities.

So too are their similarities with Grafman's MKU work (also discussed in the INTRODUCTION). In fact, here the similarities are striking. Reviewing the requirements for planning knowledge dictated by Grafman's neuropsychological work, we see these all arising in the APE model. To wit,

- Grafman's model demands a memory of complex planning information that is used in guiding long-term behavior; APE encodes this directly in the higher level schemata.
- Grafman requests hierarchically ordered schemata that are used to represent this information; APE directly models this in its multilevel approach.
- Grafman describes schemata processing that is activated and/or affected by environmental stimuli. APE was designed to permit environmental change (like the unexpected appearance of the ice cube) to effect the high-level schematas causing them to be temporarily set aside (as happens to the dirty sock task during handling the ice cube) or indefinitely suspended.
- The MKU model assumes that multiple schemata with differing temporal extents must be active in parallel. APE provides parallel processing of planning knowledge across a wide range of schemata some which last for short times, others which span longer intervals. In addition, the multiple level approach allows several competing "dominant" schemas to cooperate in

use of low-level competences for problem solving, again similar to the approach used in the MKU model.

- Finally, Grafman expects activation effects that occur both in the choice of the memory schemata to use and in monitoring the processing during the execution of those schemata. In APE, it is exactly such mechanisms that provide the information flow (although in a slightly more symbolic form than expected by Grafman), although these details were not discussed in this paper.

Again, however, I caution that these similarities, although encouraging, are not in themselves sufficient to let us claim that the AI models are themselves neuropsychologically plausible models. There are many differences in implementation, representation, and supervisory control that need to be explored and resolved before serious testable models could be developed. However, it is clear that interesting parallels exist between these models. In fact, I would say these parallels are significantly more striking than the similarities with the so-called neurobiologically plausible models espoused by many in the neural networks community.

It is hoped that this short paper may help others to better understand the AI literature and to begin the pursuit of models that can be constrained both by our knowledge of neuropsychology and our knowledge of the information processing constraints on planning systems—including the human planner.

SUMMARY

In this paper, some of the features of models of planning emerging from the area of artificial intelligence (AI) are explored. The goal of this exposition is to explain how researchers are getting machines to attack problems that appear to be similar to those handled in the human prefrontal cortex. In particular, I tried to explain some of the features of AI models that might help explain how planned behavior can occur, with an eye toward examining the specific information-processing constraints necessary for computational models of planning. I described how some AI researchers are converging on a model in which (1) a memory of complex planning information is used in guiding long-term behavior, (2) hierarchically ordered schemata are used to represent this information, (3) activation spreading-like effects occur both in the choice of the memory schemata to use and in monitoring the processing during the execution of those schemata, (4) schemata processing is activated and/or affected by environmental stimuli, and (5) multiple schemata with differing temporal extent are active in parallel. A specific AI planning model, developed in conjunction with Dr. Lee Spector of Hampshire College, was also presented; it was shown how it uses the features above to give rise to interesting planning behaviors for robotic systems.

ACKNOWLEDGMENTS

Portions of this paper come from proposals and/or unpublished manuscripts that contained contributions by Jordan Grafman, Lee Spector, and Drew McDermott.

REFERENCES

1. STUSS, D. & D. BENSON. 1984. Neuropsychological studies of the frontal lobes. Psychol. Bull. **95:** 3–28.
2. DUNCAN, J. 1986. Disorganization of behavior after frontal lobe damage. Cogn. Neuropsychol. **3:** 271–290.
3. MILNER, B., M. PETRIDES & M. SMITH. 1985. Frontal lobes and the temporal organization of memory. Hum. Neurobiol. **4:** 137–142.
4. PETRIDES, M. 1985. Deficits on conditional associative-learning tasks after frontal and temporal lobe lesions in man. Neuropsychologia **23:** 601–614.
5. SALMASO, D. & G. DENES. 1982. Role of the frontal lobes on an attention task: A signal detection analysis Percept. Mot. Skills **54:** 1147–1150.
6. WARRINGTON, E. 1985. A disconnection analysis of amnesia. Ann. N.Y. Acad. Sci. **444:** 72–77.
7. MILNER, B. 1963. Effects of different brain lesions on card sorting. Arch. Neurol. **9:** 90–100.
8. MILNER, B. 1964. Behavioral effects of frontal lobectomy in man. *In* The Frontal Granular Cortex and Behavior. J. Warren & K. Akert, Eds. McGraw-Hill. New York.
9. GOLDING, E. 1981. The effects of unilateral brain lesions on reasoning. Cortex **17:** 31–40.
10. CICERONE, K., R. LAZAR & W. SHAPIRO. 1983. Effects of frontal lesions on hypothesis sampling during concept formation. Neuropsychologia **21:** 513–524
11. SHALLICE, T. & M. EVANS. 1978. The involvement of the frontal lobes in cognitive estimation. Cortex **14:** 294–303.
12. SHALLICE, T. 1982. Specific impairments of planning. Philos. Trans. R. Soc. Lond. Med. Ser. **B298:** 199–209.
13. SCHACTER, D. 1987. Memory, amnesia, and frontal lobe dysfunctions. Psychobiology **15:** 21–36.
14. GHENT, L., J. MISHKIN & H. TEUBER. 1962. Short-term memory after frontal lobe injury in man J. Comp. Physiol. Psychol. **55:** 705–709.
15. STUSS, D., E. KAPLAN, D. F. BENSON, W. S. WEIR, S. CHIULLI & F. F. SARAZIN. 1982. Evidence for the involvement of orbitofrontal cortex in memory functions: An interference effect. J. Comp. Physiol. Psychol. **6:** 913–925.
16. NORMAN, D. & T. SHALLICE. 1982. Attention to action: Willed and automatic control of behavior. Tech. Rep. No. 99. Center for Human Information Processing. University of California, San Diego CA.
16A. NORMAN, D. & T. SHALLICE. 1986. *In* Consciousness and Self Regulation: Advances in Research, Vol. IV. R. J. Davidson, G. E. Schwartz & D. Shapiro, Eds. Plenum Press. New York.
17. SHALLICE, T. 1988. From Neuropsychology to Mental Structure. Cambridge University Press. Cambridge, UK.
18. SCHANK, R. 1982. Dynamic Memory. Cambridge University Press. Cambridge, UK.
19. GRAFMAN, J. 1989. Plans, Actions and Mental Sets: The Role of the Frontal Lobes. *In* Integrating Theory and Practice in Clinical Neuropsychology. E. Perecman, Ed.: 93–138. Lawrence Erlbaum Associates. Hillsdale, NJ.
20. GRAFMAN, J. 1991. Script generation as an indicator of knowledge representation in patients with Alzheimer's disease. Brain Lang. **40:** 344–358.
21. SPECTOR, L. & J. GRAFMAN. 1994. Planning, neuropsychology, and artificial intelligence: Cross-fertilization. in F. Boller & J. Grafman, Eds. Handbook of Neuropsychology, Vol. 9: 377–392. Elsevier, North-Holland. Amsterdam.
22. GRAFMAN, J., A. SIRIGU, L. SPECTOR & J. HENDLER. 1993. Damage to the prefrontal cortex leads to decomposition of structured event complexes. J. Head Trauma Rehabil. **8(1):** 73–87.
23. GREEN, C. 1969. The application of theorem proving to question-answering systems. PhD thesis. Stanford University, Stanford, CA.
24. FIKES, R. & N. NILSSON. 1971. Strips: A new approach to the application of theorem proving to problem solving. Artif. Intel. **5:** 189–208.

25. FIKES, R., P. HART & N. NILSSON. 1972. Learning and executing generalized robot plans. Artif. Intel. 3(4).
26. SACERDOTI, E. 1977. A Structure for Plans and Behavior. American Elsevier Publishing Company, Inc., New York.
27. TATE, A. 1977. Generating project networks. Proc. Int. J. Conf. AI 5: 888–893.
28. WILKINS, D. 1988. Practical Planning: Extending the Classical AI Planning Paradigm. Morgan Kaufmann Publishers. San Francisco, CA.
29. CHAPMAN, D. 1985. Planning for conjunctive goals. Tech. Rep. 802. MIT AI Lab. Cambridge, MA.
30. ALTERMAN, R. 1988. Adaptive planning. Cogn. Sci. 12:
31. HAMMOND, K. 1990. Explaining and repairing plans that fail. Artif. Intel. 45(1–2): 173–228.
32. HENDLER, J. 1987. Integrating marker-passing and problem solving: A spreading activation approach to improved choice in planning. Lawrence Erlbaum Associates. Hillsdale, NJ.
33. DEAN, R. & D. MCDERMOTT. 1987. Temporal data base management. Artif. Intel. 32(1):
34. SIMMONS, R. 1992. The roles of associational and causal reasoning in problem solving. Artif. Intel. 53(2–3): 159–208.
35. KAMBHAMPATI, S. & J. HENDLER. 1992. A validation structure based theory of plan modification and reuse. Artif. Intel. 54: 1–65.
36. BROOKS, R. 1986. A robust layered control system for a mobile robot. IEEE J. Robotics Automation RA-2:
37. AGRE, P. & D. CHAPMAN. 1987. Pengi: An implementation of a theory of activity. Proc. Am. Assoc. AI 6: 268–272.
38. GEORGEFF, M. & A. LANSKY. 1986. Procedural knowledge. Proc. IEEE Spec. Issue on Knowledge Representation 74(10).
39. KAELBLING, L. & S. ROSENSCHEIN. 1990. Action and planning in embedded agents. In New Architectures for Autonomous Agents: Task-level Decomposition and Emergent Functionality. P. Maes, Ed. MIT Press. Cambridge, MA.
40. SANBORN, J. & J. HENDLER. 1988. Monitoring and reacting: Planning in dynamic domains. Int. J. AI Eng. 3(2): 95–102.
41. FIRBY, R. 1987. An investigation into reactive planning in complex domains. Proc. Am. Assoc. AI 6.
42. GAT, E. 1991. Reliable goal-directed reactive control of autonomous mobile robots. PhD thesis. Virginia Polytechnic Institute and State University. Blacksburg, VA.
43. SPECTOR, L. 1992. Supervenience in dynamic-world planning. PhD thesis. Dept. Computer Science, University of Maryland. College Park, MD.
44. ALBUS, J. 1991. Outline for a theory of intelligence. IEEE Trans. on Systems, Man, and Cybernetics 21.
45. SPECTOR, L. & J. HENDLER. 1992. Planning and control across supervenient levels of representation. I. J. Intel. Cooperat. Inf. Sys. 1(3–4): 411–449.

Planning and Script Analysis following Prefrontal Lobe Lesions[a]

ANGELA SIRIGU,[b,c] TIZIANA ZALLA,[b,d] BERNARD PILLON,[b]
JORDAN GRAFMAN,[e] BRUNO DUBOIS,[b] AND YVES AGID[b]

[b]INSERM U289
Hôpital de la Salpêtrière
Paris, France

[d]CREA
Ecole Polytechnique
Paris, France

[e]Cognitive Neuroscience Section
National Institutes of Health
Bethesda, Maryland

INTRODUCTION

Everyday life activities are directed, implicitly or explicitly, toward the achievement of specific goals. They often involve extended sequences of actions that are temporally and hierarchically organized. In order for these sequences to be executed in a smooth and coordinated manner, the mind must anticipate the future course of actions and events. In short, our behavior must be guided by a *plan*. This paper will focus on two main questions: How are plans represented in the brain? and What is the role of the frontal lobes in planning?

Although it is a common observation that patients with damage to the frontal lobes often experience considerable difficulties in managing and planning common everyday situations,[1–4] it is not clear yet what the role of the frontal cortex is in representing and organizing complex action schemas. What are the neuropsychologically relevant dimensions of planning and how are they represented in the frontal lobes? Is the frontal cortex involved in the actual storage of plans? Do the prefrontal areas essentially control and monitor the execution of action sequences or do they intervene in the early stages of plan elaboration? Do they play a more important role in dealing with novel tasks[5] than in highly familiar situations where well-rehearsed routines can be applied?

In the two studies[6,7] that will be reviewed here, the planning abilities of patients with selective lesions in the prefrontal cortex were analyzed in terms of the information processing taking place while a plan of action is being formulated. The view presented is that frontal lesions cause impairments of the knowledge necessary for

[a] This research was supported by the European Community Human Capital and Mobility fellowship to A.S.

[c] Address correspondence to Dr. Angela Sirigu, INSERM Unité 289, Hôpital de la Salpêtrière, 47, Boulevard de l'Hôpital, 75013 Paris, France.

assembling a plan, independent of any executive impairment in carrying it through its execution. Two main arguments in favor of this hypothesis are that (1) although frontal subjects have intact access to contextual information used in planning a sequence of actions, they fail to appreciate the temporal order of actions and their importance with respect to a given objective; and (2) they are impaired at verifying the internal consistency of an action sequence and in maintaining clear boundaries between distinct sequences.

The theoretical framework adopted for analyzing planning impairments postulates that event and action sequences can be represented in memory in the form of mental entities, which we refer to as *scripts*.[8-12] Grafman[13,14] has proposed that the frontal cortex is involved in the neural representation of script-like structures that serve as vehicles for representing complex acts. The following description attempts to outline the main features of the script concept.

Two aspects of a script can be distinguished a priori: syntax and contents. Scripts have a relatively simple syntax which represents a succession of events bounded by an initial state (an internal or external trigger) and by a final state (corresponding to the achievement of a goal). Individual acts are thus primarily defined by their position in a sequence, but other dimensions can be important as well. Different actions have different priority levels because not all actions in a script are equally important. For example, when getting up in the morning and preparing to go to work, one can skip breakfast if running late, but can hardly omit getting dressed. The strength of the representation of an action sequence can vary, from highly frequent sequences with a low activation threshold to rarely performed sequences, which sometimes must be assembled anew, probably drawing upon analogical representations to help one process on-line schemas. How often an action is executed in a particular context and how instrumental it is in bringing about a desired result will jointly determine the strength of the representation of this action in a plan. How often it is performed at a particular point in the sequence will determine how strongly its temporal order in the plan is represented. Thus, there can be a continuum of familiarity, from highly rehearsed routines to unfamiliar or novel plans with corresponding determinate sequential progressions.[13,14]

The informational structure or contents of a script is similar to what can be found in associative networks and refers to spatial and temporal contextual elements, sometimes in the form of external trigger events, self-initiated actions, or the consequences of prior actions. Elements of scripts are thought to be related to one another much like items of a semantic network, with various degrees of association strength. An action that takes place with high frequency in a given context will appear "semantically closer" to the central theme, that is, it will be activated faster, at a lower threshold, than a rarely performed one. The strength of association between an action and a "goal" determines how prototypical that action is for a given script.[10]

SCRIPT KNOWLEDGE IN PATIENTS WITH FRONTAL LOBE DAMAGE

In a first study of script knowledge,[6] we analyzed the performance of patients with frontal lobes lesions, all of whom had focal lesions predominating in the anterior medial and dorsolateral prefrontal regions. These patients were compared with patients with lesions of the posterior cortical regions and normal controls on performance in a script generation task. Subjects were requested to evoke, without any time limits, as many actions as possible belonging to a particular action theme. Before starting they were shown a cue card containing the theme header, a starting point, and an end point. Following the generation phase, the subjects had to rank the actions in the correct order of their execution. Finally, they rated the importance of each action with respect to the script's stated goal on a 5-point rating scale from "least important" to "most important." The complete procedure was performed for three themes differing in degree of familiarity: preparing to go to work ("routine"), taking a trip to Mexico ("non-routine"), opening a beauty salon ("novel").

Some similarities as well as some remarkable differences were observed between the frontal subjects and the other two groups. The first set of results concerned the number of actions generated and the speed at which they were named. The second variable was included because, as no time limit was imposed, different subjects could produce the same number of actions but employ different amounts of time to do so. No differences between the three subject groups were found in either total number of actions or evocation speed (FIG. 1A and B). There were differences in the rapidity of access to actions from the routine, non-routine, and novel conditions in all groups (FIG. 1B), which seem to validate the role of familiarity in the ability to evoke script information.

The distribution of actions along a gradient of centrality was examined by assigning each action evoked by normal subjects a coefficient of frequency that corresponded to the proportion of subjects who evoked that action. The frequency distribution that was thus obtained showed that a small number of actions (generally less than 10) were evoked by a large majority of subjects. These can be considered the most central or *prototypical* actions for this script (FIG. 2). Frequency scores were obtained in a similar manner within the posterior and the frontal groups. In order to compare the distributions obtained in the three groups, correlations between those distributions were computed. Consistently high correlation coefficients were obtained for the three types of activities (ranging from .79 to .93), implying that the same actions tended to be evoked with the same relative frequency in normals, posteriors, and frontals.

This first set of results thus indicates that the size of the information domain, the speed of access to it, and the content that is retrieved seem to be quite similar for frontal patients, posterior patients, and normal controls. The information necessary for evoking and assembling a plan of action is therefore not impaired following frontal lesions. Contrasting results were obtained concerning the organization of script information, which was reflected in three variables: (1) Number of *out-of-sequence* actions. These were determined independently by three judges asked to score as a sequence error both a physically impossible ordering (e.g., drinking coffee before preparing it) and an illogical ordering (e.g., preparing an inauguration party for the beauty salon before constructing it). (2) Number of *boundary* errors, defined as either a failure to reach the stated end point of the script (early closure) or failure to stop at the end point (late closure). (3) Priority setting, assessed through subjective judgments of action importance.

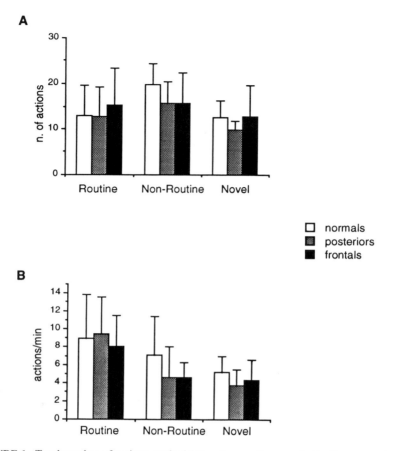

FIGURE 1. Total number of actions evoked (**A**) and evocation speed of actions per minute (**B**) in normal subjects and posterior and frontal patients and for the three type of activities (routine, non-routine, novel).

The results showed that none of the posterior patients or normal subjects made any errors of script sequence or script boundaries. In contrast, the majority of patients with frontal lesions committed both types of errors (sequence, 80%; boundary, 70%). Boundary errors were mostly of the early closure type. The histogram in FIG. 3 shows the mean number of sequence errors in frontal patients and a tendency for an increase in the number of such errors with decreasing familiarity. Most of these errors were of the logical type.

Judgments of priority level were obtained by asking subjects to rate each action on a 5-point rating scale from "least important" to "absolutely essential." The data were analyzed for all actions that were reported by 60% or more of the subjects in each group. Eleven of the 15 actions thus selected showed significant

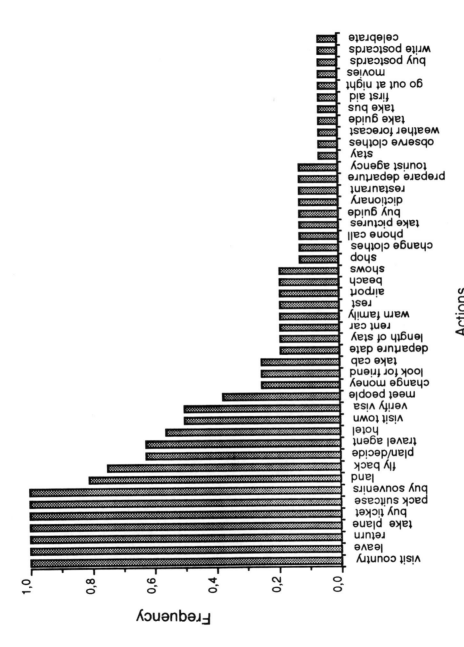

FIGURE 2. Frequency distribution of actions in normal subjects for the non-routine activity.

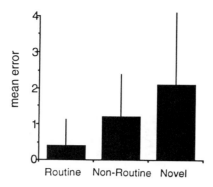

FIGURE 3. Mean number of sequence errors in frontal patients for each script. Error bars are equal to one standard deviation. (From Sirigu *et al.*[6] Reprinted with permission from *Cortex.*)

group differences in mean action importance. Judgments made by frontal patients systematically deviated from those made by posteriors and normals, who did not differ from each other. For example, frontals gave relatively low priority to "packing suitcase," whereas they overestimated the importance of buying souvenirs with respect to the other two groups of subjects (FIG. 4). Incidentally, the fact that normal subjects give a relatively low priority rating to a prototypical script element indicates that action frequency and action importance are not equivalent dimensions. An action can be evoked by a large number of subjects, making it a prototypical script event, even when it is not highly instrumental in achieving a desired objective. Similar patterns of underestimation or overestimation were found for the other scripts as well.

SCRIPT SORTING AND ORDERING

In a second study,[7] the ability of frontal lobe patients to analyze action sequences in terms of their internal organization or syntax was further investigated with tasks using standardized script material. We tested the same groups of patients and normal controls who participated in the study described above. The subjects were shown a set of 20 cards, each describing verbally a different action drawn from everyday activities such as the different steps in washing one's hair, starting a car, going to the movies, etc. Each action was associated with one of four distinct sequences. The subject's task was (1) to sort actions according to the script to which they belonged and (2) to order the actions in the proper order of execution within the script. Three different sets of actions were shown, which corresponded to three different task conditions. In conditions A and B, individual script headers were supplied along with the set of 20 action descriptions displayed on individual cards. Condition B differed from condition A by the presence of distractors—that is, actions which did not belong to any of the scripts and which thus had to be discarded. Two types of distractors were used: (1) actions that were semantically close to the script's theme, but did not fit into the logical and temporal unfolding of the sequence of events, and (2) actions that were semanti-

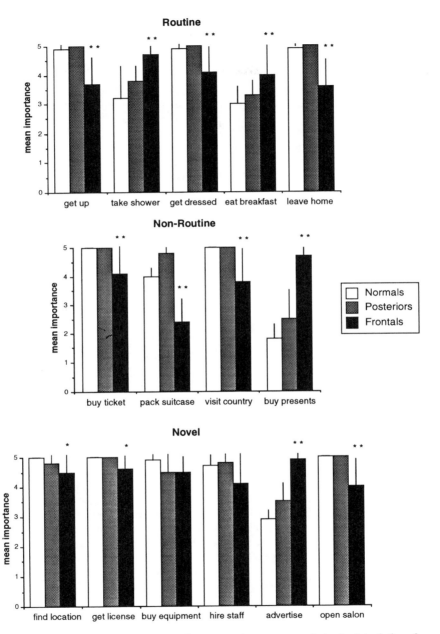

FIGURE 4. Judgments of importance. Histograms show means and standard deviations for judgments of importance (maximum = 5) for normal subjects and posterior and frontal patients for a selected set of actions (see text for criteria) in each of the three scripts. Statistically significant differences indicated above the columns: ** at the $p < .01$ level, * at the $p < 0.5$ level. (From Sirigu *et al.*[6] Reprinted with permission from *Cortex*.)

cally distant, whose contents were clearly incongruent with any of the action sequences. Condition C contained no distractors, but in contrast to the first two conditions, script headers were not supplied, and subjects had to identify how many distinct sequences were present and what each script was about.

The results showed that as in the script generation task, difficulties in temporal ordering were a hallmark of the frontal impairment. Collapsing across conditions, we found only one normal subject and one posterior patient made a single sequence error each, whereas all frontal patients committed sequence errors (mean error per subject, 5.3). Other types of errors were observed in these patients which never occurred in the other two groups:

1. Sorting errors were scored when an action was attributed to the wrong script. Displaced actions usually appeared when two scripts could compete to some degree for the same item. These errors were found in the totality of frontals (mean error per subject, 3.6). For example, certain patients transposed the action "insert the ignition key" from the sequence "starting the car" into a script about riding the elevator. Although private elevators frequently require the use of a key, it would not be called an *ignition* key. This might lead to the conclusion that frontal patients overlook such cues because of attentional or mild semantic impairments. This is unlikely, however, because at the end of the experiment the examiner systematically reviewed with the subject each of the erroneous decisions. Even with such a procedure, the patients did not modify their initial choice and usually went on to motivate it.

2. Frontal patients frequently included distractors into an action sequence (mean error per subject, 3.2), in particular if the distractor was semantically close to the theme of the script and when the action appeared somewhat plausible in a given context, such as inserting the item "ask for the check" in a script about buying ice cream. This action is congruent with the concept of eating out, but although it is appropriate when sitting at a restaurant table, it would not be done at an ice-cream parlor setting such as is depicted in the other actions. More importantly, an adequate logical transition did not exist for inserting that request at any point in the sequence. In the face of semantic ambiguities, it is likely that normals or posteriors use such "syntactic" criteria as a basis for including or rejecting a particular item.

3. In condition C, frontal patients failed to segment properly the four different scripts: 6 of 10 subjects fused together two or more scripts under a single theme header. Here again, the difficulty did not stem from poor semantic analysis, because the subjects were quite able to identify locally the theme of the individual sequences. Rather, they seemed unable to maintain the cognitive distance between different action clusters and to recognize the script boundaries. For instance, one patient fused the script "boiling an egg" with the script "riding the elevator" and gave the following header: "going back home after work and preparing dinner." Another combined two different scripts, riding the elevator and buying the newspaper, in order to form a single one. The unifying theme proposed was "go up in the elevator and go down again to buy the newspaper." The two-stage ride deviates from the actual action sequence and was obviously "filled in" by the patient in order to accommodate the logic of the scenario.

Finally, the difficulties experienced by frontal patients in processing distractors

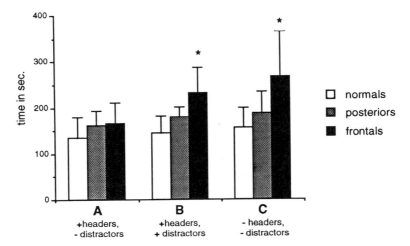

FIGURE 5. Mean time employed for script sorting and ordering in the different conditions by normal subjects and posterior and frontal patients. (**A**) Scripts with headers and without distractors; (**B**) scripts with headers and distractors; and (**C**) scripts without headers and without distractors.

and identifying script boundaries were reflected in the total time spent in sorting and ordering actions (FIG. 5). Normals and posteriors employed about the same amount of time regardless of the task condition. Frontals, however, showed significant increases in conditions B and C, which might reflect the sensitivity of conditions that make strong demands on the ability to perform a syntactic analysis of action sequences.

DISCUSSION

The findings from these two studies suggest that the frontal lobes play an important role in processing knowledge used in planning action sequences. The performance of frontal patients in script generation and in script analysis showed specific impairments in certain aspects of this knowledge, whereas other aspects appeared to be spared. The main distinction that emerges bears on the organization versus the contents of scripts. Frontal lesions seem to affect principally the former. A simplistic interpretation of this pattern of results is that prefrontal regions are only involved in processing the temporal relations of events whose contents are stored elsewhere, presumably in the posterior associative areas and in the temporal lobes. An alternative view is that information used in planning a course of action is stored in a distributed manner, although different brain areas may represent this information in ways which emphasize different properties. For instance, semantic networks in the posterior cortical regions may be well suited for encoding prototypical script events along with their related contextual information. The maintenance of a general chronological orientation in the sequences produced by frontal patients suggests that the intact cortical regions contain some degree of information about temporal order. The retrieval of an event from long-term memory might in fact produce activation spread, reaching the representations of other events and actions normally occurring in close temporal contiguity with that event. However, the presence of numerous sequence errors also implies that these associative networks are unable to represent temporal order reliably, perhaps because they permit both parallel and sequential activation of the different script events.

The importance of intact frontal lobe function for the maintenance of chronology suggests that this area encodes scripts in a manner that emphasizes sequential ordering of action. It should be pointed out that in contrast with previous studies which have shown difficulties in temporal ordering in frontal patients,[15,16] the results presented here did not involve learning novel sequences or monitoring sequentially presented stimuli in working memory. The tasks that elicited these deficits merely required the subjects to retrieve information from long-term memory. This raises as-yet-unanswered questions regarding how sequences are encoded and what schema is used to represent sequences in prefrontal cortex.

Do prefrontal patients experience difficulties in recognizing the cues that mark temporal order? In a sentence, temporal order need not match the order of propositions because it is given by the grammatical structure. "I looked at the posted menu, selected my favorite flavor, then ordered the ice cream" is equivalent to "I ordered the ice cream after having selected my favorite flavor from the menu." Would prefrontal patients, who are not agrammatic, recognize the identity between the sequence of temporal events described by those two sentences, yet fail to determine whether they represent a conceptually correct sequence of events? Sequence reversal such as putting "order the ice cream" before "select the flavor" are actually observed in the performance of frontal patients. This could imply an impairment in the capacity to retrieve these script elements in the correct temporal order, a failure to recognize that one must identify one's desires before formulating a request, or both. In fact, it is not clear whether sequences merely represent a temporal succession of events, or whether the underlying logical rules and cause/effect relations which the sequence must obey are encoded as well.

The coding of sequences is a problem which computational approaches attempt to solve, and recent simulations suggest that temporal order and conditional rules which govern sequential behavior may both be represented implicitly in specialized neural networks. A recent model proposed by Guigon et al.[17] was shown to learn short motor sequences through the use of hierarchically organized arrays of cells which emulate "working memory" response profiles described in primate prefrontal cortex.[18] In this model sustained neuronal discharges orient the flow of activity in the network through a gating mechanism that serves to promote appropriate actions while blocking inappropriate ones. Whether similar principles could encode more complex and elaborate sequences of actions such as those that prefrontal patients have difficulties with is an issue that has not yet been addressed.

Other findings from our studies indicate that more than temporal ordering is affected following frontal lobe damage, and point to the existence of higher-level conceptual impairments. Sequence processing might be but one of the many facets of degraded script representations. The incapacity to correctly assign priority levels to actions reveals a specific difficulty in relating the significance of individual actions to a stated goal. This could reflect a deficit in mean-ends analysis and/or weakened representation of the formulated intention, leading to an evaluation of actions for their own sake. For instance, prefrontal patients could be considering that an action is important simply because it is pleasurable or because it is habitually performed in a given context, regardless of its true usefulness.

Another aspect of script analysis that is impaired in such patients is the capacity to maintain internal coherent action sequences. In the first study,[6] boundary violations were reflected in failures of script closure, that is, in the inability to terminate a script at the appropriate end point. In the second study, boundary impairments appeared under various forms. Intrusions from other scripts and from deliberately planted distractor elements suggest that boundaries between simultaneously activated script representations have become permeable. The same explanation can account for the tendency, observed in several patients, to fill in the gaps and search for a hidden logic, linking the different sequences in the situation where no script header was supplied. Although task instructions emphasized the fact that the set of actions contained distinct sequences, of the three sorting conditions, condition C was the most open-ended one[4] because subjects were not supplied with explicit "bins" to put actions into and did not know how many such bins there should be. If explicitly instructed to do so, normal subjects could probably produce story themes similar to those given by prefrontal patients, but would likely recognize their farfetched nature given the obvious conceptual gaps between the four action sequences. This was not the case with frontal patients, who spontaneously provided global headers they found perfectly adequate. Following the above line of interpretation, such filling in behavior would be expected to occur when simultaneously activated sets of representations cannot be kept in separate working memory clusters, and their boundaries consequently appear fuzzy.

In conclusion, evidence has been presented that prefrontal regions could play a critical role in planning and organizing behavior by acting as a site for storing and activating temporally ordered sequences of actions and events. In addition, these regions could be important in maintaining coherent working memory representations of simultaneously activated intentions and action programs. This function is likely to be crucial in everyday life situations which most acutely typify the case where parallel, multilevel plans often need to be elaborated, initiated, and coordinated.

REFERENCES

1. SHALLICE, T. 1982. Specific impairments of planning. Philos. Trans. R. Soc. Lond. B **298:** 199–209.
2. STUSS, D. T. & D. F. BENSON. 1984. Neuropsychological studies of the frontal lobes. Psychol. Bull. **95.**
3. ESLINGER, P. J. & A. DAMASIO. 1985. Severe disturbances of higher cognition after bilateral frontal lobe ablation: Patient EVR. Neurology **35:** 1731–1741.
4. SHALLICE, T. & P. BURGESS. 1991. Deficits in strategy application following frontal lobe damage in man. Brain **114:** 727–741.5.

5. SHALLICE, T. 1988. From Neuropsychology to Mental Structure. Cambridge University Press. Cambridge.
6. SIRIGU, A., T. ZALLA, B. PILLON, J. GRAFMAN, Y. AGID & B. DUBOIS. 1995. Selective impairments in managerial knowledge following prefrontal cortex damage. Cortex 31(2): 301–316.
7. SIRIGU, A., T. ZALLA, B. PILLON, J. GRAFMAN, Y. AGID & B. DUBOIS. Encoding of sequence and boundaries of scripts in prefrontal lesions. Cortex. In press.
8. SCHANK, R. 1982. Dynamic Memory: A Theory of Reminding and Learning in Computers and People. Cambridge University Press. Cambridge, MA.
9. BOWER, G. H., J. B. BLACK & T. J. TURNER. 1979. Scripts in memory for text. Cogn. Psychol. 11: 177–220.
10. GALAMBOS, J. A. & L. J. RIPS. 1982. Memory for routines. J. Verb. Learn. Verb. Behav. 21: 260–281.
11. MANDLER, J. M. 1984. Stories, Scripts, and Scenes: Aspects of Schema Theory. Erlbaum. Hillsdale, NJ.
12. ABBOTT, V., J. B. BLACK & E. E. SMITH. 1985. The representation of scripts in memory. J. Mem. & Lang. 24: 179–199.
13. GRAFMAN, J. 1989. Plans, actions, and mental sets: Managerial knowledge units in the frontal lobes. In Integrating Theory and Practice in Clinical Neuropsychology. E. Perecman, Ed. Erlbaum. Hillsdale, NJ.
14. GRAFMAN, J., A. SIRIGU, L. SPECTOR & J. HENDLER. 1993. Damage to the prefrontal cortex leads to decomposition of structured event complexes. J. Head Trauma Rehabil. 8: 73–87.
15. MILNER, B., M. PETRIDES & M. L. SMITH. 1985. Frontal lobes and the temporal organisation of memory. Hum. Neurobiol. 4: 137–142.
16. JANOSWSKY, J. S., A. P. SHIMAMURA & L. R. SQUIRE. 1989. Source memory impairment in patients with frontal lobe lesions. Neuropsychologia 27: 1043–1056.
17. GUIGON, E., B. DORIZZI, Y. BURNOD & W. SCHULTZ. 1995. A neural correlate of learning in the prefrontal cortex: A predictive model. Cereb. Cortex 2: 135–147.
18. GOLDMAN-RAKIC, P. S. 1987. Circuitry of primate prefrontal cortex and regulation of behavior by representational knowledge. In Handbook of Physiology, Vol. 5. F. Plum & V. Mountcastle, Eds.: 373–417. American Physiological Society. Bethesda, MD.

Toward a Cognitive Account of Frontal Lobe Function: Simulating Frontal Lobe Deficits in Normal Subjects[a]

KEVIN DUNBAR[b] AND DEBRA SUSSMAN

Department of Psychology
McGill University
1205 Dr. Penfield Avenue
Montreal, Quebec, Canada H3A 1B1

Over the past 20 years, considerable progress has been made on characterizing the mental processes underlying higher-level cognition. In particular, there now exists a number of detailed models and theories of the cognitive processes underlying problem solving, reasoning, and concept acquisition.[1-3] While these models were being developed, there also emerged a literature indicating that patients with frontal lobe damage exhibit a wide variety of deficits in reasoning, problem solving, and concept acquisition.[4-6] Surprisingly, little attempt has been made to link the cognitive research with the brain-based research. One of the reasons for this is that there has not, as yet, been a specification of the cognitive processes that underlie higher-level cognition and how higher-level cognitive processes are related to the attentional and working memory deficits implicated in frontal patients. The goal of the work reported in this paper is to begin to articulate the mechanisms that mediate higher-level cognition and specify their relationship to the deficits observed in patients with frontal lobe injury.

Perhaps the most striking and consistent impairment documented in frontal lobe cases is the difficulty patients encounter on a variety of reasoning tasks.[7,8] In one task—the Wisconsin Card Sorting Test (WCST)—the patient is shown four cards placed in a row, each displaying geometric figures varying in terms of color, shape, and number. The patient is then given a pack of 128 cards containing exemplars from the same categories as those represented in the four cards on display. He or she is told that the examiner has a particular *undisclosed* sorting criterion in mind (for instance, color) which has to be *discovered* by assigning each card to one member of the target set. The examiner indicates whether the response is right or wrong, and the patient must use this information to minimize the number of placement errors. Frontal patients show a clear impairment on this task relative to patients of comparable IQ with left or right posterior lesions. Researchers have found that (1) frontal patients achieve fewer categories than controls; (2) they make more perseverative errors than controls, and (3) they tend to make more perseverative than nonperseverative errors. It should be noted that

[a] This research was supported by funds provided to K.D. by a grant from the Fonds de la recherche en santé du Québec, and a grant from the Natural Sciences and Engineering Research Council of Canada (OGP0037356).
[b] Corresponding author.

some researchers have found that some frontal patients show little or no impairment on the WCST and have failed to find differences in performance between frontal patients and patients with other types of brain damage.[9,10] Furthermore, researchers have found nonfrontal patients and normal controls can show perseveration on the WCST.[11] Despite these findings, the WCST is still widely used as a diagnostic tool to measure frontal injury.

A number of different explanations have been offered for performance on this task. Milner[5] argued that frontal patients perseverate because they have an inability to overcome previously reinforced responses. More recently, researchers have offered cognitive reasons for the performance of frontal patients. For example, Shallice and his colleagues have argued that frontal patients have a deficit in the allocation and supervision of attention,[12] and Baddeley has argued that their deficit is a working memory deficit.[13] In particular, he has argued that frontal patients have a deficit in the Central Executive component of working memory—this is the component of working memory that performs mental operations and controls other working memory systems. Baddeley's model of working memory is not universally accepted; other researchers have argued for a more unitary working memory.[14,15] However, the Baddeley model makes it possible to derive a number of clear predictions regarding frontal patients and has been widely used in the literature on frontal patients. In this paper, we will use the Baddeley model because it allows us to make clear experimental predictions; we are not committed to his model of working memory.

The hypothesis that perseveration on the WCST is due to a failure of the central executive has not been directly tested. Nonetheless, this hypothesis has been used to account for the performance of patients. Furthermore, current theories of performance on the WCST do not make it possible to determine precisely how the central executive is deficient in patients with frontal deficits. Thus, a number of different types of central executive deficits might produce the same performance: Subjects might not attend to feedback, lose track of feedback, be unable to integrate information, etc. Furthermore, although classic frontal performance is consistent with a central executive deficit, it is possible that other types of working memory deficits underlie this type of performance.[16] Finally, recent research demonstrating that nonfrontal patients can show perseveration on the WCST further clouds the issue of what this task measures, and how the frontal lobes are involved in the task.[9]

One of the problems that prior accounts of the WCST have had is that the accounts have not been based on a cognitive analysis of the task. When the WCST is looked at as a classic concept attainment task in which patients must induce new concepts from sets of examples, it becomes clear that there are a number of different possible sources of perseveration.[3,17] Subjects have to keep in working memory the current hypothesis, feedback from at least the current trial, and also compare feedback to the current hypothesis on every trial. When the feedback is inconsistent with the current hypothesis, patients must be able to notice it, generate another hypothesis and compare it to the current feedback, and continue to generate hypotheses until they find an hypothesis that is consistent with the current feedback and, if possible, recent feedback. Clearly, the task involves maintaining different types of information in working memory, and conducting various computations on the feedback in order to give correct responses. Potentially, many different types of memory and/or attentional deficits could be involved in performing this task.

The goal of the research reported here was to investigate the memory mechanisms underlying perseveration. Currently, we know that frontal patients and other patients perseverate, but not what processes underlie this performance. To investigate these issues we used non-brain-damaged patients. Our hypothesis was that if working memory deficits underlie perseveration, then it should be possible to induce perseveration in normal subjects. To do this, we used a "dual task" methodology in which normal subjects were given the WCST and asked to perform a working memory task at the same time as performing the WCST. In dual-task terminology, the WCST is known as the "primary task" and the working memory task is known as the "secondary task." The secondary tasks that we used were tasks that take up different amounts and different types of working memory capacity. By manipulating the types of secondary tasks given to subjects, we can investigate whether working memory deficits do indeed underlie perseveration and, if so, what types of working memory are involved in perseveration.

The tasks that we chose were selected in terms of Baddeley's model of working memory. Baddeley has proposed that there are three main types of working memory: the central executive, the phonological loop, and the visuospatial sketch pad. The central executive is the component of working memory that coordinates and controls the maintenance and flow of information in and out of working memory. The phonological loop maintains phonologically based information in working memory. The visuospatial scratch pad maintains visual representations of information. Baddeley has devised many different tasks that selectively take up one type of working memory while sparing the other type. Thus, his framework provides a specification of the types of tasks using one type of working memory and not another. Using Baddeley's model, we designed secondary tasks that can take up different types of working memory capacity while performing the WCST. The main manipulation was whether the secondary task took up the phonological loop or the central executive. The reason for choosing tasks that took up these types of working memory capacity is that a task analysis indicates that the WCST involves both phonological memory (to store the current hypothesis, feedback, and perhaps prior instances) and the central executive (for allocating attention to, and performing operations on, the contents of the phonological loop).

EXPERIMENT 1

Three groups of subjects were tested: a control group that received the WCST alone and two experimental groups (a phonological and a central executive group). Both experimental groups heard a tape of digits and then a tone. Subjects in the phonological group had to recall all digits when they heard the tone. Subjects in the executive group had to give the sum of all numbers heard prior to the tone. The digit recall task is primarily a phonological task: Subjects have to maintain a set of numbers in memory, and this should be phonologically based. There were some executive components, in that the subjects did have to update their memory set after each digit was heard. However, the task should primarily tap phonological memory. If the WCST involves a phonological component, then the phonological task should produce a deficit in performance on the WCST. The addition task was primarily a central executive task because subjects had to update their memory, add the two digits, and store the result after each digit was heard. In this condition, there were more computations that needed to be performed than in the phonological condition, yet the memory load was minimal. It was expected that subjects in the executive condition would show performance that was more "frontal-like" than subjects in the phonological condition. That is, these subjects should achieve few categories, and show more perseverative than nonperseverative errors.

Method

Subjects. Three groups, each with 12 subjects, participated in the experiment. All were McGill University undergraduates who participated in the experiment for course credit.

Procedure. Subjects in the experimental conditions heard a tape of digits with each digit presented once every three seconds. A tone was presented randomly, once every 4, 5, or 6 digits. In the phonological condition, subjects repeated the number when they heard it. When the tone occurred, they had to repeat all numbers heard since the previous beep. In the central executive condition, subjects heard the same tape; after hearing a number, they added the number to the previous number. They added each new number until they heard a beep. After the beep, subjects said the grand total, then began adding from zero with the next set of numbers.

While performing the number recall or number addition tasks, subjects performed the WCST. The WCST was presented on a computer.[18] Subjects used a mouse to select the key card under which the stimulus card was placed. When the subject clicked under the key card, the stimulus card appeared directly below the key card, and the next card appeared at the top of the deck. As soon as the card was placed, the word *correct* (if the response was correct), or *incorrect* (if the response was incorrect) appeared under the card. This feedback stayed on the screen until the subject placed the next card. The same order of categories and cards was used as in the noncomputerized version of the WCST. Categories were given in the following order: color, form, number, color, form, number. When subjects had achieved 10 correct responses in a row, the sorting category was changed. If subjects achieved all six categories before they had used all 128 cards, the experiment was terminated. If subjects failed to achieve all six categories by the time 128 cards were used, the experiment was also terminated.

Results and Discussion

The data were automatically analyzed by the computer using the same criteria as found in the Heaton norms.[19] The data that we will focus on is number of

TABLE 1. Performance of Normal Subjects in the Three Experimental
Conditions and Performance of Frontal Patients in the Milner Study and
Heaton Norms

	Control	Phonological	Executive	Milner	Heaton
Categories (n)	6	2.3	4	1.8	3.1
Perseverative errors (n)	5.2	40	26	44.6	35.9
Nonperseverative errors (n)	14	27	27	15	18.4
Perseverative errors in first category	0.6	11.6	4.6		
Perseverative errors in second category	1.1	16	25		
Nonperseverative errors in first category	2.3	10.1	8.0		
Nonperseverative errors in second category	4	11	10		

categories achieved, number of perseverative errors, and number of nonperseverative errors. Subjects can achieve a maximum of six categories. Perseverative errors are errors in which the subject sorts according to a dimension even though
feedback indicates that this is the incorrect sorting dimension. A nonperseverative
error is an error in which the subject sorts along an incorrect dimension, and this
dimension is not the same as the previous incorrect response.

The number of categories achieved by subjects in each of the three groups
was calculated. A one-way analysis of variance (ANOVA) revealed significant
differences between the three groups in terms of number of categories completed
$[F(2,32) = 17.82, p < .001]$. Post hoc tests indicated that all three conditions
were significantly different from each other, with the subjects in the phonological
condition achieving the least number of categories. The results for this experiment
and those of Milner[5] and Heaton[19]—who used frontal patients—are given in
TABLE 1. Comparing our results to those obtained with frontal patients indicates
that subjects in the phonological condition obtained the fewest categories and
looked most like frontal patients.

The results for perseverative errors mirror those for number of categories. A
one-way ANOVA showed that subjects in the phonological condition had more
perseverative errors than the central executive and control groups $[F(2,32) =
23.59, p < .0001]$. An ANOVA of nonperseverative errors revealed a significant
effect of condition $[F(2,32) = 6.56, p < .01]$. Post hoc tests revealed that there
were no significant differences between the central executive and phonological
groups, but that both of these groups had more nonperseverative errors than the
control group. We also analyzed perseveration for the second category. The second category is the first time in which a category is changed, and should have more
perseverative errors than for the other categories. An ANOVA of the difference
between perseverative and nonperseverative errors in the second category revealed a significant effect of condition $[F(2,31) = 3.9, p < .05]$. Post hoc comparisons revealed that only subjects in the phonological condition had significantly
more perseverative than nonperseverative errors. They had more perseverative
errors than nonperseverative errors, and their absolute numbers of perseverative
errors were similar to those obtained from frontal patients.

The results of this experiment were surprising: The phonological task produced more perseveration and subjects achieved fewer categories than in the executive task. Furthermore, in the phonological task more perseverative than nonperseverative errors occurred, whereas in the executive task more nonperseverative than perseverative errors were made. These results may indicate that the locus of perseveration is not in the central executive component of working memory, but is in phonological working memory. Another possible interpretation of these findings is that neither of these tasks tapped solely the central executive or the phonological loop. The phonological task may have involved central executive components (such as updating the items maintained in the phonological loop), and the central executive task may not have been demanding enough to produce perseveration.[20] We conducted a second experiment in which subjects had to perform either a pure phonological task, or a pure central executive task to further determine the roles of these types of working memory in the WCST.

EXPERIMENT 2

Two different secondary tasks were used in experiment 2. One was an articulatory suppression task in which subjects had to say "the-the-the" continuously while performing the WCST. Baddeley and his colleagues have frequently used this task and have argued that it prevents subjects from rehearsing information in the articulatory loop.[21] For a purer version of a central executive task, subjects were given a tone detection task. In this task, subjects heard a tone, and as soon as they heard the tone, they had to press a pedal with their foot. The tone was presented randomly. This task involves dynamically allocating resources to a secondary task; it can be described as a pure central executive task or as a task in which subjects must switch attention between tasks. This task should not tap phonological memory, nor does it require the storage of information by working memory. For this task, we varied whether subjects used their right or left foot to press the key. Given that motor planning has been implicated in the left prefrontal dorsolateral cortex, we hypothesized that subjects using the right foot might show more perseveration than subjects using the left foot.

Method

Subjects. Two groups, each composed of 11 McGill University undergraduates, were paid $5.00 per subject to participate in the experiment. All subjects were right handed and stated that they were also right footed.

Procedure. In the articulatory suppression condition, subjects said "the-the-the-the" in a continuous stream while doing the WCST. No minimum speed was required as long as subjects were constantly articulating. In the tone detection task, subjects heard a beep coming from the computer at random intervals between 750 and 1850 ms (e.g., 750, 850, 950 . . . or 1850 ms). Subjects were told that as soon as they heard the tone they were to press the foot pedal.

TABLE 2. Experiment 2 Performance for the Three Experimental Conditions

	Articulatory Suppression	Left Foot	Right Foot
Categories (n)	4.3	4.9	3.9
Perseverative errors (n)	29	16	19
Nonperseverative errors (n)	23	24	24
Perseverative errors in first category	1.2	1.6	1.1
Perseverative errors in second category	19.7	6.4	18.4
Nonperseverative errors in first category	2.7	5.3	4.2
Nonperseverative errors in second category	6.5	7.1	11.6

Results

One-way ANOVAs were conducted of all the basic measures of performance. As can be seen in TABLE 2, there were no significant differences between the three groups in number of categories achieved [$F(2,30) = .81, p > .05$]; number of perseverative errors [$F(2,30) = 2.58, p > .05$]; and number of nonperseverative errors [$F(2,30) = .42, p > .05$]. Because the results of experiment 1 indicated that the bulk of perseveration occurred for the second category, we conducted further analyses of perseverative and nonperseverative errors for the second category. An effect of condition was seen on the difference between perseverative and nonperseverative errors [$F(2,27) = p > .05$]. Post hoc tests revealed significantly more perseverative than nonperseverative errors in the articulatory suppression condition. No other significant effects were found, although it should be noted that subjects in the right-foot condition did have more perseverative than nonperseverative errors, although this difference was not significant. For the left-foot condition, there was no evidence of any difference in numbers of perseverative and nonperseverative errors.

The results of this experiment indicate that at a global level no significant differences existed between subjects in the three groups. However, an analysis of errors in category 2 revealed that subjects in the articulatory suppression condition did show more perseverative than nonperseverative errors.[22] A post experiment interview with subjects indicates that after the second category they developed strategies for coordinating the two tasks. Thus, more perseverative than nonperseverative errors only showed up for the second category. There was a nonsignificant trend in the direction of more perseverative than nonperseverative errors for the right-foot condition, indicating the possibility of a central executive component to the task. The results for the second-category performance are consistent with the hypothesis that perseveration in the WCST is the result of a deficit in maintaining information in the phonological loop, rather than a central executive deficit.

EXPERIMENT 3

The results of experiments 1 and 2 indicate that it is possible to obtain perseveration when the phonological coding of information is prevented. These results make it possible to predict that patients with a deficit in phonological working memory should show perseveration on the WCST. Usually, patients with these types of deficits are not given the WCST, and the question as to whether patients with a phonological working memory deficit will show perseveration on the WCST is not asked. Experiment 3 was conducted to test this hypothesis.

We investigated this hypothesis by testing patient RoL of Belleville et al.[23] This patient has a lesion in the left temporoparietal region and has conduction aphasia. Belleville et al. have investigated this patient extensively and have argued that his main deficit is an articulatory rehearsal deficit. They found that on a variety of memory tasks his performance was similar to that of normal subjects given tasks that interfere with articulatory rehearsal. Furthermore, they found that when he was given tasks that in normal patients interfere with articulatory rehearsal, his performance showed no further decrease. Thus, this patient has a pure case of an articulatory rehearsal deficit. The findings of the first two experiments indicate that a patient such as this should also show deficits in performance on the WCST.

Method and Results

Patient RoL was administered the WCST. He obtained zero categories and showed 94 perseverative and 2 nonperseverative errors. He was administered the WCST a second time and was told that the categories will change. Even in this situation he still obtained only one category. Thus, his performance indicates that indeed an articulatory rehearsal deficit can produce perseverative errors.

SUMMARY OF SIMULATION EXPERIMENTS

The results of the three experiments reported thus far indicate that it is possible to produce frontal-like performance in normal subjects. Using a dual-task methodology, normal undergraduates formed fewer categories, made many errors, and made more perseverative than nonperseverative errors than control subjects. The performance of these subjects was very similar to that reported in the literature on frontal patients. Surprisingly, the conditions under which the most perseveration was obtained were phonological conditions. We further investigated the hypothesis that perseveration is the result of phonological deficits by testing a patient known to have a deficit in phonological processing and found that the performance of this patient was typical of that reported for frontal patients. Thus, we found further evidence for a potential phonological etiology of perseveration on the WCST.

The results of these experiments help explain why other researchers have questioned the validity of the WCST as a diagnostic tool. Recently, a number of laboratories have shown that patient populations other than frontal patients also display perseveration.[9,10] One possible reason for these other patients' perseveration is that their deficits may involve phonological working memory, and that it is deficits in phonological memory that lead to perseveration. Although the phonological deficit hypothesis can explain much of the performance in the three preceding experiments, we also found a nonsignificant trend toward perseveration when subjects were given a more pure central executive task with no memory load. These results suggest that another possible mechanism underlying perseveration is that a central executive deficit may prevent patients from maintaining information in phonological working memory and thus cause perseveration in an indirect manner. Therefore, it is still necessary to explore the role of the central executive. In the next two experiments we investigated one function of the central executive—the allocation of attention in patients with frontal deficits.

EXPERIMENTS WITH FRONTAL PATIENTS

Although many authors have argued that frontal patients have a deficit in the central executive, what the central executive actually is remains somewhat shrouded in mystery. Baddeley has argued that it controls the flow of information in and out of the phonological loop and the visuospatial sketch pad. One way of describing it would be to say that it controls the allocation of attention to specific tasks and processes. Given that many authors have implicated this type of working memory/attentional allocation in frontal deficits, the goal of the research reported here was to investigate the question of whether frontal patients do in fact have an attentional allocation deficit and precisely how this affects thinking and reasoning.

To test the hypothesis that frontal patients have a deficit in the allocation of attention, we used a variant of the Stroop test.[24,25] In the Stroop test, subjects see a word, such as the word *red* in green ink. There are two subtasks involved in the Stroop test—a color-naming task and a word-reading task.[26] In the color-naming task the subject is required to name the ink color and ignore the word. In the word-reading task, the subject is required to read the word and ignore the ink color. The typical findings are that the word interferes with ink color naming, but the ink color does not interfere with word reading. The usual interpretation of this data is that word reading is an automatic process and is involuntary, causing interference with word reading.[27] Conversely, color naming is thought to be a controlled or voluntary process, and hence does not interfere with word reading. This task has been used with frontal patients, with mixed results. Perret has shown that in color naming, frontal patients show more interference than controls.[28] However, Shallice was not able to obtain differences between frontal patients and controls on this task.[29] If Perret's results hold, then it would be consistent with the hypothesis that frontal patients cannot inhibit a well-learned or automatic process. The first goal of the research reported here was to use the Stroop test to see whether frontal patients do in fact show increased interference. Once we have obtained baseline information on the Stroop test, we can then use a novel version of the Stroop test that can be used to investigate whether frontal patients have deficits in attentional allocation.

We used a version of the Stroop test known as the picture-word interference task.[30] In this task the subjects see a stimulus such as a picture of a horse with a word typed on the picture—for example, the word "cat." In the word-reading task, subjects must read the word and ignore the picture. In the picture-naming task, subjects must name the picture and ignore the word. Just as in the standard Stroop color-naming task, picture naming is thought to be less automatic than word reading, and thus the word interferes with picture naming, but the picture does not interfere with word reading. Thus, the picture-word task is equivalent to the standard color-naming task. We used this task, rather than the color-naming task because it allows us to manipulate a wide variety of semantic and categorical variables that are not possible to manipulate using the standard color-naming task.

EXPERIMENT 4

In this experiment we used the picture-word task to determine whether frontal patients show more interference than normal subjects. A further goal of the experiment was to determine whether frontal patients are more subject to interference from words that are potential responses than control groups. Recall that one explanation for frontal deficits is that their deficit is one of inhibiting well-learned responses. If this is the case, frontal patients should not only show more interference than controls, but they should also show more interference from words that are potential responses than from words that are not potential responses. However, recent simulations by Jonathan Cohen, using the Cohen, Dunbar, and McClelland model of attention, predict that a disturbance in the mechanisms of attentional allocation should reduce the size of the response set effect, such that nonresponse set members might produce more interference relative to response set members.[26,31]

To test these predictions we varied the relationship between the pictures and the words. For example, the pictures that the patients name might be of a horse, bear, rabbit, sheep, and cat. Patients would see one of these five pictures on every trial. What would be varied is the type of word superimposed on the picture. The words that are potential responses would also be *horse, bear, rabbit, sheep,* and *cat.* Words that are not potential responses might be *dog, goat, seal, donkey.* In normal subjects words that are potential responses produce around 25 ms more interference than nonpotential responses. If the deficit that frontal patients have is one of inhibiting responses, then we would expect them to show much more interference from words that are potential responses than words that are not potential responses. If the deficit is one of allocating attention—as the Cohen, Dunbar, and McClelland model predicts[26]—then we would expect no more interference from words that are potential responses than from words that are not.

The patient population that we used were patients with frontal closed head injuries. These patients all had frontal head injuries and were similar to patients used in a number of studies of frontal lobe function. However, it should be noted that data obtained from patients with closed head injuries are more difficult to interpret than those obtained from patients with focal frontal lesions: closed head injury patients also have widespread white matter lesions. We attempted to circumvent this problem by only using patients who obtained three or fewer categories on the WCST, had an IQ in the range of 100, and obtained normal scores on naming and memory tests.

TABLE 3. Reaction Time of Subjects for the Four Conditions of the Picture-Naming Task

Incongruent same set	Incongruent different set	Control	Congruent
803	800	706	653

Method

Subjects. Five patients with frontal closed head injuries were used. All five patients obtained three or fewer categories on the WCST and had a mean IQ of 103.

Procedure. The patients were tested on a Macintosh plus computer. The stimuli were the digitized pictures of a horse, rabbit, bear, cat, and sheep.[32] There were four conditions. In the control condition, the pictures had a row of four Xs superimposed upon them. In the congruent condition, the word was the same as the picture. In the incongruent same set condition, the words were from the same set as the pictures, and the word and picture were never the same. In the incongruent different set, none of the words were from the same set as the pictures. The words were *dog, mouse, donkey, goat,* and *seal.* Subjects were given a block of 120 trials. Each block consisted of 30 trials of each of the four types of stimuli, randomly intermixed. Each trial consisted of a subject seeing a fixation point in the middle of the screen for 150 ms; then the picture-word stimulus appeared. The stimulus stayed on the screen until the subject named the picture or three seconds had elapsed. Reaction time was measured from the onset of the picture-word stimulus to the onset of the verbal response.

Results and Discussion

Block 1 was considered to be a block of practice trials that introduced the subjects to the response set and was not analyzed. A one-way ANOVA was conducted on reaction time for blocks 2–4. There was a significant difference between conditions [$F(3,15) = 16.7, p < .001$]. As can be seen from TABLE 3, subjects did show interference in both the incongruent same set and incongruent different set conditions. However, as predicted by recent simulations using the Cohen, Dunbar, and McClelland model,[26,31] no difference was found between same set and different set conditions. Furthermore, the amount of interference that the patients showed was between 94 and 97 ms. This was within the range reported for normal subjects.

Overall, the patients in this experiment showed neither more interference than normal subjects nor any more interference from words that are potential responses than from words that are not potential responses. The results suggest that these patients did not have a deficit in inhibiting responses. The results are consistent with the Cohen, Dunbar, and McClelland model of attention, indicating that these patients have a deficit in attentional allocation. These data are also consistent with those recently reported by Vendrell *et al.*[33] Using the Stroop test, they found that frontal patients do not show more interference than controls. Having obtained this baseline information, we can now turn to a more direct test of whether the deficit that frontal patients have is one of the allocation of attention and begin to answer the question of how this leads to deficits in performance on higher-level cognitive tasks.

EXPERIMENT 5

The goal of the research reported in this experiment is to determine whether frontal patients do indeed have a deficit in the allocation of attention. Recently, we conducted a number of experiments in which we investigated how normal subjects allocate attention.[34] We used a version of the Stroop test in which subjects do not know whether their task is to name an ink color or read a word until they hear a tone. We used conditions in which the tone indicating which task to perform occurs either at the same time as the Stroop stimulus, or 400 ms prior to the Stroop stimulus. In both of these conditions, subjects demonstrated that it takes them time to allocate attention to the task and that, unlike in the normal version of the Stroop test, ink color interferes with word reading. This task makes it possible to investigate directly the allocation of attention, and should make it possible to investigate attentional allocation in frontal patients.

We developed a picture-word version of the allocation task for use with frontal patients. In this task, patients do not know whether the task that they must perform is a word-reading or picture-naming task until they hear a tone. Subjects hear a tone 400 ms before the picture-word stimulus appears. The tone indicates which task to perform. Note that subjects have to wait until they hear the tone before they begin allocating all their attention to one task rather than the other. Thus, the task is concerned with one of the core components of the central executive—allocating mental capacity to a task. When the task is given to frontal patients, a number of outcomes are possible. First, subjects might not be able to allocate their attention appropriately. In particular, patients may allocate attention to the most automatic process—word reading. If this is the case, patients should make many errors in the picture-naming task and show increased interference with picture naming. If patients have this type of deficit, they should also have few errors in word reading, and little interference with word reading. A second potential outcome is that frontal patients will not be able to allocate attention appropriately and will randomly pick which task to perform. This outcome would occur if their deficit is one of allocating attention. A third possibility is that, as in experiment 4, patients will be able to execute both tasks with only a small error rate and be similar to normal subjects.

Method

Subjects. A different set of five subjects, from the same population as the previous experiment, were used. These subjects were also administered the experiment 4 version of the picture-word tasks, after they had been given experiment 5.

This manipulation was conducted to ensure that the patients showed the same effects as in experiment 4, which they did.

Procedure. The stimuli were the pictures of a horse, rabbit, bear, sheep, and cat. The words were also *horse, bear, rabbit, sheep,* and *cat.* There were three types of stimuli: congruent, incongruent, and control items. Congruent items were where the words and pictures were the same (e.g., the word *horse* on a picture of a horse). Incongruent items were where the words were different from the picture (e.g., the word *cat* on a picture of a horse). Control items for the picture-naming task consisted of the pictures with a row of Xs. For the word-reading condition, control items consisted of a word surrounded by a geometric figure. The experiment was a 2 × 2 design with factors of task (color naming or word reading) and congruency (congruent, incongruent, or control). There were 144 trials: 72 picture naming and 72 word reading. There were 24 congruent, 24 incongruent, and 24 control trials. On each trial subjects saw a fixation point for 500 ms; the screen went blank, and 100 ms later they heard one of two tones. The tone lasted for 100 ms. The picture-word stimulus occurred 400 ms after the offset of the tone, and the patient had to name the picture or read the word, depending on what type of tone occurred. A high-pitched tone indicated that the task was to name the picture, and a low-pitched tone indicated that the task was to read the word.

Results and Discussion

Two ANOVAs were conducted—the first was on reaction-time data and the second on error data. Both ANOVAs were 2 × 3 with factors of task (picture naming or word reading), and congruency (congruent, incongruent, or control). The reaction-time ANOVA revealed no differences between picture naming and word reading nor between the three levels of congruency. The reason why there were no effects becomes clear when we look at the error data. There was a main effect of congruency, with subjects performing at chance [$F(2,8) = 27.39$, $p < .01$]. A graph of this effect is shown in FIG. 1. Here it can be seen that in the incongruent condition for both picture naming and word reading, subjects made errors on almost 50% of the trials. Thus, on half the picture-naming trials the patients were reading the word, and on half the word-reading trials they were naming the pictures. In the congruent condition, given that the word and the picture were the same, it did not matter which dimension the subject responded to; the response would always be correct, and fewer errors occurred. In the control condition the irrelevant dimension was not easily nameable, and thus did not produce as large a number of errors as in the incongruent condition.

Overall, the results of this experiment indicate that frontal patients do indeed have a deficit in attentional allocation. When there was uncertainty as to what was the correct task to perform and the patients had to dynamically allocate attention to tasks, subjects chose tasks at a level close to chance. These data are thus consistent with the hypothesis that frontal patients have a deficit in allocating attention on the basis of constantly changing incoming information.

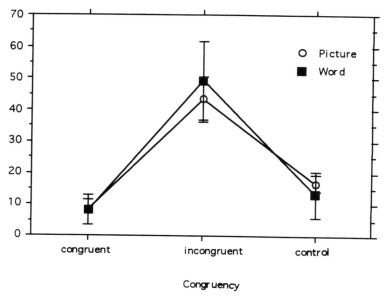

FIGURE 1. Percentage of errors for frontal patients in the task-switching version of the picture-word interference task.

GENERAL DISCUSSION

The results of the five experiments reported in this paper indicate that a complex set of interactions exist between lower-level cognitive processes, such as those involved in working memory and attentional allocation, and the higher-level cognitive processes that they subserve. By analyzing a complex task such as the WCST, it was possible to determine that the task involves both the temporary storage of information in a phonological store and the shifting of attention to move information in and out of this store. By manipulating normal subjects' ability to manipulate information in and out of the phonological loop, it was possible to produce frontal-like performance. Furthermore, it was possible to predict frontal-like performance in a patient with a deficit in phonological working memory. The results of these experiments not only indicate what components of the task are relevant to the production of the hallmark behavior of perseveration, but also help to explain why many other patients with no frontal deficits also display perseveration on the WCST: They may have working memory and/or attentional deficits.

The attentional allocation experiments reported in this paper indicate that frontal patients do indeed have a deficit in the allocation of attention. When patients had to dynamically switch attention from one task to another, their ability to perform the appropriate task dropped to levels of chance. This inability to allocate attention dynamically may be at the root of patients' difficulties on the WCST and other tasks (e.g., planning, estimating, etc.). In the case of the WCST, an inability to switch attention may mean that subjects do not update the feedback information in the phonological store, and perseveration then occurs. What this type of analysis indicates is that to truly understand the nature of frontal deficits we must go beyond simple task descriptions and discover the dynamic properties underlying complex tasks. As the results of the experiments reported here show, an analysis of the dynamics of a task helps reveal the mechanisms underlying frontal deficits and how together these mechanisms make up higher-level cognition.

The results of the experiments go beyond merely concluding that the frontal lobes are concerned with attentional allocation and working memory. Specifically, this research suggests that the deficits in higher-level reasoning observed in frontal patients occur when the task involves the maintenance of a temporary representation in working memory. We hypothesize that the central executive or attentional allocation system cannot update information in the temporary stores, particularly when there is more than one chunk of information to be maintained in working memory. The model presented here moves from a static account of how subjects and patients use information while reasoning to a dynamic account that stresses the importance of temporary representations used in higher-level thinking. By conducting detailed task analyses of the changing representations that subjects and patients generate while performing a task, it is possible to predict frontal-like deficits in normal subjects when they are prevented from constructing these temporary representations. The key to understanding frontal deficits is two-fold—knowing what temporary representations are involved in a task and the operations that must be performed on these representations. Theories that are solely concerned with attentional or working memory deficits without regard to the mental operations and contents of temporary representations will only provide a partial picture of the cognitive deficits underlying frontal deficits in higher-level cognition.

ACKNOWLEDGMENTS

We would like to thank Sylvie Belleville of the Université de Montréal for allowing us to test patient RoL and Howard Chertkow for providing the frontal closed head injury patients.

REFERENCES AND NOTES

1. NEWELL, A. & H. SIMON. 1972. Human Problem Solving. Prentice Hall. Englewood, NJ.
2. HOLLAND, J. H., K. J. HOLYOAK, R. E. NISBETT & P. R. THAGARD. 1986. Induction. MIT Press. Cambridge, MA.
3. KLAHR, D. & K. DUNBAR. 1988. Cognit. Sci. 12: 1–48.
4. SHALLICE, T. 1982. In The Neuropsychology of Cognitive Function. D. E. Broadbent & L. Weiskrantz, Eds. The Royal Society. London.
5. MILNER, B. 1963. Arch. Neurol. 9: 90–100.
6. DUNCAN, J. 1986. Cogn. Neuropsychol. 3: 271–291.
7. SHALLICE, T. & M. C. EVANS. 1978. Cortex 14: 294–303.

8.   FUSTER, J. M. 1980. The Prefrontal Cortex. Raven Press. New York.
9.   BECHRA, A., A. R. DAMASIO, H. DAMASIO & S. W. ANDERSON. Cognition **50**: 5–17.
10. CARAMANOS, Z. & M. PETRIDES. 1994. Soc. Neurosci. Abstr. **20(2)**: 1004.
11. GRAFMAN, J., B. JONAS & A. SALAZAR. 1990. Percept. Mot. Skills **71**: 1120–1122.
12. NORMAN, D. & T. SHALLICE. 1986. *In* Consciousness and Self-Regulation. R. J. Davidson, G. E. Schwartz & D. E. Shapiro, Eds. Plenum Press. New York.
13. BADDELEY, A. 1986. Working Memory. Clarendon Press. Oxford. UK.
14. COWAN, N. 1993. Memory & Cognition **21(2)**: 162–167.
15. CARPENTER, P. A., A. MIYAKE & M. A. JUST. 1994. *In* Handbook of Psycholinguistics. Morton Ann Gernsbacher, Ed.: 1075–1122. Academic Press. San Diego, CA.
16. KIMBERG, D. & M. FARAH. 1992. J. Exp. Psychol. Gen. **122**: 411–428.
17. DUNBAR, K. 1993. Cognit. Sci. **17**: 397–434.
18. DUNBAR, K. & D. BUB. 1990. Frontal assessment battery. Unpublished manuscript. McGill University. Montreal.
19. HEATON, R. K. 1984. Wisconsin Card Sorting Test Manual. Psychological Assessment Resources Inc. Odessa, FL.
20. A further explanation for these results is that the phonological task took up more memory capacity than the executive task, and that it is the taking up of working memory capacity that produces perseveration. In a recent set of experiments Dunbar and Migas (in preparation) manipulated memory load (one or two items) and type of memory load (letters, numbers, or tones) in a task in which subjects had to say whether the current stimulus was the same or different from a previous stimulus. We found more perseverative than nonperseverative errors only when phonological working memory was used. Memory load per se had an effect on total number of errors.
21. BADDELEY, A., V. J. LEWIS & G. VALLAR. 1984. Q. J. Exp. Psychol. **36**: 234.
22. One further difference between the two tasks is that subjects must respond more frequently in the articulatory suppression task than in the tone detection task. Thus, differences obtained might be due to more frequent responding in the articulatory suppression task. We are currently investigating this hypothesis.
23. BELLEVILLE, S., J. PERETZ & M. ARGUIN. 1992. Brain & Lang. **43**: 713–746.
24. STROOP, J. R. 1935. J. Exp. Psychol. **18**: 643–662.
25. DUNBAR, K. & C. M. MACLEOD. 1984. J. Exp. Psychol. Hum. Percept. Perform. **10**: 622–639.
26. COHEN, J. D., K. DUNBAR & J. M. MCCLELLAND. 1990. Psychol. Rev. **97**: 332–361.
27. MACLEOD, C. M. 1991. Psychol. Bull. **109**: 163–203.
28. PERRET, E. 1974. Neuropsychologia **12**: 323–330.
29. SHALLICE, T. 1982. Phil. Trans. R. Soc. Lond. B298: 199–209.
30. DUNBAR, K. 1985. Unpublished PhD thesis. University of Toronto. Toronto.
31. COHEN, J. D. 1995. Personal communication.
32. SNODGRASS, J. & M. VANDERWART. 1980. J. Exp. Psychol. Hum. Learn. Mem. **6**: 174–215.
33. VENDRELL, P., C. JUNQUE, J. PUJOL, M. A. JURADO, J. MOLET & J. GRAFMAN. 1995. Neuropsychologia **33**: 341–352.
34. DUNBAR, K., J. D. COHEN & V. FERREIRA. Submitted.

Neuronal Models of Prefrontal Cortical Functions

STANISLAS DEHAENE[a,b] AND JEAN-PIERRE CHANGEUX[c]

aInstitut National de la Santé et de la Recherche Médicale
Paris, France

cInstitut Pasteur
Paris, France

In the last 10 years, considerable advances have been made toward understanding the functions of prefrontal cortex and their anatomical and neurophysiological counterparts.[1,2] Relating these behavioral and neurobiological data into a coherent picture, however, remains a challenging enterprise. The development of explicit models of prefrontal cortex architecture and functions can potentially help to bridge this gap by identifying the most relevant features of cellular and behavioral data, by testing the plausibility of hypotheses put forward to relate these data in a causal manner, by drawing attention to specific experimental predictions, and by pointing to unsolved questions.

We have tried to achieve some of these goals in the limited context of simple behavioral tests of prefrontal functions. Over the years, our modeling efforts focused successively on delayed-response tasks,[3] on the Wisconsin Card Sorting Test,[4] and on the possible contribution of prefrontal cortex to the development of numerical competence.[5] In each case, we speculated on the implementation of the task in neuronal networks, and we described computer simulations of formal neuronal networks whose properties reproduce, to some extent, the available neurophysiological and behavioral data. Although the details of the models varied, common principles of neural architecture were used for all tasks. In this review, three such principles will be discussed: (1) the distinction of levels of organization, with prefrontal circuits modulating lower-level networks, (2) the role of long-lasting neuronal activity in maintaining representations of task events, and (3) the interconnection of these representations with reward systems that compute the value associated with actions or events.

The general framework in which our work has developed is that of *neural* or *mental selectionist mechanisms*.[6,7] It stresses that organisms are not passively responsive to environmental inputs and do not absorb knowledge by instruction from an external teacher. Rather, higher organisms function in a projective mode in which hypotheses or prerepresentations are internally generated and are maintained or rejected depending on their adequacy to the situation at hand. Learning proceeds by selective elimination of spontaneously generated alternatives. Thus, behavior is not driven by quasireflex responses to stimulation, but by internal goals and by representations of past events and of future actions that may be

b Address correspondence to Dr. Stanislas Dehaene, Laboratoire de Sciences Cognitives et Psycholinguistique, Centre National de la Recherche Scientifique and Ecole des Hautes Etudes en Sciences Sociales, 54 Boulevard Raspail, 75270 Paris cedex 06, France.

relevant to these goals. In mammals, prefrontal cortical circuits seem instrumental in generating goals, in maintaining representations of goal-relevant information, and in selecting these representations as a function of their expected value for the organism. Our simulations illustrate how specialized prefrontal circuits may implement these functions.

LEVELS OF ORGANIZATION

A first key feature of our models is their organization in multiple hierarchical and parallel levels. The notion that prefrontal cortex intervenes at a level of representation higher than that of other cortical circuits is common to almost all accounts of prefrontal cortical functions. Luria[8] considered the frontal lobes as crucial for the programming, regulation, and verification of activity. According to Grafman,[9] prefrontal cortex maintains and controls the execution of complex scripts or hierarchical plans for actions. Fuster[1] and Goldman-Rakic[2] have also emphasized the role of prefrontal cortex in modulating lower-level sensory-motor contingencies using working-memory representations of the organism's intentions and past knowledge. Finally in the Norman-Shallice theory,[10] prefrontal cortical areas together form a supervisory attentional system that can inhibit or select lower-level automatized thought or action schemata.

Our models[3-5] have implemented these ideas by introducing a layered architecture with multiple parallel mappings between hierarchical representations of sensory inputs and of intended motor outputs. At least three levels of processing have been distinguished: a direct mapping between sensory data and corresponding motor actions, an indirect mapping mediated by a working memory of past events, and another indirect mapping holding a representation of the rules of the task at hand. The last two indirect mappings, which are assumed to rely on prefrontal areas, modulate and select actions triggered at the lowest level (FIG. 1).

The functional role of such modulation is well illustrated by our model of delayed-response tasks, including the A-not-B task.[11,12] In these tasks, an object is hidden in one of two possible locations (A and B). The locations are then covered and the subject's attention is distracted for a short delay. At the end of this delay, one then measures the subject's ability to reach towards the appropriate location. When the task is made simpler by reducing the delay to zero, or by repeatedly hiding the object at the same location A, rhesus monkeys with prefrontal cortex lesions, as well as infants between 7 and 9 months of age whose prefrontal cortex is immature, succeed in reaching to the correct location. Hence, reaching to spatial locations and learning to always reach to a certain location are not dependent on prefrontal cortex, but rely on lower-level action schemata. In our simulations, these abilities were embodied in a direct sensorimotor pathway with slowly modifiable connections that linked a representation of the features of the objects to a representation of the available motor responses. This lower level of the model easily learned the reaching part of the task.

When the task is made more difficult, however, by imposing a longer delay between cuing a location and letting the subject reach to it, and by changing the location of the hidden object from trial to trial, young infants and monkeys with

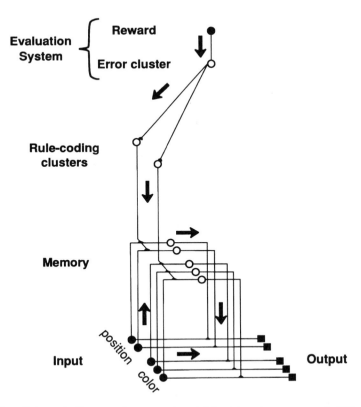

FIGURE 1. Schematic diagram of a neuronal model for delayed-response tasks,[3] illustrating a hierarchical and parallel organization with multiple levels of processing.

prefrontal lesions fail systematically. In the A-not-B task, they continue to reach towards the previously cued location A, even after the object has been shifted to location B. In other words, an immature or lesioned prefrontal cortex yields an impairment in inhibiting a previously learned response. Our simulation with the sensorimotor pathway only behaved quite similarly, making a systematic error of perseveration in reaching to location A (FIG. 2). In order to pass the test, just as neurologically intact monkeys and 12-month-old human infants do, our network had to be supplemented with a second pathway, parallel to the first, but which held a short-term memory of the cued location throughout the delay. Units at this higher level were not allowed to influence directly the motor output units, but only to modulate the connections of the lower level sensorimotor reaching pathway. They held a representation of the past location of the object and used it to bias reaching when two possible locations could be reached at after the end of the delay. These units therefore implemented a form of "working memory" which has been related to dorsolateral sectors of prefrontal cortex.[1,13]

At an even higher level of representation in our models, units that we called

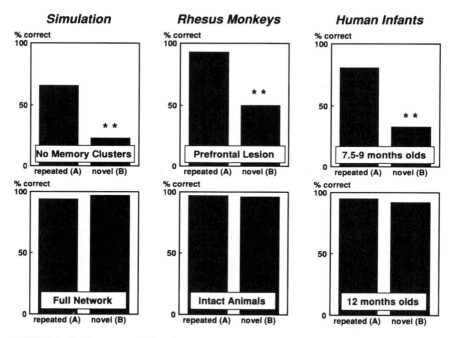

FIGURE 2. Performance of the simulated delayed-response model (*left*) as compared to actual data from rhesus monkeys (*middle*) and human infants (*right*) (data from ref. 12). The model with lesioned memory clusters, like monkeys with prefrontal lesions and 7.5–9-month-old infants, is able to reach to a hidden object after a delay when the object is repeatedly hidden at the same location, but not when the object is switched to a novel hiding location (*top graphs*). The full network model, like intact animals and older infants, reaches correctly to the hidden object in both cases (*bottom graphs*).

rule-coding clusters were allowed to modulate entire sets of connections at the lower levels (see also ref. 14). Their activation therefore drastically affected information processing. For instance, when the rule-coding cluster coding for "color" was activated, color information, rather than spatial information, was paid attention to and stored in the circuit memory. Changing the activity pattern over rule-coding clusters allowed for a very fast change in the rules used by the system, a performance analogous to that of normal human adults in the Wisconsin Card Sorting Test.[15,16] This part of the system therefore effectively performed functions attributed to the "central executive,"[17] "supervisory attentional system,"[10] or "attention for action" system[18] postulated by psychologists to underlie flexible task switching and controlling. Anatomically, this level may rely on orbitofrontal cortex,[19] the anterior cingulate,[18] and other areas forming a prefrontolimbic network.[20]

Our emphasis on levels of complexity should not imply that the connectivity in our models is purely hierarchical and pyramidal. The classical view that prefrontal cortex is an end-point in cortical processing is not tenable.[20] In our models, multi-

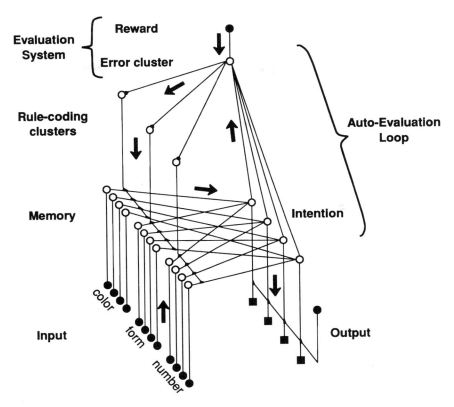

FIGURE 3. Schematic diagram of a neuronal model capable of solving the Wisconsin Card Sorting Test.[4] Note the central role of the evaluation system (*top*), which can selectively inactivate inappropriate rules at the lower levels (*left*), and can itself be internally activated by upcoming intentions via an auto-evaluation loop (*right*).

ple anatomical loops integrate prefrontal representations, together with sensory and motor representations, into parallel circuits for processing of color, form, location, or number information (FIGS. 1 and 3). This bears some similarity to the known parallel cortico-cortical circuits linking prefrontal cortex with multiple areas such as posterior parietal, anterior and posterior cingulate, and occipital and superior temporal areas.[20] Recent observations have revealed parallel functional circuits for the representation of object identity and location information in distinct prefrontal areas.[21] Working memory for object identity, on the one hand, rests on the prefrontal area of the inferior convexity, in relation with the occipitotemporal "what" pathway. Working memory for object location, on the other hand, rests on dorsolateral prefrontal cortex, in close anatomical relation to the occipitoparietal "where" pathway. This anatomical organization is similar to the maintained segregation between color and location information at all levels of processing in our models (FIGS. 1 and 3).

LONG-LASTING NEURONAL ACTIVITY

It has been known for at least 20 years that prefrontal neurons can maintain a sustained level of firing for extended periods of time.[22] In our models, as in some others,[23] this is seen as a critical and specific property of prefrontal areas that enables them to hold on-line representations of past events, future intentions, and rules of behavior. We have simulated long-lasting firing using local recurrent excitatory connections within clusters of neurons coding for a given feature (e.g., the color red). These clusters coarsely model the known columnar organization of cortical areas. Theoretical analyses and simulations show that such clusters may possess two levels of activity that are stable in time. Either most neurons in the cluster are inactive, or most neurons fire at a sustained rate. In the latter case, neurons keep a sustained or "remanent" activity because they reactivate each other through fast recurrent connections. Simulations[4] indicate that the temporal activity profiles of neurons within bistable clusters resemble those seen in actual recordings (e.g., ref. 13).

It should nevertheless be stressed that our attribution of long-lasting neuronal activity to local recurrent connections is a strictly theoretical hypothesis that awaits experimental confirmation. Alternative approaches attribute long-lasting firing to single-cell membrane properties, to distant recurrent loops with other brain areas, either cortical or subcortical,[24,25] or altogether disregard long-lasting firing as an important and specific property for the simulation of prefrontal functions.[26,27] Indeed, cells in many areas such as posterior parietal cortex or basal ganglia have also been recorded to keep a sustained level of firing during extended periods of time. In our interpretation, however, this could be due to a propagation of activation originating from local circuits forming neuronal clusters within prefrontal areas. Clearly, further research will be needed to decide between the single-cell, local circuit, and distant loop interpretations of sustained firing. Until then, our working hypothesis is that the ability to keep a sustained level of firing in the absence of sustained inputs from other areas is a specific property of prefrontal circuits that stems from strong local recurrent connections and that is not seen in other cortical regions.

What *function* does sustained firing serve? Goldman-Rakic,[2] Fuster,[1,22] and others have provided convincing evidence that prefrontal cell activity encodes a representation of past or future events. In our models, these events can be of several types. Consider for instance the model capable of solving the Wisconsin Card Sorting Test and depicted in FIG. 3. The cards that have to be sorted are encoded along three dimensions, according to the color, number, and form of the symbols on the card. Different assemblies of memory clusters are allocated to each of these parameters. Throughout a trial and the succeeding intertrial interval, these clusters hold in their activation pattern a memory of the parameters of the input card, long after it has been removed from sight. Activation from the memory clusters is then transmitted to an intention network that codes for the stack in which the network will place the input card. Hence, units at this level code for an anticipation of subsequent motor outputs ("intention") rather than for a memory of past inputs. Neurophysiologically, both types of units have been recorded in prefrontal cortex:[28] during the delay period of delayed-response task, some neurons fire only after certain types of cues were presented (e.g., red cues), whereas other units fire only before certain types of movement are made (e.g., rightward movements).

Importantly, the memory and intention clusters in our models can be completely isolated from actual inputs and outputs. Memory units can maintain a sustained level of firing in the absence of their original inputs. Likewise, intention unit activity is not propagated to motor activators unless a "go" signal is received. The effect of this "go" signal is to potentiate the intention-to-motor connections and therefore to release a preprogrammed motor command. Before the "go" signal is received, the representations held in memory and intention units function as a "mental model" or "working memory space" that can be used to freely manipulate hypotheses independently of current input-output contingencies.

In the card sorting model, a third type of unit also shows long-lasting activation: the rule-coding clusters. Here, long-lasting firing is used to maintain on-line the behavioral rule which is currently being applied and which specifies how the lower-level network will sort the input cards. The Wisconsin Card Sorting Test imposes two contradictory requirements on the rule-coding system. First, a rule must be discarded as soon as it is found not to apply well to the present situation. Second, a successful sorting rule, once found, must be maintained and applied systematically across several trials. According to our model, prefrontal cortex is ideally suited for meeting these demands because rules can be represented as stable activity patterns over rule-coding clusters rather than as slowly modified connection weights. The bistable property of neuronal clusters makes it possible to keep a rule active as long as it is useful, and yet to immediately turn the corresponding circuit off if the sorting rule must be changed.

FIGURE 4 shows how the different kinds of units with long-lasting firing in our model are activated on two consecutive trials of the Wisconsin Card Sorting Test. Even before the first trial starts, a rule-coding cluster is already active. It codes for the sorting rule that the system is going to try first. Upon presentation of a card to be sorted, input units (not shown) are activated and the corresponding memory clusters therefore switch to an active state. The sorting rule is applied, leading to the activation of an intention cluster coding for the upcoming response of the network. When the "go" signal is received, activity is allowed to propagate from intention to output units which execute the intended response. Feedback is then received from the experimenter. On the first trial depicted in FIG. 4, feedback is positive and therefore the active rule-coding cluster is maintained throughout the duration of the trial. On the next trial, feedback is negative. The active rule-coding cluster is therefore turned off and another one is activated, thus implementing the switch from one sorting rule to another.

REWARD AND AUTO-EVALUATION SYSTEMS

The example of the Wisconsin Card Sorting Test illustrates the critical role that reward systems play in the architecture of our models. Most real organisms do not acquire information about the environment via a teacher that specifies desired levels of neuronal activity, as in the backpropagation algorithm. Rather,

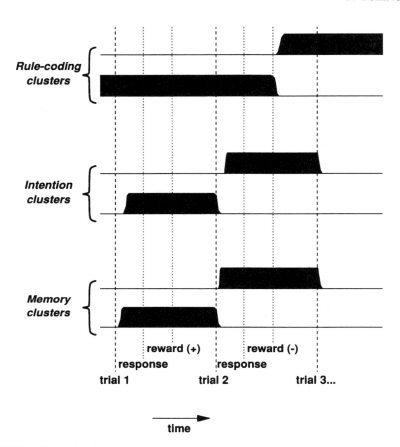

FIGURE 4. Example of long-lasting activity in memory, intention, and rule-coding clusters during two simulated trials of the card sorting task. Negative reward during the second trial induces a change in the activity of rule-coding clusters.

they are exposed, often with some delay, to the positive or negative consequences of their actions, and they learn to anticipate future rewards and to adapt their representations and goals in order to optimize these rewards. Hence, the development of adequate *value systems,* which can evaluate internal representations and use this evaluation to direct behavior, is an essential part of learning and decision making.[3–5,7,19,29] Prefrontal cortex is richly interconnected with limbic areas such as the anterior cingulate as well as with subcortical nuclei, which have been postulated to provide information about the relevance and value of behavior. Furthermore, prefrontal cell activity is often modulated by the relevance, or value, of the situation to the organism. Hence, some sectors of prefrontal cortex obviously play an important role in evaluative functions.

In our models, the interaction between the representations held on-line in prefrontal cell activity and their evaluation in limbic and/or subcortical circuits has been modeled as a bidirectional pathway. On the one hand, external rewards such as food or punishment, which are received from the environment, can be transmitted to the appropriate representations and yield an immediate modification of behavior (external evaluation). On the other hand, the same circuitry can also be activated internally, with similar consequences on behavior, because the system has learned to anticipate that a given situation is likely to result in a negative or positive reward (internal evaluation or auto-evaluation).

External Evaluation

In our model, external evaluation works as follows. The system, as a result of being in a certain activity state—for instance, with an active "color" rule cluster—performs a certain motor action (e.g., sorting a card by color). If the experimenter decides that this action was incorrect, negative reward is provided to the network. In turn, the reward input activates an error-coding cluster which signals that the network has performed an error. This error signal then has two effects on the rest of the network: a slow diffuse effect and a fast focal effect. First, the error signal is broadcast via diffuse neuromodulatory systems to all areas of the network, where it enables slow and diffuse modifications of connection strengths. The Hebbian rule that we use for synaptic modifications destabilizes recent neural activity if it led to negative reward, and stabilizes it if it led to positive reward, thus slowly increasing the chances of obtaining positive rewards in the future.

In parallel, the error signal is also sent to a targeted network, the rule-coding clusters, where it yields a fast desensitization of currently active synapses. A tentative molecular mechanism has been proposed for such desensitization.[4] A diffuse neuromodulator signaling recent negative reward (e.g., a catecholaminergic input), when occurring in conjunction with a molecular marker of recent postsynaptic activity such as an elevated intracellular concentration of calcium, would induce a reversible allosteric transition of postsynaptic receptor molecules toward a slow, desensitized state (FIG. 5). Whatever the exact molecular mechanism, the result of this fast focal effect of reward is to turn currently active rule-coding clusters back to an inactive state, thus letting other rule-coding clusters compete for the control of behavior. In the terminology of learning by selection, the rule-coding network functions as a *generator of diversity*. Spontaneous fluctuations in activity lead one rule-coding cluster to take control and inhibit the others. Subsequent negative rewards ensure the elimination of inadequate active clusters until, after several trials, one is found to yield only positive rewards.

In simulations of the rule-coding cluster network, we found ranges of parameters for which the occurrence of one or two consecutive erroneous trials was sufficient to trigger an internal change in the sorting rule used. This is comparable to the performance of normal adult subjects in the Wisconsin Card Sorting Test, who rapidly switch to a new sorting rule when the previous one is found incorrect. When we lesioned either the reward network or the rule-coding network, however, perseverations were observed: the system continued to use the same sorting rule

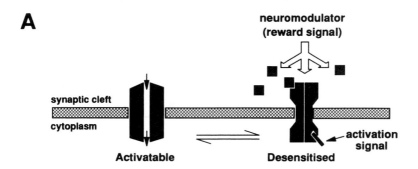

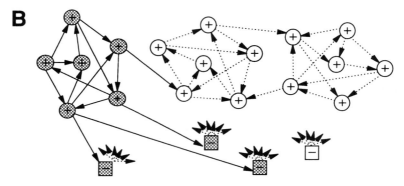

FIGURE 5. Tentative mechanism for the shift in rule-coding cluster activity when negative reward is received (the "generator of diversity"). (**A**) The simultaneous occurrence, on a given postsynaptic site, of a diffuse neuromodulator signaling recent negative reward and of a postsynaptic marker of recent cell activity, such as intracellular calcium, triggers an allosteric transition of postsynaptic receptor molecules towards a desensitized state (ion channel closed). (**B**) This molecular mechanism has the effect of depriving currently active neurons from supporting inputs from neighboring neurons belonging to the same cluster. The cluster therefore shifts from a stable active state to a stable inactive state, releasing other clusters from lateral inhibition and allowing them to compete for the control of behavior.

for several trials in a row, even after it was negatively rewarded several times. Hence, the lesioned network mimicked the perserverative behavior observed in patients with frontal lesions.[15,16]

Perseverations were observed in our model after many sorts of simulated lesions, including weakening the reward input, weakening the influence of the error signal on the rule-coding network, weakening or destroying the connections originating from rule-coding clusters, or eliminating the rule-coding clusters altogether. Hence, we would expect many different types of frontal and/or subcortical lesions to affect card sorting performance. We also found that our simulation performed poorly (but without perseverating) when the rule-coding layer was extended to include rules other than the three basic color, form, and number rules. This may, to some extent, account for the failure of some normal subjects in the task.[16] Our contention is that the two sorts of failure have very different origins: normal subjects fail because they tend to try out complex sorting rules before having exhausted the simplest ones, whereas frontal patients fail because of an impairment in changing the current sorting rule in the face of negative reward.

Internal Evaluation or Auto-Evaluation

The ability to evaluate behavior internally and to anticipate future errors was also provided to the card sorting network by introducing modifiable connections from the intention units to the error cluster (FIG. 3). These connections, which formed an *auto-evaluation loop,* were able to learn when a pattern of activity over intention clusters had been associated with negative reward. If, later on the same trial, the same intention recurred, the error-coding cluster was spontaneously activated via the auto-evaluation loop, with the consequence that the sorting rule was immediately changed without actually having to try it on the environment.

Auto-evaluation, in conjunction with the previously described ability of memory and intention clusters to remain isolated from external inputs and outputs, provides our simulation with an internal work space in which representations can be manipulated and rules can be tried out until a satisfactory one is found. A precise sequence of neuronal activity is predicted (FIG. 6). When negative reward is received, it triggers a change in rule-coding cluster activity and a new sorting rule becomes active. This new rule, when applied to the memorized features of the input card, yields a new pattern of activity over intention clusters. If this pattern is again recognized by the auto-evaluation loop as likely to be negatively rewarded, the error cluster is internally activated, and the whole cycle starts overs until a more satisfactory intention is found.

The notion of auto-evaluation and its relation to prefrontal cortex has now begun to receive experimental support. Damasio and colleagues[19,30,31] have studied patients who experience severe difficulties in decision making in everyday life and whose deficit is traceable to an impairment in evaluating whether a given image, situation, or plan has a positive or negative outcome. Because their auto-evaluation of ideas and plans is impaired, these patients do not know how to select a course of action other than by chance or by attempting to list all the events that could happen. Anatomically, these patients have lesions of the orbitofrontal cortex, which is a good candidate for a component of the auto-evaluation loop because of its strong connectivity with the limbic system.

In our model, the auto-evaluation loop is used exclusively for the internal detection of erroneous intentions. Recently, an electrophysiological correlate of such error-detection has been observed in normal humans.[32–34] In several reaction time tasks, a sharp focal negativity was recorded from medial frontal scalp electrodes only on trials in which the subject made an error. This error negativity occurred with a very short latency (about 70 ms) after the response was made, ruling out sensory feedback and suggesting that errors were internally monitored in parallel to the execution of the response. Anatomically, dipole modeling suggested that the generator of the error effect was located in the anterior cingulate cortex. Single-

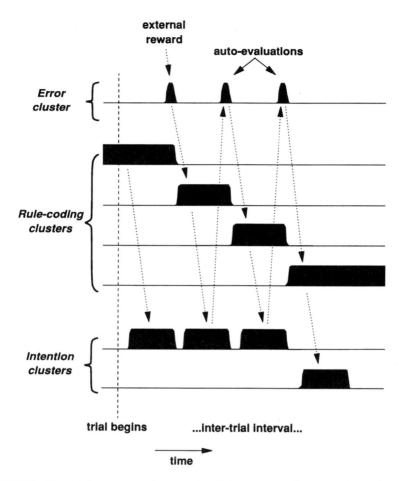

FIGURE 6. Simulated sequence of neuronal activity corresponding to an internal test of several rules. At the beginning of a trial, an intention is tried out and external negative reward is received. This sets up a cyclical sequence of activity in which (1) a new rule-coding cluster becomes active; (2) this leads to the activation of an intention cluster; (3) the current intention is recognized as being the same one that previously led to negative reward; and (4) the error cluster is activated via the auto-evaluation loop and the process repeats. The testing cycle stops when a rule is found which leads to a different intention, one that is not known to yield a negative reward.

cell recordings in monkeys have also revealed anterior cingulate cells that fire when the animal makes an error or when an expected reward fails to be delivered.[35] It is not known yet whether the anterior cingulate contributes to error detection, error correction, or both. However, its strong connectivity with multiple areas of prefrontal cortex fit well with its involvement in an anterior auto-evaluation circuit.

CONCLUSION AND FUTURE PROSPECTS

According to our models, three aspects of frontal lobe circuitry are critical to an understanding of its contribution to cognitive functions. First, prefrontal areas are involved in hierarchically organized nested circuits that modulate lower-level sensory and motor circuits. Second, prefrontal circuits can sustain a long-lasting neuronal activity, which enables them to maintain over time representations of past events, anticipations of future events, and putative goals or rules for behavior, and to manipulate these representations in a purely internal manner. Third, prefrontal representations can be rapidly selected or eliminated based on an evaluation of performance by reward systems. Frontolimbic circuits forming an auto-evaluation loop endow the organism with a capacity to evaluate behavior internally instead of having to wait for external reinforcement.

The three properties of modulation of lower levels, representation detached from input-output contingencies, and auto-evaluation fit well with views of the frontal lobe as a "central executive" or "supervisory system"[10,17] that evaluates and controls cognitive processing. Nevertheless, our models of this supervisory system remain highly simplified. From the anatomical point of view, an important direction for future modeling will be to incorporate more realistic data on the anatomy and connectivity of known brain areas. From the functional point of view, tasks that are known to depend on the supervisory functions of prefrontal cortex, but cannot be handled by present network architectures, should be addressed in future simulations.

For instance, some prefrontal lesions are known to affect the ability to retrieve temporal-order information and use it to guide behavior.[1] Our models cannot address this issue yet because although they incorporate a mechanism for maintaining on-line representations of past events, the order in which these events occurred is not represented explicitly. Indeed, we know of no neuronal model of temporal-order judgments that has attempted to account for prefrontal impairments in the time domain. However, models for the role of frontal and subcortical areas in the production of temporal sequences of actions[23-25] might probably be extended to account for relative order judgments.

Another function not properly addressed by current models is the planning of a future sequence of actions. A classical test of planning is Shallice's Tower of London test,[36] a puzzle with pegs and movable disks in which the patient must find the shortest sequence of moves for achieving a given configuration of the disks. Solving the test requires the exploration of a tree of possible moves by trial and error. Normal subjects decompose the problem into a hierarchical sequence of subgoals; patients with prefrontal lesions may have a specific impairment in managing this subgoal hierachy.[37] Auto-evaluation probably plays an important role in the process of subgoal selection by permitting the elimination of moves that diverge from the main goal. However, other components are also needed which have not yet been incorporated in models. Most notably, how could a hierarchy of goals and subgoals be represented within a neural network? And how could neural activity progress through a sequence of goals with automatic backtracking when errors or impasses are found? As our knowledge of prefrontal functions increases, these questions stand out as important unsolved problems that will have to be addressed by theorists and neurobiologists alike.

REFERENCES

1. FUSTER, J. M. 1989. The Prefrontal Cortex. 2nd edit. Raven. New York.
2. GOLDMAN-RAKIC, P. S. 1987. Circuitry of primate prefrontal cortex and regulation of behavior by representational knowledge. *In* Handbook of Physiology. F. Plum & V. Mountcastle, Eds. Vol. 5: 373–417. American Physiological Society. Bethesda, MD.
3. DEHAENE, S. & J. P. CHANGEUX. 1989. A simple model of prefrontal cortex function in delayed-response tasks. J. Cognit. Neurosci. 1: 244–261.
4. DEHAENE, S. & J. P. CHANGEUX. 1991. The Wisconsin Card Sorting Test: Theoretical analysis and modelling in a neuronal network. Cereb. Cortex 1: 62–79.
5. DEHAENE, S. & J. P. CHANGEUX. 1993. Development of elementary numerical abilities: A neuronal model. J. Cognit. Neurosci. 5: 390–407.
6. CHANGEUX, J. P. & S. DEHAENE. 1989. Neuronal models of cognitive functions. Cognition 33: 63–109.
7. EDELMAN, G. 1987. Neural Darwinism. Basic Books. New York.
8. LURIA, A. R. 1966. The Higher Cortical Functions in Man. Basic Books. New York.
9. GRAFMAN, J. 1989. Plans, actions, and mental sets: Managerial knowledge units in the frontal lobes. *In* Integrating Theory and Practice in Clinical Neuropsychology. E. Perecman, Ed.: 93–138. Erlbaum. Hillsdale, NJ.
10. SHALLICE, T. 1988. From Neuropsychology to Mental Structure. Cambridge University Press. Cambridge, MA.
11. PIAGET, J. 1954. The Construction of Reality in the Child. Basic Books. New York.
12. DIAMOND, A. & P. S. GOLDMAN-RAKIC. 1989. Comparison of human infants and rhesus monkeys on Piaget's A-not-B task: Evidence for dependence on dorsolateral prefrontal cortex. Exp. Brain Res. 74: 24–40.
13. FUNAHASHI, S., C. J. BRUCE & P. S. GOLDMAN-RAKIC. 1989. Mnemonic coding of visual space in the monkey's dorsolateral prefontal cortex. J. Neurophysiol. 61: 331–349.
14. COHEN, J. D., K. DUNBAR & J. McCLELLAND. 1990. On the control of automatic processes: A parallel distributed processing model of the Stroop effect. Psychol. Rev. 97: 332–361.
15. MILNER, B. 1963. Effects of brain lesions on card sorting. Arch. Neurol. 9: 90–100.
16. NELSON, H. E. 1976. A modified card sorting test sensitive to frontal lobe defects. Cortex 12: 313–324.
17. BADDELEY, A. 1986. Working Memory. Oxford University Press. New York.
18. POSNER, M. I. & S. DEHAENE. 1994. Attentional networks. Trends Neurosci. 17: 75–79.
19. DAMASIO, A. R. 1994. Descartes' error: Emotion, reason, and the human brain. G. P. Putnam. New York.
20. GOLDMAN-RAKIC, P. S. 1988. Topography of cognition: Parallel distributed networks in primate association cortex. Annu. Rev. Neurosci. 11: 137–156.
21. WILSON, F. A. W., S. P. O'SCALAIDHE & P. S. GOLDMAN-RAKIC. 1993. Dissociation of object and spatial processing domains in primate prefrontal cortex. Science 260: 1955–1958.
22. FUSTER, J. M. 1973. Unit activity in prefrontal cortex during delayed-response performance: Neuronal correlates of transient memory. J. Neurophysiol. 36: 61–78.
23. GUIGON, E., B. DORIZZI, Y. BURNOD & W. SCHULTZ. 1995. Neural correlates of learning in the prefrontal cortex of the monkey: A predictive model. Cereb. Cortex. 5: 135–147.
24. BERNS, G. S. & T. J. SEJNOWSKI. How the basal ganglia make decisions. *In* Neurobiology of Decision-Making. A. R. Damasio, Ed. Springer Verlag. Berlin. In press.
25. DOMINEY, P., M. ARBIB & J. P. JOSEPH. A model of cortico-striatal plasticity for learning oculomotor associations and sequences. J. Cognit. Neurosci. In press.

26. COHEN, J. D. & D. SERVAN-SCHREIBER. 1992. Context, cortex, and dopamine: A connectionist approach to behavior in schizophrenia. Psychol. Rev. **99:** 45–77.
27. LEVINE, D. S. & P. S. PRUEITT. 1989. Modelling some effects of frontal lobe damage—novelty and perseveration. Neural Networks **2:** 103–116.
28. NIKI, H. & M. WATANABE. 1976. Prefrontal unit activity and delayed response: Relation to cue location versus direction of response. Brain Res. **105:** 79–88.
29. FRISTON, K. J., G. TONONI, G. N. REEKE, O. SPORNS & G. M. EDELMAN. 1994. Value-dependent selection in the brain: Simulation in a synthetic neural model. Neurosci. **59:** 229–243.
30. DAMASIO, A. R., D. TRANEL & H. DAMASIO. 1990. Individuals with sociopathic behavior caused by frontal damage fail to respond autonomically to social stimuli. Behav. Brain Res. **41:** 81–94.
31. ESLINGER, P. J. & A. R. DAMASIO. 1985. Severe disturbance of higher cognition after bilateral frontal lobe ablation: Patient EVR. Neurology **35:** 1731–1741.
32. DEHAENE, S., M. I. POSNER & D. M. TUCKER. 1994. Localization of a neural system for error detection and compensation. Psychol. Sci. **5:** 303–305.
33. FALKENSTEIN, M., J. HOHNSBEIN, J. HOORMANN & L. BLANKE. 1990. Effects of errors in choice reaction time tasks on the ERP under focused and divided attention. *In* Psychophysiological Brain Research. C. H. M. Brunia, A. W. K. Gaillard & A. Kok, Eds.: 192–195. Tilburg University Press. Tilburg, the Netherlands.
34. GEHRING, W. J., B. GOSS, M. G. H. COLES, D. E. MEYER & E. DONCHIN. 1993. A neural system for error detection and compensation. Psychol. Sci. **4:** 385–390.
35. NIKI, H. & M. WATANABE. 1979. Prefrontal and cingulate unit activity during timing behavior in the monkey. Brain Res. **171:** 213–224.
36. SHALLICE, T. 1982. Specific impairments of planning. Phil. Trans. R. Soc. London B **298:** 199–209.
37. GOEL, V. & J. GRAFMAN. Are the frontal lobes implicated in "planning" functions? Interpreting data from the tower of Hanoi. Neuropsychologia. In press.

Re-examining the Role of Executive Functions in Routine Action Production[a]

MYRNA F. SCHWARTZ[b]

Moss Rehabilitation Research Institute
1200 West Tabor Road
Philadelphia, Pennsylvania 19141

In Higher Cortical Functions in Man,[1] Luria wrote:

> Actions in relation to objects require a series of successive links, and these must be in the proper order. It is this sequence that is disturbed in patients with a lesion of the frontal lobes; an action that has become firmly established by previous experience disintegrates into a series of isolated fragments. (p. 237)

This passage continues with examples of patients with extensive frontal lobe lesions whose attempts to light a cigarette were fragmented, disorganized, and perseverative. Such difficulties were further compounded if the patient was asked to perform an act that was less familiar (lighting a candle) that had some elements in common with the other, more habitual action.

> In these instances the patient could not retain the plan of the required action and was easily distracted by the more firmly established motor stereotype. Having lit the candle he would put it into his mouth, or perform the habitual movements of smoking a cigarette with it, or break it and throw it away (as he usually did with a match), etc. . . . The plan of the action, formed in response to the instruction, readily disintegrated and was replaced by isolated, fragmentary acts. Comparison between the effect of the completed action and its intention was also lost. (pp. 237–238)

Although many of Luria's teachings on the frontal lobe syndrome have been incorporated into contemporary theories, the notion that simple, routine behaviors like lighting a cigarette fall within the purview of the frontal lobes would find few adherents today. On the contrary, a consensus exists among contemporary theorists that frontal executive functions play little role in the performance of routine, everyday skills:

> On the model, well-learned cognitive skills and cognitive procedures do not require the higher level control system. Higher level control only becomes necessary if error correction and planning have to be performed, if the situation is novel, or temptation must be overcome.
> —Norman and Shallice[2]

> The prefrontal cortex is the anatomical basis for the function of control. . . .
> The frontal lobes are imperative at the time a new activity is being learned

[a] This work was supported by National Institutes of Health Grant No. 1R01 NS31824-02.
[b] e-mail: mschwar@vm.temple.edu.

and active control is required; after the activity has become routine, however, the frontal participation is no longer demanded.

—Stuss and Benson[3]

The structure of behavior formed by the agency of prefrontal cortex contains enough variable and uncertain elements to be treated by the organism as new, even though its elements may be old and familiar. . . . Thus, the automatic or instinctual series of acts, however complex, is not within the purview of the prefrontal cortex.

—J. Fuster[4]

The supporting evidence is compelling: Focal lesions restricted to the frontal lobes which cause disorganization and error in nonroutine behavior leaves routine behavior intact. Luria's counter-examples come from patients with bilateral frontal tumors or massive frontal hematomas and thus are subject to dismissal as arising from general cerebral dysfunction and dementia.[5]

In this paper, I wish to re-examine the role of frontal executive functions in routine action production along lines that are more sympathetic to Luria's position. My observations will be drawn from two sources: the spontaneous action slips of everyday life, and the breakdown of routine action organization in traumatic brain injury and other injuries involving, but not limited to, the frontal lobes. In previous work, we have used Luria's term, "frontal apraxia," to refer to this breakdown of routine action organization. Here, we adopt a more neutral designation, suggested by Tim Shallice: action disorganization syndrome (ADS). The ADS is discussed in the second part of this paper. Part I focuses on spontaneous action slips in non-brain-damaged individuals.

SPONTANEOUS ACTION SLIPS

Action slips are the nonverbal analogs of slips of the tongue: they are behaviors that deviate from what the actor intended. Like slips of the tongue, action slips provide a window onto the organization of planning and production systems (e.g., refs. 6–10). Drawing primarily on such evidence, investigators have reached a consensus framework, which Sellen and Norman[11] recently summarized as follows:

Most researchers in the field agree on a hierarchically organized system containing multiple levels of representation. At the highest level is the representation of conscious goals and desires. At the lowest levels are representations of the details of the particular actions to be executed. With regard to the issue of control, we have evidence of a broad but important distinction. There are two main modes of control: an unconscious, automatic mode best modeled as a network of distributed processors acting locally and in parallel; and a conscious control mode acting globally to oversee and override automatic control. Automatic and conscious control are complementary: the unconscious mode is fast, parallel, and context-dependent, responding to regularities in the environment in routine ways, whereas the conscious mode is effortful, limited, and flexible, stepping in to handle novel situation. (p. 318)

Readers who follow the frontal lobe literature will have encountered these ideas in Norman and Shallice's theory of attention and action.[2,12–14] The distributed

TABLE 1. Action Slips as Novel Creations

Omission	
Intended:	Undress; get into shower
Did:	Got into shower (with clothes on)
Exchange	
Intended:	Put *cigarette* in mouth; strike *match*
Did:	Put *match* in mouth; struck *cigarette*
Substitution	
Intended:	Hold *toothbrush* under running water
Did:	Held *toothpaste tube* under running water
Intended:	Shake salt *onto food*
Did:	Shook salt *into tea*
Intended:	Peel *oranges*
Did:	Peeled *can of meatballs*

processors are known by such terms as "demons," "automatisms," and "schemas"; the fast, parallel, unconscious mode of control is "contention scheduling"; the conscious, limited capacity controller is "supervisory attention." Regarding action slips, the claim is that supervisory attention is called upon to prevent or correct errors when the automatic control mode will not suffice, which is primarily in cases where a behavior that is habitual in a given context must be suppressed in favor of a novel behavior. Failure to apply supervisory attention at such instances leads to strong habit intrusions,[7] alternatively called "liberated automatisms"[15] or "capture errors."[10]

> I (M.S.) am in the habit of brushing my teeth several times a day, and more often than I intend. It often happens that I go into the bathroom to take something from the closet or cabinet only to find myself at the sink with toothbrush and toothpaste in hand.

This a capture error, a liberated automatism. But not all action slips show this bias toward the familiar. Consider the examples in TABLE 1, taken from the Manchester diary study (note A).[7,16–17] Omission errors depart from the routine by the deletion of a critical step. Exchange errors distort the structure of a familiar sequence by a transposition of arguments from two successive actions. Substitutions replace an argument of the action with something that affords similar actions or is located nearby. In contrast to the tooth-brushing example, peeling a can of meatballs is presumably a "novel creation," and not part of the normal action repertoire; and so, too, for the other errors in TABLE 1.

A variety of explanations have been offered to account for such novel creation errors. For example, Baars and colleagues[18–20] have produced exchange and substitution errors in the laboratory by inducing in their subjects competing action plans and limited time to respond. The idea is that plan competition encourages movement errors among lower-level constituents of the plans. An entry in the Manchester study reads:

> When I leave for work in the morning, I am in the habit of throwing two dog biscuits to my pet corgi and then putting on my earrings. One morning, I

threw the earrings to the dog and found my self trying to attach a dog biscuit to my ear.

Presumably, the two plans were simultaneously active in the mind of the actor and in competition for control of the effectors, which promoted the transposition of the lower-level constituents (i.e., earrings [theme of transport-to-ear] transposed with biscuits [theme of throw-to-dog]).

Above, I referred to such movable constituents as "arguments." This follows from the view that schemas specify slots or variables to be filled by a process of selection. On this view, argument substitutions can also arise from competition among a set of candidates that meet specified "calling conditions" on slot fillers.[9,21] The more precisely specified the calling conditions, the less likely are substitutions; however, in contention scheduling there is a natural tendency toward underspecification,[21,22] which predisposes to substitutions.

> I (M.S.) was doing some calculations in front of the TV and wanted to change the station. I picked up my calculator, aimed it at the TV, and began pressing the buttons.

On the "underspecification" account of this error, the mental representation of the remote control device elaborated at the moment of reaching provided an acceptable match to the representation of the calculator delivered by my perceptual/semantic system.

From such considerations, it appears that routine action production involves a more highly constructed process, with greater potential for error, than appeared at first blush. The requirement is for the constituents of action plans—for example, goal, action, and argument schemas (note B)—to be bound together in temporary assemblies; but with competition at each level of constituent structure there is the potential for faulty selection within level and erroneous or rapidly fading linkages across levels.

Here, then, is the key point: If routine action production is as prone to error as this, and if it falls to supervisory attention to monitor for errors and correct them before they are overtly expressed, then the supervisory attention system is playing a more active role in routine action production than is generally appreciated.

It is often said that routine activities are carried out "automatically." According to the Norman and Shallice theory, this means with minimal involvement of supervisory attention. However, this does not rule out a key role for attention in the broader sense of that term, that is, in the functional sense of task-directed information pick up;[23] in the neurophysiological sense of temporary and contingent closure of some communication channels and selective opening of others;[24] and in the cognitive sense of selecting actions in accordance with goal requirements, and objects and spatial locations in accordance with action requirements.[24–26] Indeed, attention, in this broader sense, may be said to serve precisely those selection and binding operations that routine action depends on. Are prefrontal structures implicated in attention in this broader sense? As I read the literature on anterior attention systems, the answer is yes (26–30) from which I conclude that the role of prefrontal systems in routine action production extends well beyond the monitoring, or novelty promotion functions attributed to supervisory attention.

The working memory functions of prefrontal cortex[31,32] may also be implicated in routine action production, as when a current goal must be maintained in an active state during the search for, or preparation of, materials needed to serve the action plan. As this implies, the demands for working memory vary with task, context, and personal habits, and so, too, for the attentional demands. If you are accustomed to carrying out your grooming activities at a sink cluttered with jars, tubes, bottles, and a variety of implements, the attentional requirements for selecting the right object and the right location will be greater than if the sink is clear. If the order of your morning routines varies from day to day, there will be more competition among plans, and more potential for argument exchanges, than if the order is fixed. And, if you must locomote some distance, say to an upstairs bathroom, to execute these activities, you run a greater risk of having the intention fade from working memory before you get there.

Even so, the demands on prefrontal attention and working memory systems will generally be less for routine activities than they are for activities that are not highly practiced. First, the very process of routinization imposes constraints on selection operations and goal-action-object linkages.[9,10] Moreover, routine actions such as those I have been discussing rarely require bridging long temporal dependencies,[4] and the working memory requirements are minimized by the concreteness of the tasks,[32] that is, the fact that they involve operations on real objects, rather than second- or third-order representations.[33] The point is not to deny that routine tasks are less demanding of prefrontal executive functions; rather, it is to argue that there is no clear demarcation of novel and routine that justifies attributing executive functions to one but not the other. The routine activities of everyday life are certainly low on the continuum of executive demands, but they are represented on that continuum nonetheless.

THE ACTION DISORGANIZATION SYNDROME

In the Drucker Brain Injury Center of MossRehab Hospital, we work with individuals recovering from traumatic brain injury (TBI), primarily closed head injuries incurred in motor vehicle accidents. Such accidents impact significantly on the functions served by the frontal lobes. Disorders of executive functions are well-known sequelae of TBI, and individuals with TBI are prominently represented in studies of the dysexecutive syndrome. What is less well recognized is that a sizable number of individuals recovering from TBI pass through a phase in which they are prone to errors and other disruptions in executing even the simplest, most routine tasks of everyday life.[34,35] These patients look very much like Luria's frontal apraxics. (Recall that we have relabeled the syndrome ADS: action disorganization syndrome.) If Luria was correct in his view that ADS represents an extreme form of the frontal executive disorder, it would pose a second challenge to the view that executive functions are not involved in routine action production.

In our initial studies of the ADS, we simply set up a video camera in the hospital's rooms and dining halls and recorded the patients as they performed their morning routines. We observed each patient over several days and, in some cases, months, recording events like these:

> *Patient H.H.*:[22] At the breakfast tray: spoons butter into coffee; attempts to pour from closed juice container; at the sink: perseveratively opens and closes the water tap.
> *Patient J.K.*:[36] At the breakfast tray: pours dry cereal into coffee mug; at the sink: attempts to shave without plugging in electric shaver; spreads shaving cream on toothbrush.

From these early observational studies we developed an *action coding system,* which describes the temporal and hierarchical structure of the task as it is performed by the patient, and which quantifies the degree of disorganization and the frequency and types of error.[22]

In subsequent studies,[37,38] we moved to somewhat less naturalistic settings but with the focus still on familiar, pragmatic tasks. Borrowing from the literature on ideational apraxia, we had patients perform tasks like *making a pot of coffee* and *preparing a letter to mail* under standardized conditions, and we examined performance as a function of task and of patient etiology (e.g., TBI; unilateral brain damage).

More recently, we expanded this procedure into what we call the Multi-Level Action Test (MLAT). The MLAT assesses performance on three different tasks—preparing a slice of toast with butter and jam, wrapping a package, and preparing and packing a child's lunch box. Each task is performed under conditions that vary in their cognitive and executive demands: with and without foils in the array; alone or in combination with other tasks; with and without a requirement of searching through a drawer for essential items. Patients with a variety of neurological injuries are being tested. Administration and scoring procedures have been developed that can be uniformly and reliably applied to all types of patients.

From these lines of investigation have come a number of findings that any adequate theory of the ADS will have to account for:

1. There is substantial variability in how patients with ADS go about their supposedly routine tasks from day to day, and in the likelihood of success at each step. Actions carried out normally on one day may be omitted or seriously distorted on the next.

2. Performance varies also as a function of task and context. For example, Schwartz *et al.*[38] found that patients with ADS, regardless of etiology, were likely to make primarily argument substitution errors in preparing a pot of coffee but primarily sequence errors in packing a lunch box. Analysis of the preliminary data from our MLAT study shows that patients with mild-to-moderate TBI make more errors executing a single task when foils are present, and they make more errors executing two tasks when required to search through a draw for essential items (FIG. 1).

3. All of the error types that have been documented in collections of spontaneous action slips can be observed as well in patients with ADS (TABLE 2). Yet there are also important differences between patients' errors and spontaneous action slips. Patients commit errors even when it appears that they are attending

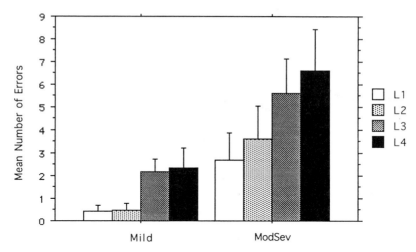

FIGURE 1. Mean error score (± 1 standard error) for patients with traumatic brain injury run on the Multi-Level Action Test (MLAT). The severity classification is based on the Functional Independence Measure (FIM). Moderate–severe patients ($n = 10$) had FIMs in the range 13 to 85; mild patients ($n = 13$) had FIMs in the range 86 to 130. All subjects executed all four MLAT levels: On level 1 they performed a single task with no foils present; on level 2, a single task with foils; on level 3, two tasks; on level 4, two tasks with a search-through-drawer requirement. Tasks and order of levels were counterbalanced across subjects.

closely to the task. Moreover, their errors are more blatant, and they may persist for long periods without being corrected. Indeed, patients do not always acknowledge their errors when they are pointed out to them. Thus, although spontaneous action slips qualify as "actions not as intended," it is less clear that patients' errors do.

The following excerpts illustrate some of these characteristics of errors in patients with ADS. These excerpts all come from a single patient, C.R., as she performed the MLAT tasks.

C.R. exhibited transcortical sensory aphasia and ADS after an episode of anoxia. An MRI study was negative; SPECT scans with technetium-HMPAO demonstrated decreased tracer uptake in the anterior and temporal lobes bilaterally, as well as dorsolateral prefrontal cortex, left greater than right.

Task: *Prepare one piece of toast with butter and jam, and a cup of instant coffee with milk and sugar.* C.R. started out as most controls do, inserting the bread in the toaster and preparing the coffee during the time that the bread was toasting. When the coffee was made, she returned to the toast, spread butter, then *repeated the sugaring of coffee.* This error involved the perseveration of the complete sugaring sequence: a heaping teaspoon followed by a half teaspoon, exactly as she had done seconds earlier.

Task: *Pack a child's lunchbox with sandwich, snack and juice (foils are present).* In making the sandwich, C.R. used *raw hot dogs* (a foil) as a substitute for lunch meat, and *spatula* (a foil) as a substitute for the knife. She first attempted to slice the hot dog with the spatula, then corrected to the knife. After spreading the sliced hot dog on the sandwich bread, she attempted to

TABLE 2. Examples of Errors Committed by Patients Performing the Multi-Level Action Test

Capture	
Intended(?):	Prepare sandwich; pack sandwich
Did:	Prepared sandwich; ate sandwich
Omission	
Intended(?):	Fill thermos; seal thermos
Did:	_____; sealed (empty) thermos
Exchange	
Intended(?):	Seal thermos; seal mustard
Did:	Put mustard lid on thermos; put thermos lid on mustard
Substitution	
Intended(?):	Tear piece of *Scotch tape* from roll; use to fasten gift wrap
Did:	Tore strip of *stamps* from stamp roll; used to fasten gift wrap
Addition	
Intended(?):	Put present in gift box
Did:	Put present and bows in gift box
Anticipation	
Intended(?):	Pack sandwich, cookies & thermos; close lunchbox
Did:	Packed sandwich; closed lunchbox after each item packed
Perseveration	
Intended(?):	Toast bread; apply butter; apply jelly
Did:	Toasted bread; applied butter; toasted bread (i.e., buttered toast)

apply mustard with the spatula, which would not fit into the jar opening. She then switched again to the knife. The substitution of hot dog for lunch meat was not corrected; nor was there any sign that she detected the error.

Task: *Wrap a present as a gift.* C.R. successfully wrapped the gift box, but omitted inserting the gift. When it came to applying the bow, she experienced difficulty removing the paper backing and wound up pulling off the whole adhesive strip. As most of our subjects do who find themselves in this situation, she proceeded to create a roll of Scotch tape with which to stick the bow on the present. Having made the tape roll, however, she applied it instead to the bottom of the *tape dispenser,* which she had just put down. She then pressed the *tape dispenser* onto the top of the present, looked the whole assembly over, and indicated that she was satisfied.

Task: *Pack a lunchbox and a child's schoolbag.* C.R. created a sandwich with lunch meat, then opened the mustard jar. Situated next to the sandwich was a set of colored markers, which was to be packed in the schoolbag. She extracted the blue marker from the set, removed the top, and *colored the lunch meat* in the open sandwich. She did this slowly and in a quite deliberate fashion, following which she replaced the top on the marker, and returned it to its set. At this point, she closed the sandwich, then opened it again to check on the contents, then closed the mustard jar.

This error involves replacing one action (spreading mustard on sandwich) with another that is much less likely in that context (coloring a sandwich with magic marker). Arguably, it was due to faulty or incomplete specification of the goal (e.g., "apply color to the lunch meat"). If so, it explains why C.R.

failed to detect the error: the outcome (colored lunch meat) provided an adequate match to the specified goal.

4. The neuropsychological profiles of patients with ADS tend to be quite complex. Most patients (C.R. included) perform abnormally on tests assessing both posterior and frontal cognitive functions. However, one should not jump to the conclusion that the ADS is merely a reflection of global dementia or confusion. There is generally more specificity to the testing profile that would be expected on this account.

Schwartz et al.[36] report on a patient with closed head injury, in whom an MR scan revealed multiple focal lesions located in left inferior posterior parietal lobe, right orbital and dorsolateral frontal lobe, and the temporal lobes bilaterally. The patient presented with ADS, including a marked tendency to use the wrong object for a given action, or the wrong action for a given object. He was anomic and had a severe anterograde amnesia. He was also impaired on tests of sustained attention and gestural praxis (note C). Although there was some evidence of impaired access to semantic memory, he generally performed quite well on tests that assessed his knowledge of the types of objects utilized in routine, everyday tasks. For example, on a test requiring the matching of objects on the basis of shared function, his performance was in the range of normal controls. He also performed without error when required to discriminate correct from incorrect object use and also when required to arrange photographs to convey the sequential organization of routine tasks. Visual perceptual functions were intact.

THEORETICAL INTERPRETATION OF THE ACTION DISORGANIZATION SYNDROME

The account of routine action planning set forth in the first section suggests three alternative accounts of the ADS: a disorder of supervisory attention; a disorder of contention scheduling; or a disorder of the schemas upon which contention scheduling operates.

ADS as a Disorder of Supervisory Attention

In the original formulation of the Norman and Shallice theory, a severe disorder of supervisory attention results in unmodulated contention scheduling (see refs. 14 and 39). Depending on the task and the context, this might manifest as distractibility, utilization behavior, and capture errors; or, alternatively, stuck-in-set perseverations. But the full-blown ADS, with its abundance of novel creation errors, was not predicted by the theory, and indeed was viewed as incompatible with it.[40] Currently, Shallice and colleagues[41] are working on a reformulation of the theory that fractionates supervisory attention into multiple components and assigns it a more extensive role in contention scheduling. The evidence from spontaneous action slips reviewed in the first of this paper supports such a move. With regard to the ADS, the point is this: If supervisory attention participates in contention scheduling in such a way as to support or monitor the selection and binding of constituents of action plans, then it is indeed possible that a severe disorder of supervisory attention might give rise to the full variety of errors seen in the ADS. The variability in performance from day to day and as a function of task demands would be readily accommodated by this account, as would the resemblance to spontaneous action slips. The major difficulty is that to date, there are no reports of patients with impairments restricted to the supervisory attention system (or its presumed equivalent, the central executive component of working memory)[42,43] who demonstrate the full-blown ADS. As my colleagues and I have emphasized, the ADS seems rather to be associated with more complex neuropsychological profiles.

ADS as a Disorder of Contention Scheduling

In an early series of papers,[22,40] my colleagues and I argued that the ADS reflects a specific disorder in routine action planning, attributable to the failure to activate low-level action schemas from high-level goal specifications (see refs. 9 and 27 for related accounts). This is equivalent to a disorder of contention scheduling in which the activation of low-level schemas by parent schemas is impaired while the triggering of such schemas by perceptual input systems, so-called bottom-up activation,[44] continues to operate.

The contention scheduling account of ADS has a number of problems. First, it sheds no light on the relation between errors in ADS and spontaneous action slips. Second, it ignores the attendant neuropsychological deficits in patients with ADS. Third, it fails to explain why it is that the ADS often evolves into a more typical frontal lobe syndrome (e.g., ref. 22). Why do we not see ADS in patients with normal frontal lobe functions?

ADS as a Disorder of the Knowledge/Memory Substrate for Routine Action Production

Earlier, I suggested that routine action production requires attention to achieve selection and binding operations, but that in the normal system these attentional requirements are minimal due to learned associations between goals and actions, actions and objects, and so forth. These learned associations are what make up the action schemas on which contention scheduling operates. Neurologically, they are instantiated in connections within posterior representational systems, and between these systems and prefrontal and premotor systems. We know this from the various apraxia syndromes that arise from parieto-occipital and parietotemporal lesions, especially of the left hemisphere. One such syndrome, ideational apraxia, bears a close relation to the ADS. Ideational apraxics are unable to demonstrate the correct use of objects out of context, and when asked to carry out familiar actions on sets of objects (e.g., to light a candle with a match, or to prepare a letter for mailing), they make substitution errors, omissions, and sequence errors.[45,46] This raises the possibility that the ADS, too, is caused by disruption of posterior circuits that represent gesture-motor programs, serial-order knowledge, and/or knowledge of object function and usage, all of which have been said to play a causal role in ideational apraxia (for review, see ref. 47).

The idea that ADS is caused by breakdown of posterior knowledge and action schemas encounters similar problems as the contention scheduling account: it ignores the relation between ADS and spontaneous action slips, and it fails to explain the prominence of frontal pathology and frontal symptomatology in the ADS. Moreover, experts in ideational apraxia generally agree that this disorder is expressed only under artificial testing conditions and not in real-life settings (refs. 46, 48, and 49; but also see ref. 50), whereas ADS is highly disruptive of real-world behavior. What accounts for this difference?

THE UNIFIED HYPOTHESIS

In recent works,[36,47] my colleagues and I have formulated a new hypothesis regarding origins of the ADS that overcomes the deficiencies of the alternative accounts while incorporating aspects of each one. According to this "unified hypothesis," damage to posterior schemas is necessary, but not sufficient to bring about the ADS. It is not sufficient because the damage can be compensated for by, for example, slowing down, engaging in prolonged search, and problem solving one's way through the task. This is why ideational apraxics can generally perform well in familiar contexts.

The second condition that is necessary, but again not sufficient, is damage to supervisory attention (which should be read here as shorthand for frontal attention and working memory systems). Damage to supervisory attention is not sufficient because, as discussed earlier, a system operating with knowledge and action schemas *intact* requires only minimal involvement of supervisory attention.

What is necessary to produce the ADS is a combination of these two disorders. The posterior representational disorder compromises the automaticity of routine action production such that selecting actions, ordering them, filling their argument slots, etc., all become more attention demanding. Contention scheduling is no longer the effective mode of control; in effect, the patient ceases to be an expert in the performance of routine actions, and instead functions like a novice. Compensation is possible, as I have indicated, but it requires supervisory attention. If supervisory attention is impaired as well, the compromised selection, ordering, and argument-binding operations will not be compensated for, but rather will manifest in errors and behavioral fragmentation.

Thus, the unified hypothesis asserts that the necessary conditions for this syndrome are twofold: first, a disruption of posterior representational systems compromises the schematic or automatic mode of routine action production, such that planning and execution become more demanding of attentional resources. Second, a deficit in supervisory attention impairs the system's ability to compensate for these increased attentional demands.

The unified hypothesis explains all the characteristics of the ADS enumerated above.

• Spontaneous action slips and errors in patients with ADS are alike in that both involve disruption of the selection and binding operations that underlie routine action planning. In non-brain-damaged individuals, these disruptions are momentary and reversible. In the patients, they are chronic and enduring. Paying attention does not alleviate errors in patients because with an impaired supervisory attention system, the allocation of attention is inadequate or insufficient to compensate for the posterior representational deficit.

• The evolution from ADS to the frontal executive syndrome is the natural consequence of re-establishing familiar routines (and consequently reducing the demands on the impaired supervisory attention). Also, partial recovery of supervisory attention will favor simple, familiar tasks over complex, novel ones.

• That a combination of anterior and posterior defects is needed to produce the ADS explains why it tends to occur in etiologies associated with diffuse and widespread cerebral damage: closed head injury, anoxia, Alzheimer's disease. The unified hypothesis predicts that damage to knowledge and action schemas alone will not produce the ADS; nor will damage to supervisory attention alone. This is consistent with the literature: neither posterior syndromes nor anterior syndromes have the ADS as a recognized feature. But the literature is largely anecdotal. There are no studies that explore how specific brain impairments affect the performance of routine actions when context and task demands are systematically varied. Our MLAT study is designed to fill this knowledge vacuum.

CONCLUSIONS

Earlier I commented that if it were true, as Luria suggested, that ADS represents an extreme form of the frontal executive syndrome, this would pose a second challenge to the conventional view that executive functions are not involved in routine action production. The unified hypothesis entails a weaker claim, and one that is not inconsistent with the conventional view (including the original Norman and Shallice theory). This is because in the unified hypothesis, a supervisory attention disorder is not sufficient to produce the ADS unless it occurs in combination with lesions that disrupt the schema substrate for contention scheduling. Contention scheduling in the normal system could still operate in complementary fashion to supervisory attention, as the conventional view would have it. However, I believe that the evidence from spontaneous action slips forces a rethinking of this view, in favor of a more continuous gradient between automatic and control modes.

The unified hypothesis poses at least as many questions as it answers. Fortunately, most of them are empirically testable. For example, precisely what combination of deficits is necessary to produce the ADS? Here and elsewhere[36,47] we emphasized damage to posterior knowledge and action schemas. But posterior *attention* systems may also be crucial, as well as the systems of the basal ganglia that have been attributed a key role in the automatic execution of learned motor plans.[51] Similarly, as alluded to earlier, it may be necessary to recast the supervisory attention system in ways that can better account for the multiplicity of attentional and mnemonic processes served by the frontal lobes. These are matters we plan to pursue in coming years. The message we have sought to impart here is that the mundane activities of everyday life present far richer opportunities for exploring these matters than the conventional view would have it.

NOTES AND REFERENCES

A. I am indebted to Prof. J. Reason for allowing me to review the original diaries. The intended/did format used in TABLE 1 represents my own reconstruction of the diary entries. The classification of the errors is also mine.

B. A complete enumeration of the constituents, or units, of action plans would have to include representations of the direction of movement, the effectors, and the number of times the movement is repeated, in addition to the nature of the action, the objects of the action, and their respective locations. See ref. 20 for relevant evidence.

C. J. K.'s attentional functions were evaluated as part of a large study of attentional deficits in traumatic brain injury conducted at the Moss Rehabilitation Research Institute by Dr. John Whyte.

1. LURIA, A. R. 1966. Higher Cortical Functions in Man. Basic Books. New York.

2. NORMAN, D. A. & T. SHALLICE. 1980. Attention to action: Willed and automatic control of behavior (CHIP No. 99). University of California, San Diego.

3. STUSS, D. T. & D. F. BENSON. 1986. The Frontal Lobes. Raven Press. New York.

4. FUSTER, J. M. 1989. The Prefrontal Cortex (2nd edit.). Raven Press. New York.

5. CANAVAN, A. G. M., I. JANOTA & P. H. SCHURR. 1985. Luria's frontal lobe syndrome: Psychological and anatomical considerations. J. Neurol. Neurosurg. Psychiatry 48: 1049–1053.

6. BAARS, B. J. 1992a. Experimental Slips and Human Error: Exploring the Architecture of Volition. Plenum. New York.

7. REASON, J. T. 1984. Lapses of attention in everyday life. In Varieties of Attention. R. Parasuraman & D. R. Davies, Eds.: 515–549. Academic Press. Orlando, FL.

8. REASON, J. T. 1990. Human Error. Cambridge University Press. Cambridge, UK.

9. MACKAY, D. G. 1985. A theory of the representation, organization and timing of action with implications for sequencing disorders. In Neuropsychological Studies of Apraxia and Related Disorders. E. A. Roy, Ed.: 267–308. North-Holland. Amsterdam.

10. NORMAN, D. A. 1981. Categorization of action slips. Psychol. Rev. 88: 1–15.

11. SELLEN, A. J. & D. A. NORMAN. 1992. The psychology of slips. In Experimental Slips and Human Error. Exploring the Architecture of Volition. B. J. Baars, Ed. Plenum. New York.

12. NORMAN, D. A. & T. SHALLICE. 1986. Attention to action: Willed and automatic control of behavior. In Consciousness and Self-Regulation, Vol. 4. R. J. Davidson, G. E. Schwartz & D. Shapiro, Eds. Plenum. New York.

13. SHALLICE, T. 1982. Specific impairments of planning. Philos. Trans. R. Soc. Lond. B29: 199–209.

14. SHALLICE, T. 1988. From Neuropsychology to Mental Structure. Cambridge University Press. Cambridge, UK.

15. BAARS, B. J. 1992b. The many uses of error: Twelve steps to a unified framework. In Experimental Slips and Human Error. Exploring the Architecture of Volition. B. J. Baars, Ed. Plenum. New York.

16. REASON, J. T. 1979. Actions not as planned: The price of automatization. In Aspects of Consciousness. Vol. 1. Psychological Issues. G. Underwood & R. Stevens, Eds.: 67–89. Academic Press. London.

17. REASON, J. T. & K. MYCIELSKA. 1982. Absent Minded? The Psychology of Mental Lapses and Everyday Errors. Prentice-Hall. Englewood Cliffs, NJ.

18. BAARS, B. J. & M. T. MOTLEY. 1976. Spoonerisms as sequencer conflicts: Evidence from artificially elicited errors. Am. J. Psychol. **89:** 467–484.
19. BAARS, B. J., M. T. MOTLEY & D. G. MACKAY. 1975. Output editing for lexical status in artificially elicited slips of the tongue. J. Verb. Learn. Verb. Behav. **14:** 382–391.
20. MATTSON, M. E. & B. J. BAARS. 1992. Laboratory induction of nonspeech action errors. *In* Experimental Slips and Human Error. B. J. Baars, Ed. Plenum. New York.
21. REASON, J. T. 1992. Cognitive underspecification: Its variety and consequences. *In* Experimental Slips and Human Error. Exploring the Architecture of Volition. B. J. Baars, Ed. Plenum. New York.
22. SCHWARTZ, M. F., E. S. REED, M. W. MONTGOMERY, C. PALMER & M. H. MAYER. 1991. The quantitative description of action disorganization after brain damage: A case study. Cogn. Neuropsychol. **8:** 381–414.
23. GIBSON, E. & N. RADER. 1979. The perceiver as performer. *In* Attention and Cognitive Development. G. A. Hale & M. Lewis, Eds. Plenum. New York.
24. ALLPORT, A. 1987. Selection for action: Some behavioral and neurophysiological considerations of attention and action. *In* Perspectives on Perception and Action. H. Heuer & A. F. Sanders, Eds.: 395–420. Lawrence Erlbaum Associates. Hillsdale, NJ.
25. ALLPORT, A. 1990. Visual attention. *In* Foundations of Cognitive Science. M. I. Posner, Ed.: 631–682. MIT Press. Cambridge, MA.
26. DUNCAN, J. 1993. Selection of input and goal in the control of behaviour. *In* Attention: Selection, awareness and control. A. Baddeley & L. Weiskrantz, Eds. Clarendon Press. Oxford, UK.
27. DUNCAN, J. 1986. Disorganization of behaviour after frontal lobe damage. Cogn. Neuropsychol. **3:** 271–290.
28. HEILMAN, K. M. & E. VALENSTEIN. 1972. Frontal lobe neglect in man. Neurology **22:** 660–664.
29. MESULAM, M-M. 1981. A cortical network for directed attention and unilateral neglect. Ann. Neurol. **10:** 309–325.
30. POSNER, M. I. & M. E. RAICHLE. 1994. Images of Mind. Sci. Am. Library. New York.
31. KIMBERG, D. Y. & M. J. FARAH. 1993. A unified account of cognitive impairments following frontal lobe damage: The role of working memory in complex, organized behavior. J. Exp. Psychol. Gen. **122:** 411–428.
32. GOLDMAN-RAKIC, P. S. 1987. Circuitry of primate prefrontal cortex and regulation of behavior by representational memory. *In* Handbook of Physiology: The Nervous System, Vol. 5. F. Plum, Ed.: 373–417. American Physiological Society. Bethesda, MD.
33. HOLYOAK, K. J. 1995. Forms of reasoning. Insight into prefrontal functions. Ann. N.Y. Acad. Sci. This volume.
34. MAYER, N. H., D. KEATING & D. RAPP. 1986. Skills, routines, and activity patterns of daily living: A functional nested approach. *In* Clinical Neuropsychology of Intervention. B. P. Uzzell & Y. Gross, Eds.: 205–222. Martinus Nijhoff. Boston, MA.
35. MAYER, N. H., E. S. REED, M. F. SCHWARTZ, M. W. MONTGOMERY & C. PALMER. 1990. Buttering a cup of hot coffee: An approach to the study of errors of action after brain damage. *In* The Neuropsychology of Everyday Life: Assessment and Basic Competencies. K. Cicerone & D. Tupper, Ed.: 259–283. Kluwer Academic Publishers. Boston, MA.
36. SCHWARTZ, M. F., M. W. MONTGOMERY, E. J. FITZPATRICK-DESALME, C. OCHIPA, H. B. COSLETT & N. H. MAYER. Analysis of a disorder of everyday action. Cogn. Neuropsychol. In press.
37. BUXBAUM, L. J., M. F. SCHWARTZ, H. B. COSLETT & T. G. CAREW. 1995. Everyday action and praxis in callosal apraxia. Neurocase **1:** 3–17.
38. SCHWARTZ, M. F., E. J. FITZPATRICK-DESALME & T. G. CAREW. 1995. The multiple objects test for ideational apraxia: Etiology and task effects on error profiles (Abstract). J. Int. Neuropsychol. Soc. **1:** 149.
39. SHALLICE, T., P. W. BURGESS, F. SCHON & D. M. BAXTER. 1989. The origins of utilisation behaviour. Brain **112:** 1587–1598.

40. SCHWARTZ, M. F., N. H. MAYER, E. J. FITZPATRICK & M. W. MONTGOMERY. 1993. Cognitive theory and the study of everyday action disorders after brain damage. J. Head Trauma Rehabil. **8:** 59–72.

41. STUSS, D. T., T. SHALLICE & M. ALEXANDER. 1995. A multidisciplinary approach to anterior attentional functions. Ann. N.Y. Acad. Sci. This volume.

42. BADDELEY, A. D. 1986. Working Memory. Clarendon Press. Oxford, UK.

42. BADDELEY, A. D. 1993. Working memory or working attention? *In* Attention: Selection, Awareness and Control. A. Baddeley & L. Weiskrantz, Eds. Clarendon Press. Oxford, UK.

44. ROY, E. A. 1983. Neuropsychological perspectives on apraxia and related disorders. *In* Memory and Control of Action. R. A. Magill, Ed.: 293–320. North-Holland. Amsterdam.

45. POECK, K. & G. LEHMKUHL. 1980. Ideatory apraxia in a left-handed patient with right-sided brain lesion. Cortex **16:** 273–284.

46. DERENZI, E. & F. LUCCHELLI. 1988. Ideational apraxia. Brain **111:** 1173–1185.

47. SCHWARTZ, M. F. & L. J. BUXBAUM. Pragmatic action. *In* Apraxia. L. J. G. Rothi & K. M. Heilman, Eds. Lawrence Erlbaum. Hillsdale, NJ. In press.

48. DE RENZI, E., A. PIECZURO & L. A. VIGNOLO. 1968. Ideational apraxia: A quantitative study. Neuropsychologia **6:** 41–52.

49. LIEPMANN, H. 1905. The left hemisphere and action. Translations from Liepmann's Essays on Apraxia, D. Kimura (Trans.), 1980. University of Western Ontario. London, Ontario.

50. POECK, K. 1985. Clues to the nature of disruptions to limb praxis. *In* Neuropsychological Studies of Apraxia and Related Disorders. E. A. Roy, Ed: 99–110. North-Holland. Amsterdam.

51. MARSDEN, C. D. 1982. The mysterious motor function of the basal ganglia: The Robert Wartenberg Lecture. Neurology **32:** 514–539.

Similarities and Distinctions among Current Models of Prefrontal Cortical Functions

JORDAN GRAFMAN[a]

Cognitive Neuroscience Section
Medical Neurology Branch
National Institute of Neurological Disorders and Stroke
National Institutes of Health
Bethesda, Maryland 20892

INTRODUCTION

In their monograph, Plans and the Structure of Behavior, Miller, Galanter, and Pribram[1] commented on the relationship of the frontal lobes to cognitive planning. They noted that

> the effects of frontal ablation or lobotomy on man are surprisingly subtle. Very few of the usual psychometric tests turn up any deficits at all. One that frequently shows a deficit is the Porteus Maze, a paper and pencil labyrinth that would seem to require some planning. It should not be difficult to devise many more tests of planning ability and to use them on these patients. Clinical observation of their behavior would encourage us, at least in some cases, to expect that such tests would succeed in diagnosing the patient's difficulties. Such a patient is apt to fall apart when some minor detail goes awry in the Plan he is executing. If he is preparing dinner when the trouble occurs, he may not be readily capable of reshuffling the parts of the Plan. Segments of the Plan may simply be omitted—the vegetables are served raw—or the whole dinner may be lost. Even if those speculations prove to be wrong in detail, the notion that the frontal "association areas" are intimately linked to the limbic systems in the transformation and execution of plans is worth pursuing. Clinical and laboratory investigations that investigate how rather than what behavior is changed by frontal lesions have hardly begun.

A generation of investigators has belatedly come to the same conclusions although the exact framework chosen to investigate planning and other functions of the human frontal lobes is quite varied. A number of different models of the functions of the prefrontal[2] cortex have been proposed in this *Annals* and other recent monographs. Many of these models share certain *common* traits (such as "keeping information/knowledge stored in posterior cortex active for a limited period of time"). On the other hand, discussing their *distinctive* qualities (such as models that incorporate temporal or serial order processing versus those that do not) can help researchers devise experiments, designed to test model-based

[a] Address correspondence to Jordan Grafman, Ph.D., Cognitive Neuroscience Section, NIH/NINDS/MNB, Building 10, Room 5S209, 10 Center Drive MSC 1440, Bethesda, Maryland 20892-1440.

337

alternative hypotheses, that can serve to select the most promising of the models for further investigation. The purpose of this paper is to provide a brief review of the distinctions and similarities of currently prominent models of the functions of the human prefrontal cortex. By doing so, I hope to illustrate the strengths and weaknesses of these models, their testability using conventional psychological and computational methods, and their face validity in light of 150 years of observation and testing of patients with damage to the human prefrontal cortex and more recent studies using functional neuroimaging methods. The paper concludes with a relatively lengthy description of the framework I have adapted to investigate the functions of the human prefrontal cortex which stresses the importance of specifying a cognitive architecture.

DETERMINANTS OF AN APPROPRIATE MODEL

Mapping models of a cognitive process(es) to the human brain requires selecting an appropriate computational level or domain with which to accomplish the mapping. This is currently a problem receiving much discussion in the neuroscience and neuroimaging literature.[3-5] For example, if an investigator is concerned with identifying the role of the prefrontal cortex in learning, should the experimental condition focus on indices of post-rehearsal remembering such as total recall or explicit and specific indices of the rehearsal and search strategy applied? This question is important to resolve because each measure implies a different set of inferences and representations (and perhaps the activation of a different set of brain regions). Thus, the investigator could potentially misunderstand the cause of activation of a set of brain structures in a neuroimaging experiment if he did not carefully control for the cognitive strategies used during the scan and therefore the level of cognitive processing.[6]

In addition to determining the appropriate level or domain of investigation, the organization of the underlying representation itself should receive some attention. For example, if word retrieval is an important function of a particular cognitive process and brain region, studying the organization of words in a lexicon or semantic store would be important. In this case, the investigator could contrast a neural network-based (involving a set of layers and a variable number of neurodes within each layer with their accompanying connection weights) versus node-based representation.[7,8] Relationships between single items (e.g., a single node or single pattern of connection weights) within such representational networks might involve psychometric features such as word frequency, association value, imagery value, or age-of-acquisition of that knowledge.[9,10]

Furthermore, distinctive characteristics of the level of processing should be specified as much as possible. For example, temporal order constraints might be different at the level of a speech sound or syntactic frame versus the level of a story event or action sequence.[11-14] Or time coding might be different at the level of a speech sound burst compared to the estimation of elapsed time during a dinner engagement.

It is a challenge to any investigator attempting model building to incorporate these variables into his model. But what happens when conventional cognitive

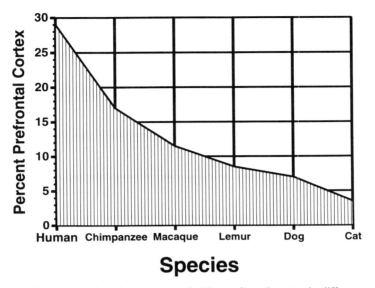

FIGURE 1. Percentage of total cortex occupied by prefrontal cortex in different species. Note the dramatic increase in the proportional space devoted to prefrontal cortex in the human compared to the other species shown in the figure.

processes appear intact in spite of damage to a significant region of the human brain—in this case, the prefrontal cortex? Investigators may choose to continue exploring knowledge structures using established psychological methods (such as the ones alluded to above) or ascribe a new sort of function to this region that cannot be easily captured by typical clinical or experimental tools. Such is the dilemma facing investigators concerned with the ascription of functions to the human prefrontal cortex, which occupies approximately 30% of the total cortical space (FIG. 1). Investigators entering this challenging area of neuropsychological research have to decide whether they simply should posit another form of knowledge structure that is stored in human prefrontal cortex or devise a new type of process; they have to determine the specifications of that process in terms that convey the cognitive attributes it must employ; and they have to specify the underlying cognitive architecture of that representation and its properties.

IDENTIFYING MODELS THAT MEET THE STANDARD

For many years, a select group of researchers in neuropsychology struggled to conceptualize the cognitive deficits and mood-state changes in patients with prefrontal cortical lesions (see refs. 15–17 for a review of this literature), but the majority of neuropsychologists have preferred to investigate the more intuitive and easily specified cognitive architectures of the lexicon, objects, and space. However, more recently, enough knowledge has accrued that several brave individuals and teams have attempted to lay out their conceptions of prefrontal lobe function in a way that begins to be amenable to verification and falsification. The frameworks offered by Shallice and associates,[15,18–20] Goldman-Rakic,[21,22] Fuster,[23] Stuss and Benson,[17] Luria and Tsvetkova,[24] Damasio and colleagues,[25–34] and Schwartz and co-workers[35] exemplify this effort. Each has approached the functions of the prefrontal cortex from a somewhat unique perspective. I will briefly outline their ideas below. Later, my own model of prefrontal lobe knowledge representation will be described in some detail.

In reading about these frameworks in this paper and in their original presentations, several methodological questions should be kept in mind. Does the researcher conceive of a level of knowledge representation within the prefrontal cortex? If so, what are the characteristics of that knowledge, and what are the implications of activation of that knowledge for attentional and memory processes? Is there an explicit attempt to map these cognitive structures and processes to brain? If so, at what level? Does the model provide testable hypotheses? What is the replicability and reliability of the results that led to the development of the model? What methods can be used to test the model?

NORMAN AND SHALLICE'S FRAMEWORK

Norman and Shallice have advocated a model of attentional control that nicely dovetailed with some views of the role of the prefrontal cortex in behavior.[15,18–20,36,37] In their model, they proposed that two basic "control" mechanisms determined how we monitor our activities. One mechanism, called the *Contention Scheduler*, operated via automatic and direct priming of stored knowledge either by stimuli in the environment or conceptual thought. For example, if you see a red light at a street corner, the red light is directly associated with the command stop, the traffic rule that specifies you must stop for a red light, and punishment in the form of a ticket or accident if this rule is disobeyed. This simple stimulus (red light) arguably not only evoked a rather simple response (stopping the car), but also activated a complex schema (driving regulations) automatically.

The second mechanism was called the *Supervisory Attention System* (SAS) and reflected conscious awareness (operating within working memory limitations) of internal knowledge states that could set the priorities for action despite contrary or absent environmental stimuli. Because this stored knowledge reached consciousness, it could override the automatic contention scheduling mechanism.[38,39] For example, if the rules governing social behavior require that a visitor defer answering a phone when it rings in another person's office, the activation of those rules should override the automatic contention scheduler which might signal to the subject that they need to answer a ringing telephone.[40]

Dividing the attention system between automatic contention scheduling and controlled supervisory mechanisms seemed to make sense and accounted for a great deal of data regarding attention and action failures in patients with prefrontal lobe lesions. That is, such patients have a general tendency to be over-responsive to the automatic demands of the environment (suggesting intact contention scheduling?), which can be seen in their impulsivity and rule-breaking behaviors. Paradoxically, these inappropriate behaviors can sometimes be viewed as appropriately performed fragments of behavior which takes place in an inappropriate context. Occasionally, the fragment of behavior reflects a more primitive urge such as excessive anger or aggressive sexual overtures which cannot be viewed as normal under any circumstances.

These two attentional mechanisms reflect other dichotomies in the psychological literature. The contention scheduler is automatic, implicit, and easily activated. The SAS is controlled, explicit, but also easily activated. The homeostasis between the two attentional control systems is critical to maintaining conventional behavioral interactions with the environment. The SAS, more than the contention scheduler, interacts with anterior brain systems that include large-scale knowledge units. Recently, Shallice has utilized the Memory Operation Packet (MOP) conception favored by Schank[41] to describe such large-scale knowledge units, but other alternatives to conceptualizing such large-scale knowledge units exist including schemas, scripts, frames, and plans. In any case, when damage occurs to this knowledge base, then the SAS cannot operate effectively in order to override, at times, the contention scheduler.[19] Norman and Shallice's framework has had a significant impact on other models of memory and cognition. For example, Baddeley and Wilson[42] have included a version of the SAS as the primary mechanism operating within the Central Executive component of working memory.

GOLDMAN-RAKIC AND PRIMATE WORKING MEMORY

Perhaps no researcher has done a better job of refining the anatomical and behavioral functions of the primate prefrontal cortex than Goldman-Rakic. Recently, she has adapted a framework for examining prefrontal cortex functions based on her electrophysiological studies.[21,22,43,44] Within this framework, the prefrontal cortex serves as a *"working memory,"* which temporarily keeps active a representation of a stimulus (including its precise spatial coordinates) until a response is required (e.g., a choice-discrimination). She has demonstrated that selected prefrontal cortical neurons fire only *during the delay* between the presentation of a stimulus set to memorize and the presentation of a probe for response. It is not clear how long this firing can be maintained or whether it can be maintained if the animal performs an intervening distraction task. It is also not clear what "keeping active" a representation means here. Does this firing represent a form of image rehearsal? Is the monkey "strategically thinking" during this delay? Is this an attentional mechanism rather than a re-representation of the stimulus held in memory? What is fascinating is that the prefrontal cortical cells are specifically linked to where in space the stimulus was seen and not just to a simple memory of the stimulus itself.

Although Goldman-Rakic has not made an extensive effort to relate these findings to humans or to the kind of deficits experienced by adults with prefrontal brain-damage, she inspired Diamond to demonstrate that certain delayed response tasks are only performed well after a certain stage of prefrontal lobe development in human infants and children.[45] Furthermore, there is some evidence of prefrontal lobe involvement in memory processes in adult humans—in particular, during human working memory activity and retrieval.[47] Patients with prefrontal lobe lesions also have diminished contingent negative-variation slow waves, which have been thought to reflect interstimulus interval preparatory and rehearsal behavior.[48] So although Goldman-Rakic's model of prefrontal lobe function has not been directly tested in adult humans, it is compatible with a large set of observations in the frontal lobe literature (see Goldman-Rakic and Awh *et al.*, this volume; for a somewhat different point of view of working memory, see Della Sala *et al.* and Dunbar and Sussman, this volume).

FUSTER'S TEMPORAL PROCESSING MODEL

Based on his single-cell and cell-array recordings, Fuster[23] has proposed that the prefrontal cortex, while having multiple functions, is principally involved with representing the *"temporal structure of behavior."* Temporal structure refers to the coding of place within a sequence of actions or perceptual observations.[49] These action sequences are goal-related, that is, conceptually driven. Fuster has also argued that the prefrontal cortex, in order to encode temporal aspects of behaviors, must be involved in the formation of *"cross-temporal contingencies."* Cross-temporal contingencies can be interpreted as the ties between events that are not simply adjacent in time but related to each other because they are part of a set of actions that have a common goal. These temporal operations are unique to prefrontal cortex according to Fuster. Numerous studies have indicated that patients with prefrontal lobe lesions have particular problems with remembering the order of events as compared to their relatively intact memory for those same individual events.[49,50]

STUSS AND BENSON'S BEHAVIORAL/ANATOMICAL THEORY

Stuss and Benson have presented exhaustive neurobehavioral reviews of the frontal lobe literature in the two editions of their monograph on the frontal lobes. Although they have shied away from extensive theorizing on the topic, they have offered their own view of the role of the prefrontal cortex in behavior. They divide the functions of the frontal lobes into two groups. One group is concerned with *sequencing behaviors, forming mental sets,* and *integrating various behaviors.* The other group is concerned with more primitive processes such as *drive, motivation,* and *will.* The former group is associated with dorsolateral prefrontal cortex activation, whereas the latter group is associated with ventromedial prefrontal cortex activation. These behaviors are at the top of a hierarchy of behaviors that control a person's interactions with the world. Stuss *et al.* have now gone beyond this simple characterization of the role of the prefrontal cortex and have distinguished among a large set of attentional processes that may be subserved by prefrontal cortex. He and his colleagues are currently testing whether these independent attentional processes can be selectively impaired by prefrontal cortical lesions (see Stuss *et al.*, this volume).

LURIA'S VIEW OF PROBLEM SOLVING AND THE FRONTAL LOBE

Luria's observations of brain-damaged patients injured during wartime and suffering from brain tumors was very influential in helping neuropsychologists conceptualize brain-behavior relations. Luria was particularly interested in failures of problem solving.[24] His approach was qualitative and relied on the analysis of verbal protocols of patients trying to solve multistep arithmetic problems. *Impaired programming and regulation of behavior* was the principal deficit exhibited by patients with prefrontal lobe lesions on problem-solving tasks in Luria's view. The patients' responses were frequently impulsive, and they had difficulty switching from one type of problem-solving strategy to another. Patients who developed characteristic stuck-in-set responses often relied on these stereotypical behaviors even when they were obviously inappropriate. Patients could access fragmentary operations but could not combine them into an overall schema in order to solve a problem. Luria believed that focal lesions of the prefrontal cortex could dissociate types of problem-solving failures.

DAMASIO'S SOMATIC MARKER THEORY

Damasio and his colleagues have promoted a framework that they believe helps explain the failure of patients with prefrontal lesions to correctly select appropriate social behaviors and make social decisions.[28-32] In short, such patients fail to behave appropriately because of a *"defect in the activation of somatic markers."* This hypothesized somatic signal binds to social behaviors and helps assure their appropriateness or relevance by providing a modulating or biasing signal to the person when they have to make a social decision.[51-53] This tag could be perceived by the person as a sensation mediated by the autonomic nervous system. Such tags may be extremely valuable in both helping to select appropriate behaviors and inhibiting inappropriate behaviors. Patients with ventromedial frontal lobe lesions can often recognize and select the appropriate interpersonal behavior on forced-choice verbal tests, but fail to perform in real situations. Damasio *et al.*'s explanation is that they fail due to a lack of somatic marker intervention during social interactions. One quantitative way to estimate somatic contributions to behavior is via psychophysiological recordings during task performance. Failures in somatic activation (e.g., a diminished galvanic skin response) have been identified when patients with ventromedial lesions have to *passively* watch evocative stimuli rather than actively respond. Ventromedial frontal cortex has been implicated as a crucial member of a larger neural network devoted to the normal integration of somatic tags with stored knowledge reflecting social conduct. This approach to understanding social-conduct disorders can be advantageously linked to social-cognitive theories that have appeared in the psychological literature.[52,53]

SCHWARTZ'S ACTION FRAMEWORK

In a recent article in *Cognitive Neuropsychology* (and in this volume), Myrna Schwartz and colleagues developed a coding scheme to break down components of simple action sequences into their constituent parts that allows for a componential error analysis.[35] Such an *action coding scheme* was developed for two different but typical actions: pouring a cup of coffee and brushing teeth. Errors were coded over different temporal epochs and for uniquely defined components of behavior. Furthermore, different error types were defined including object substitutions, anticipatory errors, omissions, and execution failures. Using this approach, the disorganization of simple actions was described in a consistent, systematic fashion. Frontal apraxia, as seen in their patients, was described as a failure of top-down mechanisms concerned with activation of sequentially stored behaviors. This detailed approach to coding ongoing behavior offers a real opportunity to more precisely define and describe the breakdown in executing typical actions so often seen in patients with large frontal lobe lesions.

SIMILARITIES AND DISTINCTIONS AMONG THE MODELS

The models described above would each like to stand on their own merits. However, there are *similarities* across these models. They all operate over *extended time domains* (seconds +). They all resemble what has been called *controlled attentional processes*. That is, many of the models suggest a process, stored in prefrontal cortex, that is monitored within consciousness and responsible for shifting conceptual set. Many of the models presume that the processes they describe depend upon or are biased toward the *internal mental state* of the subject. All consider the prefrontal cortex as a *member of a distributed set of neural networks* concerned with almost all functional behaviors that require the activation of a mental model of the world (especially when aspects of that model are no longer present in the environment).

Some *distinctions* exist between these models as well. Some focus more on general attentional mechanisms (e.g., Norman and Shallice/Stuss *et al.*), whereas others focus on a specific domain of cognition (e.g., Damasio's somatic marker theory). Some frameworks focus on working memory processes (e.g., Goldman-Rakic), whereas others focus more on action set representation (e.g., Schwartz). Finally, some are interested in the notion of executive function deficits that cut across the territory of the prefrontal cortex (e.g., Baddeley), whereas others are concerned with specifying the role of specific regions of the prefrontal cortex (e.g., Fuster).

Despite their prominence in contemporary neuropsychological accounts of the functions of the human prefrontal cortex, in my view, all of these models have substantial weak points. That is, they lack an underlying cognitive architecture, have weak psychological constructs, are difficult to validate or reject, are generally observation- instead of hypothesis-driven, and almost all deny a need to specify the form of knowledge stored in the prefrontal cortex (or, as can be seen above and in many of the papers in this volume, the proposed representations are attentional processes, passive rehearsal strategies, or are denied any special cognitive status/ role other than that they manipulate knowledge that is primarily stored in posterior regions of the cerebral cortex).

In denying or minimizing a prefrontal cortical form of knowledge representation that has an underlying cognitive architecture, specific predictions about cognitive deficits cannot easily be made. A harsher view of the current level of description of the cognitive deficits that result from prefrontal lesions is that, in general, we are listening to the equivalent of Dax or Broca reporting that left-hemisphere lesions cause language deficits. Although such observations were a landmark in neurobehavioral research, they occurred well over 100 years ago. Modern neurolinguistics has advanced well beyond that stage of development in research. On the other hand, Harlow's observations of the patient Gage over 150 years ago still are relevant today because, I would argue, of our lack of progress in specifying an underlying cognitive architecture.[54–56] A new approach is needed to understand fully the nature of the cognitive functions stored in, and utilized by, human prefrontal cortex. Such an approach needs to take into consideration the characteristic deficits that have been reported in patients with prefrontal lobe lesions[57–68] while incorporating several of the creative ideas espoused by contemporary theorists in cognitive neuroscience, cognitive science, artificial intelligence, and neuropsychology.

A NOT-SO-NEW APPROACH?

Most of the current models of prefrontal cortical functions, including those reviewed above and others, suggest that the main function of the prefrontal cortex is to manipulate, in some manner, information stored elsewhere in the cerebral cortex and brain. Whether the process being referred to is working memory, attention, or serial encoding, each appears to be indicative of an as-yet-unspecified abstract algorithm or "marionette operator" coordinating the activation of information stored post centrally. Moreover, this process or set of processes appears *contentless*. This notion should give one pause. After all, inasmuch as no other area of cerebral cortex has been anointed with this elusively abstract quality, it would represent a radical departure from current thinking about the nature of representational knowledge networks in the brain.

That is, this view suggests that there may be two fundamentally different kinds of representations in the cerebral cortex. One kind of representation, the symbolic one, is currently captured by the notion of a lexicon or associative memory system that would be contained within the boundaries of a local neural network. Thus, our representation of a word or picture is stored within a particular neural network, and increasing damage to that network (from a local brain lesion or degenerative process) would make it increasingly difficult to both retrieve and make use of that knowledge (usually based upon some metric like similarity, frequency or familiarity). This kind of symbolic representation can be contrasted with one that represents operations or processes rather than symbols. Such operations are algorithms that manipulate stored knowledge. The presumption of many investigators is that these operator algorithms are stored in local neural networks within the prefrontal cortex. They would manipulate information stored in temporal, parietal, and occipital cortex as well as subcortical structures. The operator algorithms referred to above may have several aliases, including the aforementioned working memory, attention, and temporal encoding processes.

This proposal of two distinctive kinds of representation is attractive to many researchers, yet at least two risky assumptions are associated with it. It implies that we have captured all aspects and levels of knowledge within the realm of the posterior (i.e., non-prefrontal) cortex. Accordingly, it also implies that a fundamental difference should exist in the neuroanatomy, genetics, and molecular biology of the prefrontal and posterior cortices in order to accommodate two such different forms of cognitive process.[69,70] In fact, the evidence suggests the converse.

Of course, there is also the question of how much of normal and impaired human behavior these models can explain and predict. In the case of patients with prefrontal cortical lesions, they all carry "shotgun"-type explanatory power that attempts to account for a large number of cognitive and behavioral deficits on the basis of a single type of operator failure (e.g., a type of attentional deficit). I have criticized these approaches to conceptualizing the functions of the human prefrontal cortex in the past because each fails to account in detail for too many of the cognitive deficits exhibited by patients with prefrontal lobe lesions.[71] They also fail to account for how normal subjects process plans,[72-74] themes,[75] schemas,[40,76] frames,[77] case-based scenarios,[78] scripts,[36,79-82] etc.

There is an alternative approach to understanding the functions of the prefrontal cortex. That is, to suppose that it serves a function similar to that of other regions of cerebral cortex. In other words, why assign nonsymbolic operations to the prefrontal cortex if you can suggest that a specific kind of symbolic representation might be stored there? This is a more parsimonious approach (within the context of previous cognitive neuroscience programs to understand the functions of posterior cortex) than the dichotomous representational approach described above. Of course, the cerebral cortex is not laid out in a haphazard fashion and to argue for a kind of representation that would be stored in prefrontal cortex, one must also put that representation into the broader context of forms of representational knowledge and evolutionary development (remember that in humans the prefrontal cortex has reached its apogee and is clearly the area of cortex that has shown the greatest proportional development across species).

The most parsimonious approach to building a model of the cognitive architecture of knowledge stored in the prefrontal cortex would be to adapt an architecture similar to that used in other representational domains. Thus, items stored in such an architecture would be interrelated on the basis of similarity, frequency, category membership, association values, etc.[81,83] The more related an item is to another item using any one of the metrics, the more likely that such items would be neighbors in a psychological space. The boundaries encompassing such a domain-specific psychological space would probably be fuzzy to accommodate cognitive plasticity during learning or following brain damage.

Within these cognitive architectures, a *unit* of knowledge represents a *single* assembly of information such as an edge, word, meaning, form, location in space, or syntactic frame. Across cognitive architectures there appears to be an evolutionary trend from architectures in which knowledge units are representing a single aspect or feature of a stimulus event and can be activated for very brief periods of time (such as an "edge detector") to units which represent a *series of events* that are activated for longer durations of time (such as an syntactic frame). This

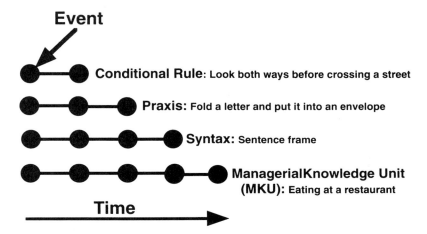

Event

Conditional Rule: Look both ways before crossing a street

Praxis: Fold a letter and put it into an envelope

Syntax: Sentence frame

ManagerialKnowledge Unit (MKU): Eating at a restaurant

Time

FIGURE 2. Structured Event Complexes (SECs). In the framework I have adapted, the Managerial Knowledge Unit is presented as the latest stage of development in memory units and is at the top of the hierarchy of structured event complexes.

trend is also apparent phylogenetically with lower species dominated by informa-tion processing components in which the units of representation are weighted toward the singular aspects of events with rapid onset and offset times, whereas higher species are dominated by components in which units of representation are weighted toward the sequential aspects of events with long-duration onset and offset times.

This evolutionary development in knowledge representation predicts that *single units* of memory would be capable of storing a *Structured Event Complex* (SEC) that varies in the number of individuated events it encapsulates (FIG. 2).[84] This SEC contains macrostructure-level information relevant to the consequences of past and current behavior by virtue of its storing events that have occurred in the past and will occur in the future (an SEC could occur at many levels of cognition from word-level recognition of a set of speech sounds to a set of action events). Each SEC representation within a cognitive architecture would store both the theme and boundaries of events assigned to it and not simply represent the other features of events such as words, sentences, visual features, etc., that might be stored in other specific cognitive architectures (both spatially and functionally independent from that cognitive architecture), but which might be temporally bound together with the SEC in any given situation.[85]

Within this conception of the evolution of knowledge representation from units representing simple, single events to units representing a potentially large series of events, linguistic terms and images that indicate future and past tense and qualify the consequences of current behavior emerged and sought a place within the cerebral cortex. This ability to combine in an SEC single units of memory representing thematic and temporal aspects of event series would give humans a distinct advantage over animals who were much more prone to respond slavishly

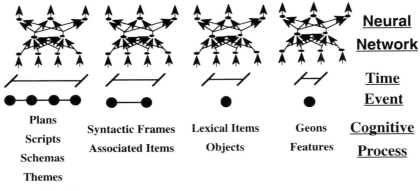

				Neural Network
				Time
				Event
Plans	**Syntactic Frames**	**Lexical Items**	**Geons**	**Cognitive**
Scripts	**Associated Items**	**Objects**	**Features**	**Process**
Schemas				
Themes				
Mental Models				

FIGURE 3. Evolution of the Managerial Knowledge Unit. The MKU is the abstract representation that subserves cognitive macrostructures such as plans, scripts, themes, mental models, and schemas. Compared to the other knowledge structures shown, these macrostructures make greater time demands on cognitive processing and require the storage of many events in order to abstract the appropriate macrolevel of knowledge across those events.

to single environmental events without being aware of, or able to conceptualize, the consequences of their actions (because of a dependency on single-event memory activation). The SEC could be established on the basis of experiencing external events or through the generation of "internal thought." It is this kind of unitized *macrostructure* knowledge—that is, the SEC—that I argue is stored in the prefrontal cortex.

Below I develop the cognitive architecture that would support an SEC, its relation with other cognitive processes, and how damage to its cognitive architecture could be responsible for many, if not all, of the higher-cognitive deficits described above and in this volume. I call the particular kind of SEC that governs our cognitive behavior the *Managerial Knowledge Unit* (MKU).

THE MANAGERIAL KNOWLEDGE UNIT

In characterizing the MKU, I will describe its cognitive architecture, its relations with other kinds of knowledge, develop testable hypotheses, and predict patterns of deficit that might be found following damage to the MKU architecture (and presumably the prefrontal cortex).

Cognitive science has long been concerned with trying to understand how people represent in memory event-series that occur in our lives.[1,86] A variety of cognitive structures have been hypothesized to account for this kind of macroknowledge. These structures include action procedures, schemas, scripts, frames, cases, and story grammars (FIG. 3). What these knowledge structures have in common is that they are composed of a set of events, actions, or ideas that when linked

The Managerial Knowledge Unit

 A structured set of events, stored as a single unit in memory in propositional/linguistic statements, imagined scenes, or real-time format, that is the underlying representation for plans, mental sets, schemas, and actions.

 A structured set of events, stored as a single unit in memory in propositional/linguistic statements or imagined scenes, that is the underlying representation for fantasies.

FIGURE 4. A simple pair of definitions of the Managerial Knowledge Unit. Note that an MKU can represent a completely self-generated fantasy that the subject was never exposed to in the world nor has the capability to perform.

together form a *knowledge unit* (e.g., a schema) containing macrostructure information such as the theme of a story. This kind of memory unit could be composed of a series of simple movements or the set of rules used to solve a physics problem. We have termed this general class of linked, unitized information the SEC. We have labeled the SEC specifically involved with cognitive planning, social behavior, and the management of knowledge the MKU. It is the MKU and its more primitive SEC precursors that I hypothesize are uniquely stored in prefrontal cortex (see FIG. 4).[87,88]

What might the informational content of an MKU be like? I suggest that an MKU is composed of a series of events (FIG. 5). There should be a typical order to the occurrence of these events. The rigidity of event order within an MKU obeys multiple constraints. Some constraints are *physical*. You cannot sip coffee from a cup unless it is first poured into the cup. Some constraints are *cultural*. In the United States, people generally shower on a daily basis in the morning before eating breakfast. Some constraints are purely *individual*. Some people brush their teeth twice in the morning—once before and once after eating breakfast. The rigidity of the event order is also dependent on the frequency of its activation. That is, a rigid event order carried out daily should have a "stronger" representation than one carried out monthly. Each MKU has a typical duration of activation, and each event that is a member of an MKU has a typical event duration.

Normative data for the *duration* of a typical MKU (e.g., the set of events that you experience from the time you wake up in the morning until you leave the house), its individual events (e.g., taking a shower), and interevent transitions are currently unavailable, but such normative data could be collected. This data should include both verbal estimates for the length of time it would take to carry out the activity, rank ordering of event time duration, and the actual timing of people carrying out the activity.

Are there kinds of events that make up a single MKU? In general, for the

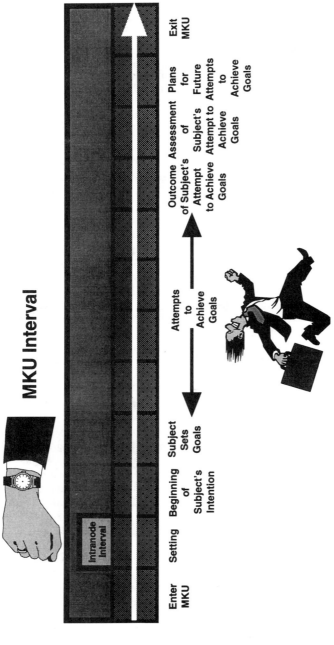

FIGURE 5. An abstract Managerial Knowledge Unit for sequential events. This MKU indicates the broad macrostructure knowledge that should be stored within the MKU, displays some of the properties of an MKU including its time duration, event durations, and variables that may help determine how rigidly the sequence of events are stored and activated. Note that recursive loops would be required to deal with reactions to unexpected interruptions during the expression of an MKU.

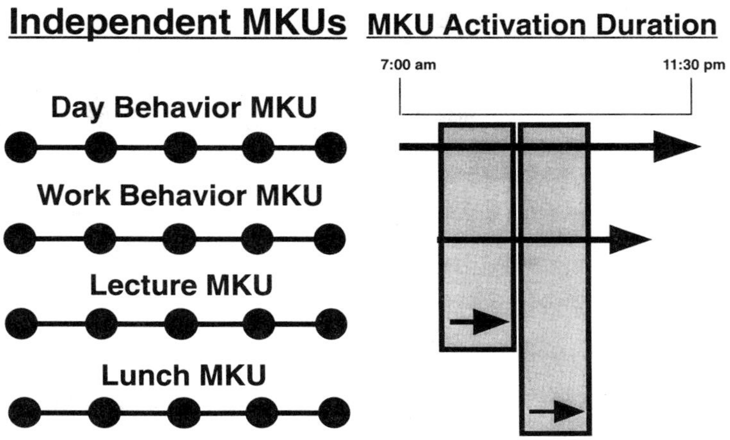

Independent MKUs MKU Activation Duration

FIGURE 6. Parallel activation of Managerial Knowledge Units. At any time during the day, one or more MKUs may be activated in parallel.

typical MKU, I suggest that there is a beginning event that specifies a setting, a following set of events that specify goals and activities to achieve those goals, and an event that signifies the setting that deactivates the MKU. Events within an MKU may have different "strength" values. That is, certain events may be more *central* or critical to the activation, execution, retrieval, or meaning of an MKU. Thus, given the assignment of events within the MKU postulated above, the MKU can serve as the underlying representation for knowledge acquired from reading a text, understanding a story, watching a street scene evolve, listening to a conversation, planning a trip, or even reacting to a physical challenge.

PARALLEL ACTIVATION

I hypothesize that a limited number of MKUs can be activated in "parallel." That is, both categorically and hierarchically distinct MKUs may be simultaneously activated. This parallel activity would, in effect, represent a cascade of activation because different MKUs have different temporal durations (e.g., eating dinner versus going out on a date). Therefore, certain MKUs could be activated and deactivated within the duration of other activated MKUs (FIG. 6). The hierarchical and categorical distinctions in MKUs to which I have alluded are next described.

MANAGERIAL KNOWLEDGE UNIT HIERARCHY

In the adult human brain, MKUs are located at the top of a hierarchy of SECs. The hierarchy can be conceived of in the following way. At the top of the hierarchy are *abstract MKUs* that simply represent event series that have a beginning, goals, actions, and an ending. This level of MKU might be instantiated when someone is exposed to an entirely novel situation. They do not represent any specific activity. One step down in the hierarchy are *context-free MKUs* that represent specific behaviors such as the events that make up eating a meal. They might be instantiated whenever someone eats a meal. Next are *context-dependent MKUs* that represent specific contexts for a behavior such as eating a meal in a restaurant (or in a kind of restaurant). One step down are *episodic MKUs* that represent a specific time and location such as eating lunch at McDonald's Restaurant. Lower in the hierarchy are SECs that include the developmental and phylogenetic precursors of the MKU, including representations specifying *rules* (e.g., wait to be seated in a restaurant by the hostess), *conditional paired–associative responses* (e.g., don't begin eating until your date has been served), *procedures* (e.g., using a knife and fork to cut a steak), and *skills* (e.g., precise carving of a turkey). Thus, I would predict that some redundancy is present in representations because simple events or behavioral fragments could potentially be preserved even when an MKU was inaccessible. Procedures and visuomotor skills most likely depend upon a cortico–basal ganglia–cerebellum loop that uses the frontal cortex and cerebellum to encode sequential movements and the basal ganglia to store them.[89–94] Furthermore, this hierarchy is built from the bottom up. That is, the more abstract and context-free MKUs emerge only after several episodic and context-dependent MKUs have been formed. The abstract and context-free MKUs are formed on the basis of MKU structural and thematic similarities that are evident across a large family of MKUs. This hierarchical description has developmental implications for the emergence of the MKU, which are presented later in this paper.

CATEGORY SPECIFICITY

Given that MKUs represent a form of knowledge, such as other kinds of knowledge (e.g., lexical), it is probable that categorical distinctions exist within the MKU cognitive architecture. Two potential categories of MKU knowledge that have already been mentioned in this paper are social behavior and abstract-symbolic reasoning. Broadening the number of categorical distinctions in MKU knowledge would not be difficult. For example, sexual behavior,[95] appetitive behavior, social behavior,[96] mechanical knowledge, and symbolic problem solving[97] could all qualify as candidate categories of MKUs (FIG. 7). Additional categorical subdivisions may also exist. For example, within the category of sexual behaviors, there might be categories for dating behavior, marriage behavior, seduction behavior, etc. Social behavior, in particular, might be idiosyncratically stored in an individual (e.g., given order and content constraints) and be particularly suited to single-case design study.

Thus, parallel activation of MKUs in both a hierarchical and categorical sense is potentially possible. Both within-category context-free (events making up eating behavior) and episodic (eating at a self-service restaurant) MKUs could potentially be activated in parallel as could MKUs representing different categories of knowl-

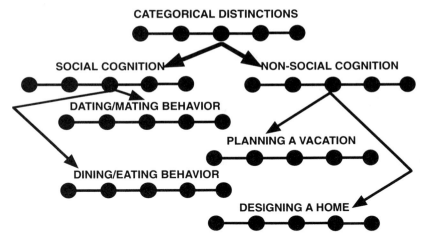

FIGURE 7. Some examples of possible category-based distinctions in representation of Managerial Knowledge Units.

edge (MKUs representing tutorial lecture behavior and social conduct rules for relating to a student of the opposite sex).

MANAGERIAL KNOWLEDGE UNIT METRIC RELATIONS

What might the metric relations in a cognitive architecture made up of MKUs be? There is no a priori reason why certain metric relations between units of memory would not be similar across knowledge domains (FIG. 8). Therefore, such

Metric Relations in an SEC/MKU
Cognitive Architecture
Frequency
Similarity
Semantic-Abstract-Associative Relations
Category Specificity

FIGURE 8. Some predicted metric relations that an Managerial Knowledge Unit cognitive architecture should have.

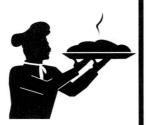

- # Eating
- ## Eating at home
- ### Eating at a restaurant
- #### Eating at the Parkway Deli
- #### Eating at Galileo
- #### Eating at French Restaurants
- ##### Eating at Le Marmiton
- ###### Eating at Au Pactole

FIGURE 9. Managerial Knowledge Units—*Frequency* as an attribute. As in other cognitive networks, the frequency of an MKU activation will determine its accessibility after brain injury. In this case, eating-at-home behavior should be better preserved than behavior when eating at Au Pactole (in Paris).

matrices as *frequency* of exposure or use, *similarity,* and *associative strength,* which are relevant to the semantic storage of words, are also candidate matrices in the case of the MKU cognitive architecture. MKUs that are more frequently activated should also have the lowest thresholds for activation. For example, in the domain of eating behaviors, eating at home might have a higher frequency rating compared to eating at a Turkish restaurant (FIG. 9). In the case of a patient with a prefrontal lobe brain lesion, we would predict that the patient would behave more appropriately at home than in a Turkish restaurant. That is, the "eat at home" MKU is more "retrievable" after brain damage by virtue of its higher frequency ratings.

Associative relations between MKUs would also determine the spread of activation (FIG. 10). MKUs that were most similar within- and across-categories of MKUs would be more strongly related. Therefore, when one MKU among these associatively related MKUs were to be activated, those MKUs within this immediate associative network (i.e., the MKU neighbors) would be more likely to be activated than less related MKUs (which might even be inhibited). For example, eating at home might partially activate eating at a family picnic, eating at a family party, or doing homework after dinner MKUs. It may even be the case that associatively linked MKUs provide the basis for analogical thinking[75,98] (i.e., our search for an analogy when trying to solve a problem is, in essence, an attempt to template match an underspecified abstract MKU to an already existing MKU via associative links—event to event). Some studies of patients with dementia–Alzheimer's type have found that they show hyperpriming in lexical decision tasks. The assumption is that due to a loss of cells, there is a concurrent diminish-

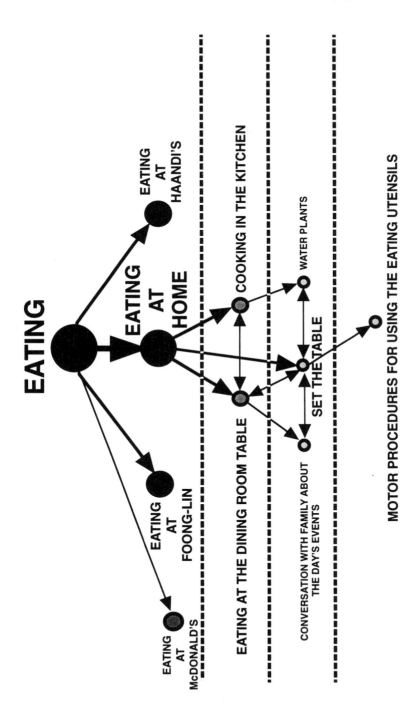

FIGURE 10. Associative spread of knowledge should occur when a Managerial Knowledge Unit is activated. Activation should be spread to *related MKUs* (e.g., eating at Haandi's) and to other events *within the MKU* (eating at the dining room table → conversation with family) as well as to *associated events* across MKUs (set the table → water the plants).

ment of an inhibitory mechanism at the lexical level. Thus, we would predict that in frontal dementia one might observe hyperpriming of specific MKUs and their bound knowledge.

ATTENTION AND THE MANAGERIAL KNOWLEDGE UNIT

Norman and Shallice[15,99] have proposed an attentional system framework that nicely "piggy-backs" on the SEC and MKU representational model (see above). One automatic selection mechanism, which they termed *contention scheduling,* results in the inhibition of unrelated MKUs or SECs once a particular MKU or SEC is activated. The unrelated MKUs or SECs would be inhibited to a degree proportional to their psychological or procedural distance from the activated MKU or SEC. This automatic mechanism allows for parallel activation of related MKUs, however. A second selection mechanism, which they called the *supervisory attention system,* helps to bias MKU or SEC selection. It has inhibitory operations to suppress strong but irrelevant (for the processing of currently activated MKUs) environmental stimuli. It also has facilitatory properties that can activate MKUs despite the absence of environmental triggers. In my view, the supervisory attention system is nothing more than a set of frequently used MKUs that are context-free and help guide us through underspecified situations. Furthermore, because the MKU is hypothesized to be part of a singular domain of knowledge representation, episodes in memory usually contain one or more MKUs that are bound together with knowledge stored elsewhere in the brain via third-party structures such as the hippocampus (FIG. 11). MKUs, as independent forms of knowledge, may be stored in an unbound fashion in patients who have episodic memory disorders, making that knowledge potentially available under conditions where implicit behavior is elicited.

DEVELOPMENT OF THE MANAGERIAL KNOWLEDGE UNIT

Thus far, I have described what may be the "mature" cognitive architecture of the MKU system. How might this cognitive architecture develop?[37,100-102] One possibility is that primitive SECs, made up of just a few events such as simple rules or, more relevantly, conditional associates, develop early in childhood and only later expand into a large multi-event MKU based on the frequency with which adjacent events occur together (and in a preferred order) in time (FIG. 12). Based on repeated exposure to an SEC, the boundaries of that event-series would become more firmly established, leading to a well-formed MKU. Another possibility is that fully formed MKUs could be stored quite early in life but only in sparse numbers and that growth in the MKU population would depend primarily on expanding life experiences (which are highly controlled when we are children and are still dependent on our cognitive capabilities in other domains, e.g., language understanding). Both possibilities are consistent with a biologically based explanation which argues that because the prefrontal cortex does not fully mature until adolescence and early adulthood, it is impossible that a rich MKU cognitive archi-

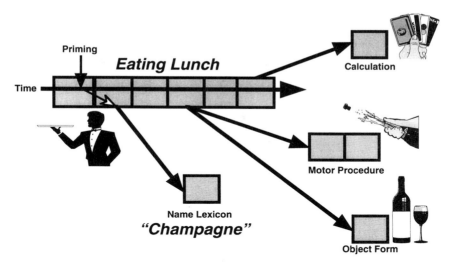

FIGURE 11. Activation of a Managerial Knowledge Unit primes bound representations. In order to form an explicit episodic memory, different memory units across the cortex must be bound together by a third-party structure (such as the hippocampus). Given the long duration activation of a multi-event MKU, it would gain priority for determining the configuration of activation across cognitive architectures. In the example shown, various events during eating lunch would prime other representations in memory such as those illustrated in the figure. Note that the onset of event A (*first rectangle*) would begin to prime the onset of event B (*second rectangle*), which in turn would begin to prime the activation of lexical unit concerned with the name champagne which would be ordered.

tecture could be developed until adolescence or adulthood regardless of the richness of experience in childhood. Also note that this hypothesis suggests that the individual and paired-events that make up an SEC are first processed as independent or paired-events, thereby creating a partial redundancy of representation where the events, event-pairs, and MKUs retain their topographical and psychological independence within the prefrontal cortex.

There is elegant primate research which suggests prefrontal lesions placed early in development do not affect performance on tasks presumably subserved by prefrontal cortex until the monkey's prefrontal cortex matures.[21,22,45] Some human data are available that supports this observation of the delayed effects of early prefrontal lesions in monkeys. Much more developmental clinical research is needed to test adequately and characterize cognitively the "delayed deficit" hypothesis.[103–105]

What might be the "usefulness" of developing an MKU form of knowledge representation in terms of evolution? One distinct advantage of having memory units in the form of SECs and concerned with plans, schemas, social rules, etc., is that they span (i.e., are activated during) time periods that can range from minutes to many hours. Thus, activating these MKUs not only activates knowledge representing the here and now (e.g., ordering food at a restaurant), but the

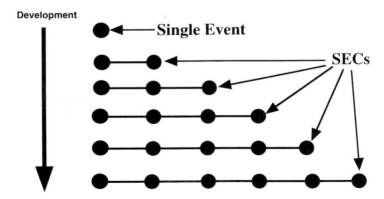

FIGURE 12. Redundancy of event representation: Ontogenetic development and partial ordering. The Managerial Knowledge Unit framework predicts that during development, single events are first encoded followed by more and more complex Structured Event Complexes (SECs) until mature MKUs become stored in adolescence. Another possibility is that a few mature MKUs can be stored very early in childhood and that development simply allows for more and more MKUs to become stored. Note that the MKU framework predicts that all these levels of knowledge are independently stored in the prefrontal cortex allowing for some redundancy in knowledge representation.

past (entering the restaurant), and the future (paying the bill). Therefore, the consequences of current behavior get linked *within a single memory unit* to behavior in the past and the future. Memories stored in this way (MKUs) allow for the development of strategies, plans, and other behaviors that could enhance survival in a competitive environment.[106] It would not be surprising if the emergence of language as a cognitive function was linked to this kind of stored knowledge. The role of language in this context would be to communicate the action, plans, consequences, and schematic memories permitted by the SEC. Syntactic frames themselves, after all, would qualify as a primitive form of an SEC.

WORKING MEMORY AND THE MANAGERIAL KNOWLEDGE UNIT

I have argued that an MKU may stay activated for minutes to hours depending on the particular event-series it represents. This poses an interesting dilemma for theories of conscious awareness and working memory. That is, by most definitions, working memory and consciousness can only keep active sets of information that contain 7+ or −2 bits. This kind of information usually appears and disappears from conscious awareness within a few seconds. Most units of memory such as objects, words, features, even sentential information can fit within this restricted boundary of working memory and consciousness (FIG. 13). I argue that the MKU that is active in real time *cannot* ever fit as a unit into working memory and consciousness. This temporal constraint may have led to the development of alternative forms of MKU representation such as verbal and written scripts, series

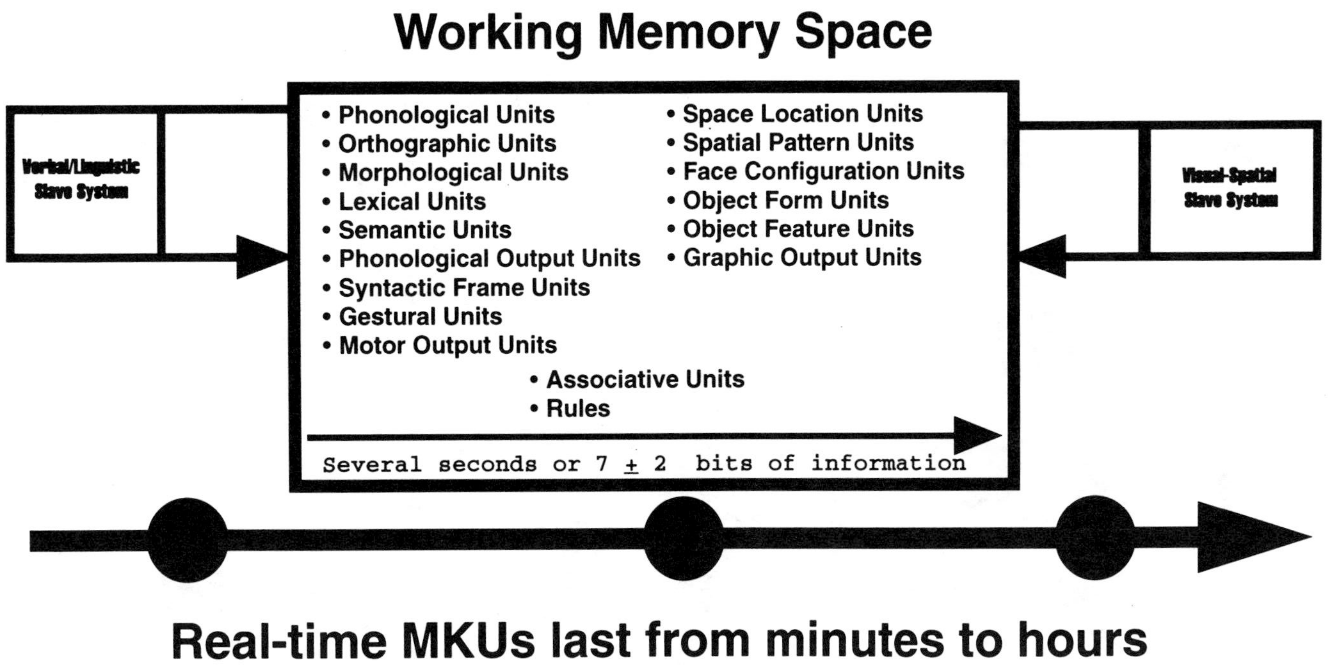

Working Memory Space

Verbal/Linguistic Slave System

Visual-Spatial Slave System

- Phonological Units
- Orthographic Units
- Morphological Units
- Lexical Units
- Semantic Units
- Phonological Output Units
- Syntactic Frame Units
- Gestural Units
- Motor Output Units

- Space Location Units
- Spatial Pattern Units
- Face Configuration Units
- Object Form Units
- Object Feature Units
- Graphic Output Units

- Associative Units
- Rules

Several seconds or 7 ± 2 bits of information

Real-time MKUs last from minutes to hours

FIGURE 13. Activated real-time Managerial Knowledge Units exceed the temporal window of working memory. Although a great many cognitive operations can be squeezed into what we consider working memory space, MKUs routinely exceed the span occupied by working memory space and therefore would be consciously impenetrable. Thus we must translate the real-time representation of an MKU into propositional listings (as in a script) or set of scenes (as in frames) in order to remember and express the nature of macrostructure knowledge.

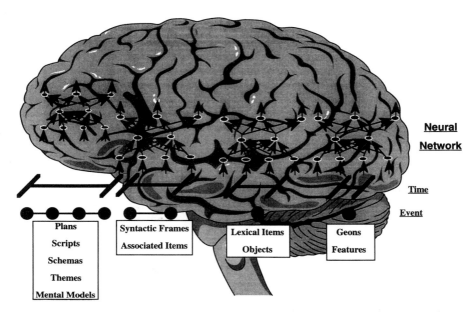

Neural

Network

Time

Event

Plans	Syntactic Frames	Lexical Items	Geons
Scripts	Associated Items	Objects	Features
Schemas			
Themes			
Mental Models			

FIGURE 14. Evolution of the Managerial Knowledge Unit. The MKU framework explicitly claims that the macrostructure knowledge and properties unique to plans, scripts, schemas, themes, and mental models are stored in human prefrontal cortex in cortical areas distinct from those storing the other forms of knowledge indicated in the figure.

of ideographs, symbolic gestural series, etc. These alternative forms of the MKU can more easily fit into the temporal constraints imposed by working memory and allow us to become consciously aware of the hidden dimensions of the SEC/MKU.

WHAT SPECIFIC FORMS OF KNOWLEDGE ARE STORED IN PREFRONTAL CORTEX?

Event and SEC boundaries must be coded. When does a specific MKU begin and when does it end? Support for permitting information to be stored across events must be obtained from the neural architecture (via sustained cell firing?). These operating constraints would lead to the storage of coarse and discrete macroknowledge structures concerned with semantics that must be processed across events (FIG. 14). For example, in order to understand the moral of a story, you must process cross-event semantics. In order to plan a vacation adequately, you must persist in performing a set of activities related to taking a vacation and so on.[107,108] Given the temporal and hierarchical organization of MKUs, they must have their own syntactic structure (e.g., a story grammar). Given their time duration, this form of knowledge, when activated, would gain prioritized control over behavior. By virtue of being bound together with other forms of knowledge (e.g., object, motor action, and spatial coordinate stores), when activated, it would supervise the activation of these other forms of knowledge.[109] Therefore, some types of attention would become the by-product of activation of this form of knowledge.

Within any representational domain (including the MKU cognitive architecture), there is great predictability in how a particular memory unit will be activated and expressed. However, in the process of binding together an MKU with other units of knowledge, there should be a fair amount of unpredictability in terms of which exact *configuration* of units across the brain will be active at any one time. For example, imagine the changing dynamics of your office in terms of which people and objects are transient and somewhat randomly appearing in time versus those that are constant in time, and try pairing all those "units of memory" with the particular set of MKUs that might be active at any time. Arguably, these "routinely" novel encoded episodes appear in unpredictable ways, are dynamic, and require people to plan reactively on a regular basis. These dynamic states may, in the long run, be best modeled by nonlinear mathematics.[110,111]

PREDICTIVE POWER OF THE SEC/MKU FRAMEWORK

The viability of this framework can be tested in many ways. There can be tests of the MKU structure itself. For example, a strong prediction would be that events within an MKU or SEC are rigidly ordered. This notion can be tested by categorizing pairs of events by physical, social, and individual constraints. Reaction times obtained during event-pair order verification tasks and production frequencies of event-pairs during script generation tasks could test this hypothesis. The MKU network structure could be tested by similar verification and production measures designed to evaluate the frequency with which an MKU header is activated, its associative strength, and the category specificity of the MKU network (e.g., you could ask a subject to generate all the activities they might do on a Saturday—this would include such things as getting dressed, eating breakfast, working in the garden, etc.). Error analyses can be used to determine whether patterns of MKU or event-activation failure correspond to proposed or obtained centrality, frequency, and MKU boundary metrics. Patients may only have difficulty in generating, verifying, or acting out low-frequency MKUs. There should be dissociations in performance between the verbal generation, visual verification, or real-time acting out of MKUs. Category-specific deficits could be expected such as a selective deficit in activating MKUs concerned with social cognition. A variety of deactivation failures may occur including difficulty in initial activation, fluctuations in activation, or premature deactivation. Such activation failures may result from a problem in maintaining appropriate modulation of the MKU knowledge domain (perhaps because of neurotransmitter deficits). Many other predictions can be made on the basis of this framework for understanding the form of knowledge that might be stored in prefrontal cortex. Such predictions indicate that the MKU and SEC framework can be rejected or verified using traditional cognitive neuropsychological methods.

CONCLUSIONS

We have already begun to use script event tasks to examine MKU knowledge in patients with Alzheimer's disease[112] and frontal lobe lesions.[113] Both the methods of assessment and error analysis that are described in the papers of Grafman et al.[112] and Sirigu et al.[113] can be used (and elaborated on) with patients with focal prefrontal lesions.[114] Real-time analysis of domain-specific MKUs (preparing a meal) can be accomplished within many rehabilitation medicine departments. Other tasks such as story understanding and memory, reasoning and remembering by analogy, and ordering events in cartoon series can all be used to assess the intactness of MKUs. Experimental tasks, such as the ones described above, can be used in conjunction with more traditional paradigms to provide a theory-based assessment of executive functions in frontal lobe–injured patients.

Prefrontal lobe damage may lead to striking behavioral deficits and/or problems in executive functions. Despite 150 years of observation and study, there has been little advance in understanding the cause(s) of these deficits. Some observers have even described executive functions as "horizontal processes" that are nonmodular with an infinite number of possible configurations of cognitive processes and therefore not amenable to traditional cognitive examination.[115] In this paper I explicitly reject the strong form of that notion and have outlined a candidate cognitive architecture for the knowledge subserved by prefrontal cortex (FIG. 15). I claim that the units of knowledge stored in prefrontal cortex are SECs with the MKU most responsible for the storage and expression of so-called executive functions. It was illustrated how the MKU cognitive architecture could break down, thereby providing a set of tests for its authenticity. Using this framework, I offered a few suggestions regarding neuropsychological assessment. Although the SEC-MKU framework may eventually be replaced by other models of prefrontal lobe functions, it is, at the least, a testable and potentially rich framework that distinguishes it from, and is an advance over, most of the other frontal lobe functional models and frameworks described above and in this volume.

Health-care professionals, family members, and acquaintances have difficulty understanding why the patient with prefrontal lobe damage who is intellectually sound, and may even have average memory, still persistently displays abnormal planning, reasoning, and social conduct. Explanations for this abnormal behavior have historically been vague. I hope that the framework(s) presented in this paper can aid in providing a coherent explanation for the kinds of knowledge that may be stored in prefrontal cortex, for the executive function deficits in patients with prefrontal lesions, and can perhaps assist in designing new tasks that can improve the evaluation of such patients.

In a paper that appeared in the journal *Brain* in 1892, Bastian[116] discussed the neural processes that subserved attention and volition. He considered the prefrontal cortex especially crucial for these operations. "Volition," he said, ". . . represents merely some phases in the association of ideas. The phenomena of volition are, therefore, not the work of any special faculty or mysterious entity, nor are they carried on in motor centres; they are merely certain exemplifications of intellect in action. . . . Anything separate to be known as will, is, in fact, a mere phantom, a kind of psychological ghost."

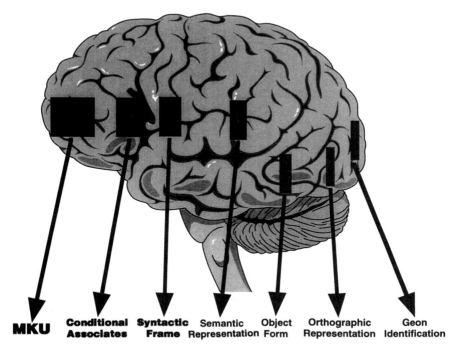

MKU   **Conditional**   **Syntactic**   Semantic   Object   Orthographic   Geon
        Associates   **Frame**   Representation   Form   Representation   Identification

FIGURE 15. Growth of the "size" of a unit of memory across the human cerebral cortex. The Managerial Knowledge Unit (MKU) framework explicitly suggests that evolution has allowed for memory units that encompass many events on a time scale of minutes to hours. This evolutionary trend appears to take on a posterior-to-anterior gradient. This increasing time scale for knowledge stored in memories allows humans to be much more aware of the consequences of their current behavior in relation to behaviors previously emitted or seen or to behaviors that are forthcoming. This awareness (which can be conveyed to others through pictorial or verbal communication or demonstrated through procedural demonstration) has obvious survival value.

The language used by Bastian is embarrassingly familiar to us today, revealing our persistent ignorance of the functions of the human prefrontal cortex over 100 years after his paper appeared. Bastian's description of "intellect in action" resembles our use of the term "working memory" as a metaphor for the actions of a central executive. Given the critical role of the prefrontal cortex in cognition in conjunction with our slow pace of understanding its functions, I anticipate that cognitive neuroscience will place central to its agenda in the twenty-first century an effort to extinguish the phantom of the prefrontal cortex and replace it with the more mundane reality of a cognitive architecture.

REFERENCES

1. MILLER, G. A., E. GALANTER & K. H. PRIBRAM. 1960. Plans and the Structure of Behavior.: 195–209. Holt, Rinehart & Winston. New York.

2. DIVAC, I. 1988. A note on the history of the term "prefrontal." IBRO News **16(2):** 5.
3. COHEN, J. D. & S. D. SERVAN-SCHREIBER. 1992. Context, cortex, and dopamine: A connectionist approach to behavior and biology in schizophrenia. Psychol. Rev. **99(1):** 45–77.
4. COHEN, J. D., S. D. FORMAN, T. S. BRAVER, B. J. CASEY, D. SERVAN-SCHREIBER & D. C. Noll. 1994. Activation of the prefrontal cortex in a nonspatial working memory task with functional MRI. Hum. Brain Mapping **1:** 293–304.
5. PASCUAL-LEONE, A., J. GRAFMAN & M. HALLETT. 1994. Modulation of cortical motor output maps during development of implicit and explicit knowledge. Science **263(5151):** 1287–1289.
6. ROLAND, P. 1993. Brain Activation.: 341–354. Wiley-Liss. New York.
7. DEHAENE, S. & J.-P. CHANGEUX. 1991. The Wisconsin Card Sorting Test: Theoretical Analysis and Modeling in a Neuronal Network. Cereb. Cortex **1(1):** 62–79.
8. GUIGON, E., B. DORIZZI, Y. BURNOD & W. SCHULTZ. 1995. Neural correlates of learning in the prefrontal cortex of the monkey: A predictive model. Cereb. Cortex **5(2):** 135–147.
9. NEISSER, U., Ed. 1987. Concepts and Conceptual Development: Ecological and Intellectual Factors in Categorization.: 317. Cambridge University Press. Cambridge, UK.
10. SMITH, E. E. & S. A. SLOMAN. 1994. Similarity-versus rule-based categorization. Memory & Cognition. **22(4):** 377–386.
11. BARRETT, A. & D. S. WELD. 1994. Partial-order planning: Evaluating possible efficiency gains. Artif. Intel. **67:** 71–112.
12. BUONOMANO, D. V. & M. M. MERZENICH. 1995. Temporal information transformed into a spatial code by a neural network with realistic properties. Science **267:** 1028–1030.
13. MINTON, S., M. DRUMMOND, J. L. BRESINA & A. B. PHILIPS. 1992. Total order versus partial order planning: Factors influencing performance. *In* Principles of Knowledge Representation and Reasoning: Proceedings of the Third International Conference (KR-92). Morgan Kaufmann Publishers. San Mateo, CA.
14. KIEN, J. & A. KEMP. 1994. Is speech temporally segmented? Comparison with temporal segmentation in behavior. Brain & Lang. **46:** 662–682.
15. SHALLICE, T. 1988. From Neuropsychology to Mental Structure. Cambridge University Press. New York.
16. LEZAK, M. 1982. The problem of assessing executive functions. Int. J. Psychol. **17:** 281–297.
17. STUSS, D. T. & D. F. BENSON. 1986. The Frontal Lobes. 2nd edit.: 1–303. Raven Press. New York.
18. SHALLICE, T., P. W. BURGESS, F. SCHON & D. M. BAXTER. 1989. The origins of utilization behaviour. Brain **112:** 1587–1598.
19. SHALLICE, T. & P. W. BURGESS. 1991. Deficits in strategy application following frontal lobe damage in man. Brain **114:** 727–741.
20. SHALLICE, T. & P. BURGESS. 1991. Higher-order cognitive impairments and frontal lobe lesions. *In* Frontal Lobe Function and Dysfunction. H. S. Levin, H. M. Eisenberg & A. R. Benton, Eds.: 125–138. Oxford University Press. New York.
21. GOLDMAN-RAKIC, P. S. 1987. Circuitry of primate prefrontal cortex and regulation of behavior by representational memory. *In* Handbook of Physiology—The Nervous System.: 373–417. American Physiological Society. Washington, D.C.
22. GOLDMAN-RAKIC, P. 1992. Working memory and the mind. Sci. Am. **267(3):** 110–117.
23. FUSTER, J. M. 1991. The prefrontal cortex and its relation to behavior. Prog. Brain Res. **87(201):** 201–211.
24. LURIA, A. R. & L. S. TSVETKOVA. 1990. The Neuropsychological Analysis of Problem Solving.: 1–230 (translation). Paul M. Deutsch Press. Orlando, FL.
25. ANDERSON, S. W., H. DAMASIO, D. TRANEL & A. R. DAMASIO. 1988. Neuropsychological correlates of bilateral frontal lobe lesions in humans. Presented at the Society for Neuroscience. Toronto.

26. ANDERSON, S. W., H. DAMASIO, R. D. JONES & D. TRANEL. 1991. Wisconsin card sorting test performance as a measure of frontal lobe damage. J. Clin. Exp. Neuropsychol. **13(6):** 909–922.
27. BECHARA, A., A. R. DAMASIO, H. DAMASIO & S. W. ANDERSON. 1994. Insensitivity to future consequences following damage to human prefrontal cortex. Cognition **50(1):** 7–15.
28. DAMASIO, A. R., D. TRANEL & H. DAMASIO. 1990. Individuals with sociopathic behavior caused by frontal damage fail to respond autonomically to social stimuli. Behav. Brain Res. **41:** 81–94.
29. DAMASIO, A. R., D. TRANEL & H. C. DAMASIO. 1991. Somatic markers and the guidance of behavior: Theory and preliminary testing. *In* Frontal Lobe Function and Dysfunction. H. S. Levin, H. M. Eisenberg & A. L. Benton, Eds.: 217–229. Oxford University Press. New York.
30. DAMASIO, A. R. & D. TRANEL. 1993. Nouns and verbs are retrieved with differently distributed neural systems. Proc. Natl. Acad. Sci. USA **90(6):** 4957–4960.
31. DAMASIO, H., T. GRABOWSKI, R. FRANK, A. M. GALABURDA & A. R. DAMASIO. 1994. The return of Phineas Gage: Clues about the brain from the skull of a famous patient. Science **264:** 1102–1105.
32. DAMASIO, A. R. 1994. Descartes' Error: Emotion, Reason, and the Human Brain.: 1–312. Grosset/Putnam. New York.
33. SAVER, J. L. & A. R. DAMASIO. 1991. Preserved access and processing of social knowledge in a patient with acquired sociopathy due to ventromedial frontal damage. Neuropsychologia **29(12):** 1241–1249.
34. TRANEL, D. & H. DAMASIO. 1994. Neuroanatomical correlates of electrodermal skin conductance responses. Psychophysiology **31:** 427–438.
35. SCHWARTZ, M. F., E. S. REED, M. MONTGOMERY, C. PALMER & N. H. MAYER. 1991. The quantitative description of action disorganization after brain damage: A case study. Cogn. Neuropsychol. **8(5):** 381–414.
36. DAVIDSON, D. 1994. Recognition and recall of irrelevant and interruptive atypical actions in script-based stories. J. Memory & Lang. **33:** 757–775.
37. AVRAHAMI, J. & Y. KAREEV. 1994. The emergence of events. Cognition **53:** 239–261.
38. COCKBURN, J. 1995. Task interruption in prospective memory: A frontal lobe function. Cortex **31:** 87–97.
39. TIPPER, S. P., B. WEAVER & G. HOUGHTON. 1994. Behavioural goals determine inhibitory mechanisms of selective attention. Q. J. Exp. Psychol. **47a(4):** 809–840.
40. ELDRIDGE, M. A., P. J. BARNARD & D. A. BEKERIAN. 1994. Autobiographical memory and daily schemas at work. Memory **2(1):** 51–74.
41. SCHANK, R. 1982. Dynamic memory: A theory of reminding and learning in computers and people. Cambridge University Press. Cambridge, MA.
42. BADDELEY, A. & B. WILSON. 1988. Frontal amnesia and the dysexecutive syndrome. Brain & Cognition **7:** 212–230.
43. FUNAHASHI, S., M. V. CHAFEE & P. S. GOLDMAN-RAKIC. 1993. Prefrontal neuronal activity in rhesus monkeys performing a delayed anti-saccade task. Nature **365:** 753–756.
44. WILSON, F. A. W., S. P. O'SCALAIDHE & P. GOLDMAN-RAKIC. 1993. Dissociation of object and spatial processing domains in primate prefrontal cortex. Science **260:** 1955–1958.
45. DIAMOND, A. 1991. Guidelines for the study of brain-behavior relationships during development. *In* Frontal Lobe Function and Dysfunction. H. S. Levin, H. M. Eisenberg & A. L. Benton, Eds.: 339–380. Oxford University Press. New York.
46. PASCUAL-LEONE, J. & J. JOHNSON. 1991. The psychological unit and its role in task analysis: A reinterpretation of object permanence. *In* Criteria for Competence: Controversies in the Conceptualization and Assessment of Children's Abilities. M. Chandler & M. Chapman, Eds.: 153–187. Lawrence Erlbaum Associates. Hillsdale, NJ.
47. MCCARTHY, G., A. M. BLAMIRE, A. PUCE, A. C. NOBRE, G. BLOCK, F. HYDER, P. GOLDMAN-RAKIC & R. G. SHULMAN. 1994. Functional magnetic resonance imaging

of human prefrontal cortex activation during a spatial working memory task. Proc. Natl. Acad. Sci. USA **91:** 8690–8694.

48. RUCHKIN, D. S., J. GRAFMAN, G. L. KRAUSS, R. JOHNSON, JR., H. CANOUNE & W. RITTER. 1994. Event-related brain potential evidence for a verbal working memory deficit in multiple sclerosis. Brain 117(Pt. 2): 289–305.

49. KESNER, R., R. P. HOPKINS & B. FINEMAN. 1994. Item and order dissociation in humans with prefrontal cortex damage. Neuropsychologia **32(8):** 881–891.

50. PETRIDES, M. 1991. Functional specialization within the dorsolateral frontal cortex for serial order memory. Proc. R. Soc. Lond. B **246:** 299–306.

51. ROLLS, E. T., J. HORNAK, D. WADE & J. MCGRATH. 1994. Emotion-related learning in patients with social and emotional changes associated with frontal lobe damage. J. Neurol. Neurosurg. Psychiatry **57:** 1518–1524.

52. WYER, J., R. S. & T. K. SRULL. 1989. Memory and Cognition in its Social Context. 1st edit.: 491. Lawrence Erlbaum Associates. Hillsdale, NJ.

53. ZAJONC, R. B. 1984. On the primacy of affect. Am. Psychol. **39(2):** 117–123.

54. HARLOW, J. M. 1848. Passage of an iron rod through the head. Boston Med. Surg. J. **39(20):** 389–393.

55. HARLOW, J. M. 1868. Recovery from the passage of an iron bar through the head. J. Mass. Med. Soc.: 329–347.

56. BARKER, F. G. 1995. Phineas among the phrenologists: The American crowbar case and nineteenth-century theories of cerebral localization. J. Neurosurg. **82(4):** 672–682.

57. ARNETT, P. A., S. M. RAO, L. BERNADIN, J. GRAFMAN, F. Z. YETKIN & L. LOBECK. 1994. Relationship between frontal lobe lesions and Wisconsin Card Sorting Test performance in patients with multiple sclerosis. Neurology **44(3 Pt. 1):** 420–425.

58. BRAZZELLI, M. *et al.* 1994. Spared and impaired cognitive abilities after bilateral frontal lobe damage. Cortex **30(1):** 27–51.

59. BRICKNER, R. M. 1934. An interpretation of frontal lobe function based upon the study of a case of partial bilateral frontal lobectomy. *In* Research Publications: Association for Research in Nervous and Mental Disease.: 259–351. Association for Research in Nervous and Mental Disease. New York.

60. DUNCAN, J., P. BURGESS & H. EMSLIE. 1995. Fluid intelligence after frontal lobe lesions. Neuropsychologia **33(3):** 261–268.

61. GLOSSER, G. & H. GOODGLASS. 1990. Disorders in executive control functions among aphasic and other brain-damaged patients. J. Clin. Exp. Neuropsychol. **12(4):** 485–501.

62. GRAFMAN, J., S. C. VANCE, H. WEINGARTNER, A. M. SALAZAR & D. AMIN. 1986. The effects of lateralized frontal lesions on mood regulation. Brain 109(Pt. 6): 1127–1148.

63. GRAFMAN, J., B. JONAS & A. SALAZAR. 1990. Wisconsin Card Sorting Test performance based on location and size of neuroanatomical lesion in Vietnam veterans with penetrating head injury. Percept. Mot. Skills **71(3 Pt. 2):** 1120–1122.

64. GRAFMAN, J., B. JONAS & A. SALAZAR. 1992. Epilepsy following penetrating head injury to the frontal lobes. Effects on cognition. Adv. Neurol. **57:** 369–378.

65. GRATTAN, L. M., R. H. BLOOMER, F. X. ARCHAMBAULT & P. J. ESLINGER. 1994. Cognitive flexibility and empathy after frontal lobe lesion. Neuropsychiatr. Neuropsychol. Behav. Neurol. **7(4):** 251–259.

66. KARNATH, H. O. & C. W. WALLESCH. 1992. Inflexibility of mental planning: A characteristic disorder with prefrontal lesions. Neuropsychologia **30(11):** 1011–1016.

67. RUECKERT, L. & J. GRAFMAN. 1994. Sustained attention deficits in frontal lobe patients. *In* Cognitive Neuroscience Society Meeting Abstracts. San Francisco, CA.

68. VENDRELL, P., C. JUNQUE, J. PUJOL, M. A. JURADO, J. MOLET & J. GRAFMAN. 1995. The role of prefrontal regions in the Stroop task. Neuropsychologia **33(3):** 341–352.

69. EBDON, M. 1993. Is the cerebral neocortex a uniform cognitive architecture? Mind & Lang. **8(3):** 368–403.

70. MIONE, M. C. & J. G. PARNAVELAS. 1994. How do developing cortical neurones know where to go? Trends Neurosci. **17(11):** 443–445.

71. GRAFMAN, J. 1989. Plans, actions, and mental sets: Managerial knowledge units in

the frontal lobes. *In* Integrating Theory and Practice in Clinical Neuropsychology. E. Perecman, Ed.: 93–138. Lawrence Erlbaum Associates. Hillsdale, NJ.

72. ALLEN, J., J. HENDLER & A. TATE, EDS. 1990. Readings in Planning.: 754. Morgan Kaufmann. San Mateo, CA.

73. PEA, R. D. & J. HAWKINS. 1987. Planning in a chore-scheduling task. *In* Blueprints for Thinking. S. L. Friedman, E. K. Scholnick & R. R. Cocking, Eds.: 273–302. Cambridge University Press. Cambridge, UK.

74. WELD, D. S. 1994. An introduction to least commitment planning. AI Magazine **15(4):** 27–61.

75. WHARTON, C. M. & T. E. LANGE. 1994. Analogical transfer through comprehension and priming. *In* Proceedings of the Sixteenth Annual Conference of the Cognitive Science Society. Lawrence Erlbaum Associates. Hillsdale, NJ.

76. CASSON, R. W. 1983. Schemata in cognitive anthropology. Annu. Rev. Anthropol. **12:** 429–462.

77. MINSKY, M. 1986. Society of Mind. Simon and Schuster. New York.

78. HAMMOND, K. J. 1989. Case-Based Planning: Viewing Planning as a Memory Task. Perspectives in Artificial Intelligence.: 277. Academic Press. Boston, MA.

79. ABELSON, R. P. 1981. Psychological status of the script concept. Am. Psychol. **36(7):** 715–729.

80. BARSALOU, L. W. & D. R. SEWELL. 1985. Contrasting the representation of scripts and categories. J. Memory & Lang. **24:** 646–665.

81. BARSALOU, L. W. 1989. Intraconcept similarity and its implications for interconcept similarity. *In* Similarity and Analogical Reasoning. S. Vosniadou & A. Ortony, Eds.: 76–121. Cambridge University Press. New York.

82. CORSON, Y. 1990. The structure of scripts and their constituent elements. Eur. Bull. Cognit. Psychol. **10(2):** 157–183.

83. MEDIN, D., R. L. GOLDSTONE & D. GENTNER. 1993. Respects for similarity. Psychol. Rev. **100(2):** 254–278.

84. GRAFMAN, J. & J. HENDLER. 1991. Planning and the brain. Behav. Brain Sci. **14(4):** 563–564.

85. GRAFMAN, J. 1994. Neuropsychology of higher cognitive processes. *In* Handbook of Perception and Cognition. D. Zaidel, Ed.: 159–181. Academic Press. San Diego, CA.

86. DEMOREST, A. P. & I. E. ALEXANDER. 1992. Affective scripts as organizers of personal experience. J. Pers. **60(3):** 645–663.

87. GRAFMAN, J., A. SIRIGU, L. SPECTOR & J. HENDLER. 1993. Damage to the prefrontal cortex leads to decomposition of structured event complexes. J. Head Trauma Rehabil. **8(1):** 73–87.

88. GRAFMAN, J. 1994. Alternative frameworks for the conceptualization of prefrontal lobe functions. *In* Handbook of Neuropsychology. F. Boller & J. Grafman, Eds.: 187–202. Elsevier Science Publishers. Amsterdam.

89. GRAFMAN, J., I. LITVAN, C. GOMEZ & T. N. CHASE. 1990. Frontal lobe function in progressive supranuclear palsy. Arch. Neurol. **47(5):** 553–558.

90. GRAFMAN, J., I. LITVAN, S. MASSAQUOI, M. STEWART, A. SIRIGU & M. HALLETT. 1992. Cognitive planning deficit in patients with cerebellar atrophy. Neurology **42(8):** 1493–1496.

91. PASCUAL-LEONE, A., J. GRAFMAN, K. CLARK, M. STEWART, S. MASSAQUOI, J. S. LOU & M. HALLETT. 1993. Procedural learning in Parkinson's disease and cerebellar degeneration. Ann. Neurol. **34(4):** 594–602.

92. PASCUAL-LEONE, A., E. M. WASSERMAN, J. GRAFMAN & M. HALLETT. The role of dorsolateral frontal lobe in implicit procedural learning. Exp. Brain Res. In press.

93. ROBERTS, R. J., JR., L. D. HAGER & C. HERON. 1994. Prefrontal cognitive processes: Working memory and inhibition in the anti-saccade task. J. Exp. Psychol. Gen. **125(4):** 374–393.

94. TYRRELL, P. J. 1994. Apraxia of gait or higher level gait disorders: Review and description of two cases of progressive gait disturbance due to frontal lobe degeneration. J. R. Soc. Med. **87:** 56–58.

95. TIIHONEN, J., J. KUIKKA, J. KUPILA, K. PARTANEN, P. VAINIO, J. AIRAKSINEN, M. ERONEN, T. HALLIKAINEN, J. PAANILA, I. KINNUNEN & J. HUTTUNEN. 1994. Increase in cerebral blood flow of right prefrontal cortex in man during orgasm. Neurosci. Lett. **170:** 241–243.

96. MILLER, L. A. 1992. Impulsivity, risk-taking, and the ability to synthesize fragmented information after frontal lobectomy. Neuropsychologia **30(1):** 69–79.

97. GOEL, V. & J. GRAFMAN. 1995. Are the frontal lobes implicated in "planning" functions? Interpreting data from the tower of Hanoi. Neuropsychologia **33(5):** 623–642.

98. JOHNSON, H. M. & C. M. SEIFERT. 1992. The role of predictive features in retrieving analogical cases. J. Memory & Lang. **31:** 648–667.

99. NORMAN, D. A. & T. SHALLICE. 1986. Attention to action: Willed and automatic control of behavior. *In* Consciousness and Self-Regulation: Advances in Research and Theory. R. J. Davidson, G. E. Schwartz & D. Shapiro, Eds.: 1–18. Plenum. New York.

100. BARON-COHEN, S., H. RING, J. MORIARTY, B. SCHMITZ, D. COSTA & P. ELL. 1994. Recognition of mental state terms. Br. J. Psychiatry **165:** 640–649.

101. CASE, R. 1992. The role of the frontal lobes in the regulation of cognitive development. Brain & Cognition **20(1):** 51–73.

102. HALFORD, G. S. 1993. Children's Understanding: The Development of Mental Models.: 521. Lawrence Erlbaum Associates. Hillsdale, NJ.

103. ESLINGER, P. J., L. M. GRATTAN, H. DAMASIO & A. R. DAMASIO. 1992. Developmental consequences of childhood frontal lobe damage. Arch. Neurol. **49(7):** 764–769.

104. ESLINGER, P. J. & L. M. GRATTAN. 1994. Altered serial position learning after frontal lobe lesion. Neuropsychologia **32(6):** 729–739.

105. LEVIN, H. S., D. MENDELSOHN, M. A. LILLY, J. M. FLETCHER, K. A. CULHANE, S. B. CHAPMAN, H. HARWARD, L. KUSNERIK, D. BRUCE & H. M. EISENBERG. 1994. Tower of London performance in relation to magnetic resonance imaging following closed head injury in children. Neuropsychology **8(2):** 171–179.

106. NICHELLI, P., J. GRAFMAN, P. PIETRINI, D. ALWAY, J. C. CARTON & R. MILETICH. 1994. Brain activity in chess playing (letter). Nature **369(6477):** 191.

107. BARRETT, A. & D. S. WELD. 1993. Characterizing subgoal interactions for planning. *In* Proceedings of the Thirteenth International Joint Conference on Artificial Intelligence. Chambery, France. Morgan Kaufmann. San Mateo, CA.

108. LEVINSON, R. 1995. A computer model of prefrontal cortex function. Ann. N.Y. Acad. Sci. This volume.

109. GRAFMAN, J. & H. WEINGARTNER. A combinatorial binding and strength (CBS) model of memory: Is it a better framework for amnesia? *In* Basic and Applied Memory Research: Theory in Context. D. Herrmann *et al.*, Eds. Lawrence Erlbaum Associates. Hillsdale, NJ. In press.

110. BARTON, S. 1994. Chaos, self-organization, and psychology. Am. Psychol. **49(1):** 5–14.

111. MCKENNA, T. M., T. A. MCMULLEN & M. F. SHLESINGER. 1994. The brain as a dynamic physical system. Neuroscience **60(3):** 587–605.

112. GRAFMAN, J., K. THOMPSON, H. WEINGARTNER, R. MARTINEZ, B. A. LAWLOR & T. SUNDERLAND. 1991. Script generation as an indicator of knowledge representation in patients with Alzheimer's disease. Brain & Lang. **40(3):** 344–358.

113. SIRIGU, A., T. ZALLA, B. PILLON, J. GRAFMAN, Y. AGID & B. DUBOIS. Selective impairments in managerial knowledge following prefrontal cortex damage. Cortex. In press.

114. LE GALL, D., G. AUBIN, P. ALLAIN & J. EMILE. 1993. Script et syndrome frontal: A propos de deux observations. Rev. Neuropsychol. **3(1):** 87–110.

115. FODOR, J. A. 1983. The Modularity of Mind.: 1–145. MIT Press. Cambridge, MA.

116. BASTIAN, H. C. 1892. On the neural processes underlying attention and volition. Brain **15(Pt. 1):** 1–34.

Analogical Transfer in Sequence Learning

Human and Neural-Network Models of Frontostriatal Function

P. F. DOMINEY,[a] J. VENTRE-DOMINEY,[a] E. BROUSSOLLE,[b]
AND M. JEANNEROD[a]

[a]Vision et Motricité
INSERM Unité 94
69500 Bron, France

[b]Service de Neurologie
Hôpital Neurologique
69003 Lyon, France

INTRODUCTION

Analogical transfer in problem solving is a fundamental aspect of human intelligence that involves exploiting knowledge about the solution for one problem to solve another.[1] In order to provide a quantifiable measure of analogical transfer in sequence learning (ATSL), we developed a novel extension of the serial reaction time (SRT) paradigm. To quantify the underlying representational and computational requirements for ATSL we extended a neurobiologically based model of primate prefrontal cortex (PFC) and basal ganglia function in visuomotor sequence learning[2] to address analogical transfer. We compared the behavior of this model with preliminary data from normal subjects and patients with frontostriatal dysfunction [idiopathic dopa-sensitive Parkinson's disease (PD)] in the ATSL paradigm.

ANALOGICAL TRANSFER PARADIGM

Reaction times (RTs) for a series of motor responses to visual stimuli are significantly reduced if the stimuli appear in a repeating sequence, as opposed to in a random order, thus demonstrating a sequence learning effect.[3] Based on this observation, the ATSL task involves pointing to targets illuminated one at a time on a touch-sensitive screen. After a target is touched it is extinguished, RT is recorded and the next target is displayed. Targets appear in blocks of two types—random and sequence. In random blocks, 120 targets are presented in random order. In sequence blocks, targets are presented in a sequence of the structure ABC$\underline{B}^1\underline{C}^2\underline{D}^3C^1D^2E^3D^1E^2F^3$ . . . of length 24 that is repeated five times for a total of 120 targets. A–H denote screen locations. Superscripts indicate analogical schema "position" where positions 1 and 2 are predictable, and position 3 unpredictable. Note, for example, how $\underline{B}$ and $\underline{C}$ are predicted respectively by the element two places behind (referred to as "n − 2"), whereas $\underline{D}$ is unpredictable (referred to as "u"). This pattern "n − 2, n − 2, u" repeats throughout the sequences, and is the underlying analogical schema.

An experimental session starts with 20 random practice targets. The recording session starts with a random block of 120 trials, followed by *three different* sequence blocks (that share the analogical schema "n − 2, n − 2, u") of 120 trials each, and a final random block of 120 trials. Partially informed subjects are told a pattern may repeat in some sequences. Fully informed subjects are additionally shown a diagram of the repeating schema before and once during the test.

A MODEL OF ANALOGICAL TRANSFER

Performance of our existing sequence learning model[2] on this task indicates sequence learning capacity alone is not sufficient for ATSL (FIG. 1A). In the updated model (FIG. 1B), instead of learning sequences of specific items, the model recognizes if elements are novel or repeated, and learns sequences of descriptions in terms of novel versus repeated elements. In this sense the sequence ABABC is the same as the sequence EFEFG. Both can be described "u, u, n − 2, n − 2, u".

HUMAN PERFORMANCE

Normal subjects display significant analogical transfer between sequence blocks in the fully informed condition (FIG. 2A), and less but still significant learning in the partially informed condition (FIG. 2B). Patients with PD appear to display impaired transfer in both conditions (FIG. 2C and D), similar to impairment in SRT of patients with PD.[4]

CONCLUSIONS

ATSL is a new, quantitative model of analogical transfer. Normal subjects and a model with capacities for (1) memory of previous elements, (2) recognition of element repetition, and (3) modulation of behavior based on this recognition can realize ATSL. Patients with PD, however, and a model that does not possess these abstract capacities are both impaired in ATSL. These capacities for abstraction are likely based in the PFC and its corresponding frontostriatal circuitry, at the head of the developmental corticofrontal hierarchy that forms progressively higher levels of representation, from muscle contraction parameters to abstract representations for goal-directed action.[5]

Our repeating sequences have length 24 (difficult even for normal subjects),[4] whereas the underlying analogical schema "n − 2, n − 2, u" has length 3. This task thus attempts to dissociate sequence learning from the induction and transfer[1] of a three-element analogical schema. The limited but existing ATSL performance of subjects with PD demonstrates an impaired capacity for analogical transfer that is at least partially independent of their impaired SRT capacity (which would be

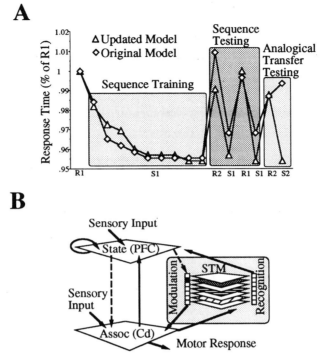

FIGURE 1. (**A**) Performance for the original and updated models of analogical transfer in sequence learning (ATSL). R1, R2 represent random blocks; S1, S2, two sequence blocks with different surface structure but shared analogical structure. R1 establishes the baseline response time. Sequence training: nine blocks of training with S1 yield standard SRT reduction in response time (RT). Sequence testing: learning demonstrated with sequence (reduced RT) and random (increased RT) blocks. Analogical transfer testing: with a new sequence (S2) that has the same analogical structure as S1. The updated model displays generalization (ATSL) to S2, whereas the original model does not. (**B**) Extension to sequence model to accommodate ATSL. Original model[2] encoded sequence state in prefrontal cortex (PFC) and learned associations between states and corresponding sequence elements. Extension is in shaded region. Layers represent 5 × 5 arrays of simulated neurons. Solid arrows, fixed connections; dotted arrows, modifiable connections. Seven short-term memory (STM) modules invariantly encode the $n-1, n-2 \ldots n-7$th previous responses. A recognition function compares the current response with these STMs. State now gets input from recognition and thus encodes both the abstract nature and the surface structure of the sequence. Modulatory neurons modulate the stored STM representations into the output. State controls this modulation. Each time a recognition occurs (that is, when sequence element is repeated), the current internal state becomes associated with the neuron in modulation that directs the recognized STM element to the output (Assoc). After training on ABABC, the model will recognize (and be able to repeat, and respond with reduced SRT) all sequences of the form 12123, or "unpredictable, unpredictable, $n-2, n-2$, unpredictable."

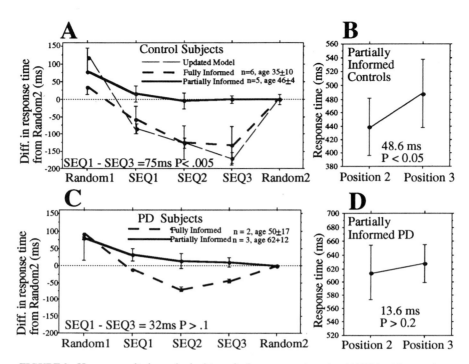

FIGURE 2. Human results in analogical transfer in sequence learning (ATSL) with a random block (Random 1), followed by three different sequence blocks (SEQ1–3), and a final random block (Random 2). (**A**) Fully informed control subjects and the updated model display significant transfer (as measured in the difference between blocks SEQ3 and SEQ1). That the three SEQ blocks are all different indicates the improvement came from learning the abstract structure common to all three. The fact that this learning does not transfer to the Random 2 block indicates that real learning has taken place, rather than simple motor facilitation. (**B**) Partially informed controls display significant learning of the analogical schema, as their reaction times in SEQ3 for position 3 elements (unpredictable) are significantly higher than those for position 2 elements (predictable). (**C**) Fully informed subjects with PD appear to display impaired transfer with respect to controls. (**D**) Partially informed subjects with PD appear to display impaired learning of the analogical schema. A three-factor ANOVA revealed the following significant effects: (1) Instruction (fully informed, partially informed), $F(1,36) = 61$, $p < .0001$; (2) Subject type (control, PD), $F(1,36) = 14$, $p < .001$; (3) Block (SEQ1, SEQ2, SEQ3), $F(2,36) = 5.5$, $p < .01$. (1 × 2) Instruction × Subject-type interaction, $F(1,36) = 5.5$, $p < .05$. Although these preliminary results indicate subjects with PD are impaired in ATSL with respect to controls, further verification with additional patients and controls is required.

of little value for sequences of length 24).[4] This implies that distinct frontostriatal systems for simple and analogical transfer sequence learning capacities may be dissociably impaired in Parkinson's disease.

REFERENCES

1. GICK, M. L. & K. J. HOLYOAK. 1983. Schema induction and analogical transfer. Cogn. Psychol. **15**: 1–38.

2. DOMINEY, P. F., M. A. ARBIB & J. P. JOSEPH. 1995. A model of cortico-striatal plasticity for learning oculomotor associations and sequences. J. Cognit. Neurosci. **7:** 311–336.
3. NISSEN, M. J. & P. BULLEMER. 1987. Attentional requirements of learning: Evidence from performance measures. Cogn. Psychol. **19:** 1–32.
4. PASCUAL-LEONE, A., J. GRAFMAN, K. CLARK, M. STEWART, S. MASSAQUOI, J.-S. LOU & M. HALLETT. 1993. Procedural learning in Parkinson's disease and cerebellar degeneration. Ann. Neurol. **34:** 594–602.
5. FUSTER, J. M. 1991. Up and down the frontal hierarchies; whither Broca's area? Commentary on Greenfield. Behav. Brain Sci. **14:** 558.

A Model of the Dynamics of Prefrontal Cortico-Thalamo-Basal Ganglionic Loops in Verbal Response Selection Tasks[a]

V. GULLAPALLI[b] AND J. GELFAND[c,d]

b Department of Mechanical and Aerospace Engineering
c Department of Psychology
Princeton University
Princeton, New Jersey 08544

We present a model of the brain mechanisms involved in verbal response selection tasks that is based on the functional anatomy of cortical and subcortical language areas, and that stresses the dynamics of prefrontal cortico-thalamo-basal ganglionic loops. Numerous studies have indicated that the left prefrontal cortex plays a role in verbal language processing.[1-5] Subcortical structures such as the thalamus and basal ganglia are also believed to participate in language function.[6,7] In addition, temporal lobe association areas are responsible for accessing cognitive or semantic representations of words. This can include Wernicke's area as well as the left posterior temporal cortex.[8,9] Finally, the anterior cingulate cortex is believed to represent information pertaining to the task that is currently being performed.[10-12]

A schematic diagram of the model showing the projections between the relevant cortical and subcortical areas is shown in FIGURE 1. The prefrontal and association cortical areas are organized as multiple groups of mutually inhibitory neurons that correspond to cortical columns.[13] These columns are indicated by groupings of neurons in the temporal association cortex and prefrontal cortex in FIGURE 1. They are not necessarily adjacent to each other in each cortical area but may be anatomically distributed. We used a distributed representation over the input cortical columns with cortico-cortical interconnections between columns formed through Hebbian learning to encode stimulus words. In this representation each column denotes a feature or category of words (e.g., colors or verbs). Within each column, each neuron denotes a particular color or verb, etc., whose excitation is associated with that word. The cingulate module stores a representation of the task (e.g., generate a color response). Phasic activity in the sensory/language cortical modules located in the temporal lobe association areas is passed on to the prefrontal cortical columns through direct projections. We presume that the output of the selection circuit projects to premotor areas, but this was not implemented here.

[a] This work was supported in part by a grant from the James S. McDonnell Foundation to the Human Information Processing Group at Princeton University and ONR Grant No. N00014-93-1-0510.

[d] Address correspondence to Dr. J. Gelfand, Department of Psychology, Princeton University, Green Hall, Princeton, NJ 08544-1010.

375

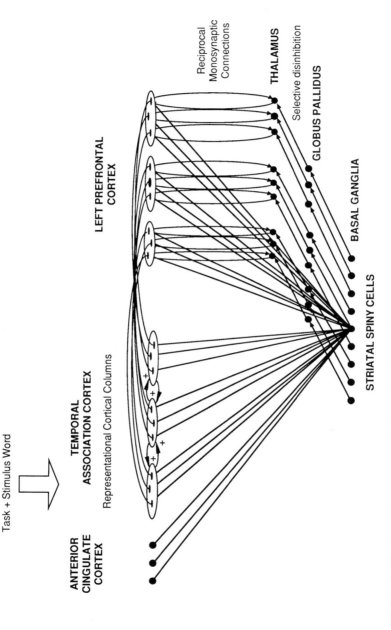

FIGURE 1. Architecture of the response selection system. For clarity, only projections to one striatal spiny cell are shown. Similar convergent projections go to each striatal neuron. The lateral inhibitory connections between neurons within each association cortex column are also not shown.

It has been proposed that reciprocal, topographic projections between the prefrontal cortex and thalamus result in local cortico-thalamic loops that, when active, may sustain activity in cortical neurons.[14-17] These loops can be activated through selective disinhibition by the basal ganglia.[18] In this model striatal spiny cells in the basal ganglia function as pattern-recognizers providing a contextual set for the prefrontal cortex. This architecture is similar to that proposed by Wallesch and Papagno.[7] However, we have implemented the specific neuronal connections and dynamics. Based on inputs from temporal association cortex and cingulate cortex, the basal ganglia selectively disinhibit the prefrontal-thalamic loops of the columns representing the word features appropriate for the task. If the task is color and the input is apple, for example, an appropriate set of features for apple is activated in the temporal association cortex based upon the dynamics of the local neuronal circuits. The prefrontal-thalamic loop for the column associated with color features would be disinhibited, thereby selecting a color response. The specific color response, however, would be determined by the projection from temporal association cortex to prefrontal cortex.

For these experiments, we selected a list of 20 words to represent. Of these, six were used as stimuli, whereas the responses could be selected from all 20. The responses were classified into four groups, namely, stimuli, color names, verbs, and miscellaneous. A separate cortical module was used to represent words in each group. Examples of the dynamic behavior of the cortico-thalamo-basal ganglionic loops under various task conditions is presented in FIGURE 2. The activity of frontal cortex neurons as a function of time is shown for three tasks. In the first time period, no task is specified and the thalamo-cortical loops are not disinhibited. The initial activity of the neurons due to stimulus word presentation decays with time. When a COLOR task is specified, the activity of neurons representing a color associated with the stimulus word is sustained through feedback in the corresponding disinhibited loops, while the activity of the other neurons decays away. Similarly, when a VERB task is specified in the third period, activity of neurons representing actions associated with the stimulus word is selectively sustained. The specific duration of activity is determined by the properties of the neurons in the loop.

This behavior observed in the model is similar to the sustained activity of prefrontal cortex neurons observed by Fuster and Goldman-Rakic in delayed-response tasks.[19,20] Thus, the prefrontal area could serve as a working memory where task-specific excitations are maintained for use by other cognitive and motor areas involved in the execution of the task. We predict that lesions that cause a lack of inhibition of the cortico-thalamic loops would result in the generation of inappropriate responses. Lesions that cause a partial or global inhibition of the thalamo-cortical loops would result in deficits in initiating responses. Deficits in shifting set would result from lesions that damage the ability to shift the modulation of thalamo-cortical loops. These deficits have been observed in prefrontal and subcortical lesion patients; however, more specific correlations are needed between the lesion sites and the resulting effects on the dynamics of these neuronal circuits in order to confirm the features of this model.

The architecture we describe here uses distributed, modular arrays for the representation and processing of information.[21,22] Little is known about the spe-

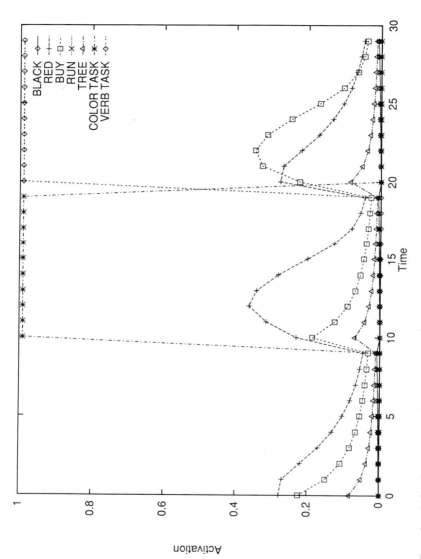

FIGURE 2. Frontal and cingulate cortex activations under three different task conditions. Examples of prefrontal cortex activation when the stimulus APPLE is presented at times 0, 10, and 20 (arbitrary units), each time with a different task (No task, COLOR, and VERB, as indicated).

cific information encoded by the cortical modules in word association areas. We postulate in our current implementation that cortical columns encode information regarding features or categories of words. Several alternative word representations organized around lexical, orthographic or phonetic attributes of words are possible and are being investigated at the present time.

ACKNOWLEDGMENTS

We acknowledge helpful discussions with James Houk, George Miller, and Nina Dronkers.

REFERENCES

1. DEMB, J., J. DESMOND, A. WAGNER, C. VAIDYA, G. GLOVER & J. GABRIELI. 1995. Semantic encoding and retrieval in the left prefrontal cortex: A functional MRI study of task difficulty and process specificity. J. Neurosci. **15:** 5870–5878.
2. KAPUR, S., R. ROSE, P. LIDDLE, R. ZIPURSKY, G. BROWN, D. STUSS, S. HOULE & E. TULVING. 1994. The role of the left prefrontal cortex in verbal processing: Semantic processing or willed action? Neuroreport **5:** 2193–2196.
3. PETERSEN, S., P. FOX, A. SNYDER & M. RAICHLE. 1990. Activation of extrastriate and frontal cortical areas by visual words and word-like stimuli. Science **249:** 1041–1044.
4. RAICHLE, M., J. FIEZ, T. VIDEEN, A. MACLEOD, J. PARDO, P. FOX & S. PETERSEN. 1994. Practice-related changes in human brain functional anatomy during nonmotor learning. Cereb. Cortex **4:** 8–26.
5. SNYDER, A., Y. ABDULLAEV, M. POSNER & M. RAICHLE. 1995. Scalp electrical potentials reflect regional cerebral blood flow responses during processing of written words. Proc. Natl. Acad. Sci. USA **92(5):** 1689–1693.
6. CROSSON, B. 1992. Subcortical Functions in Language and Memory. Guilford Press. New York.
7. WALLESCH, C.-W. & C. PAPAGNO. 1988. Subcortical aphasia. *In* Aphasia. F. Rose, R. Whurr & M. Wyke, Eds.: 256–287. Whurr Publishers. London.
8. DRONKERS, N., B. REDFERN & C. LUDY. 1995. Lesion localization in chronic Wernicke's aphasia (Abstracts). Society for Cognitive Neuroscience. San Francisco, CA.
9. WISE, R., F. CHOLLET, U. HADAR, K. FRISTON, E. HOFFNER & R. FRACKOWIAK. 1991. Distribution of cortical neural networks involved in word comprehension and word retrieval. Brain **114:** 1803–1817.
10. JANER, K. & J. PARDO. 1991. Deficits in selective attention following bilateral anterior cingulotomy. J. Cognit. Neurosci. **3:** 231–241.
11. PARDO, J., P. PARDO, K. JANER & M. RAICHLE. 1990. The anterior cingulate cortex mediates processing selection in the Stroop attentional conflict paradigm. Proc. Natl. Acad. Sci. USA **87:** 256–259.
12. VOGT, B., D. FINCH & C. OLSON. 1992. Functional heterogeneity in cingulate cortex: The anterior executive and posterior evaluative regions. Cereb. Cortex **2:** 435–443.
13. MOUNTCASTLE, V. 1978. An organizing principle for cerebral function: The unit module and distributed function. *In* The Mindful Brain. G. Edelman & V. Mountcastle, Eds. MIT Press. Cambridge, MA.
14. ALEXANDER, G., M. CRUTCHER & M. DELONG. 1990. Basal ganglia-thalamocortical circuits: Parallel substrates for motor, oculomotor, "prefrontal" and "limbic" functions. *In* The Prefrontal Cortex: Its Structure, Function and Pathology. H. Uylings, C. Van Eden, J. De Bruin, M. Corner & M. Feenstra, Eds. 119–146. Elsevier. Amsterdam.
15. GROENEWEGEN, H. & H. BERENDSE. 1994. Anatomical relationships between the pre-

frontal cortex and basal ganglia in the rat. *In* Motor and Cognitive Functions of the Prefrontal Cortex. A. Thierry, J. Glowinski, P. Goldman-Rakic & Y. Christen, Eds. Springer-Verlag. Berlin.

16. HOUK, J. 1995. Information processing in modular circuits linking basal ganglia and cerebral cortex. *In* Models of Information Processing in the Basal Ganglia. J. Houk, J. Davis & D. Beiser, Eds.: 3–9. MIT Press. Cambridge, MA.

17. SELEMON, L. & P. GOLDMAN-RAKIC. 1985. Longitudinal topography and interdigitation of corticostriatal projections in the rhesus monkey. J. Neurosci. **5:** 776–794.

18. CHEVALIER, G. & J. DENIAU. 1990. Disinhibition as a basic process in the expression of striatal functions. Trends Neurosci. **13:** 277–280.

19. FUSTER, J. & G. ALEXANDER. 1973. Firing changes in cells of the nucleus medialis dorsalis associated with the delayed response behavior. Brain Res. **61:** 79–81.

20. GOLDMAN-RAKIC, P. 1994. The issue of memory in the study of the prefrontal cortex. *In* Motor and Cognitive Functions of the Prefrontal Cortex. A. Thierry, J. Glowinski, P. Goldman-Rakic & Y. Christen, Eds. Springer-Verlag. Berlin.

21. GOLDMAN-RAKIC, P. 1988. Topography of cognition: Parallel distributed networks in primate association cortex. Annu. Rev. Neurosci. **11:** 137–156.

22. WISE, S. & J. HOUK. 1994. Modular neuronal architecture for planning and controlling motor behavior. Biol. Commun. Dan. R. Acad. Sci. **43:** 21–33.

A Computer Model of Prefrontal Cortex Function

RICHARD LEVINSON[a]

Recom Technologies Inc.
NASA Ames Research Center
Computational Sciences Division
Mail Stop 269-2
Moffett Field, California 94035

This paper describes a computer model of prefrontal cortex function which was designed by integrating the perspectives of neuropsychology and artificial intelligence (AI). The model shows how several neuropsychological theories of frontal lobe function can be combined into a single computer model. The model also extends those component theories by focusing on information processing details that glue the pieces together.

This work is motivated by the point that neuropsychology and AI describe complementary parts of a model for autonomous action. Neuropsychological models provide descriptions of how planning and reaction must be integrated for human autonomy, but the planning component is poorly understood and many information processing details have not been flushed out. In contrast, AI provides implementations of independent planning and reaction modules, but their integration is poorly understood. A computer model forces information processing issues to be addressed in detail. A computer model can also be tested more easily than models based on verbal descriptions because it produces behavior that can be compared directly with clinically observed behavior. In contrast, verbal models must be interpreted subjectively to predict and test their behavior.

NASA is interested in applying this model towards the development of autonomous instruments and spacecraft. Today's autonomous control technology is limited by executive function deficits that are similar to those found in frontal lobe patients. The control technology works well in preprogrammed situations, but it cannot reprogram itself to handle novel events. Our goal is to extend AI planning methods to simulate human executive functions in real-time closed-loop control applications. We also intend to use the model for a cognitive rehabilitation application. Earlier descriptions of the model can be found in references 1 and 2.

AN INFORMATION PROCESSING MODEL

This model is a synthesis of several neuropsychological theories which will be reviewed in the next section. The model was designed by disassembling the functional components of the neuropsychological theories and then recombining them so that the functions are grouped together based on the type of knowledge repre-

[a] e-mail: levinson@ptolemy.arc.nasa.gov

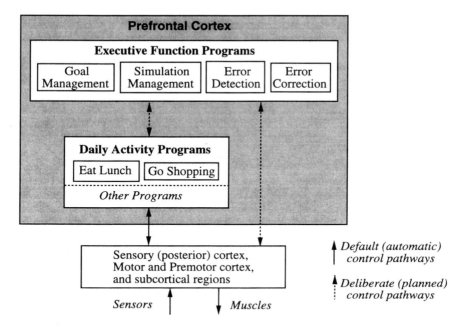

FIGURE 1. Programs stored in the prefrontal cortex.

sentation and information processing involved. Thus the model components are organized from an information processing perspective. This organizing principle shows how the information processing requirements for computer implementation have guided our model definition.

An overview of our model is shown in FIGURE 1. In this model, the prefrontal cortex stores symbolic (linguistic) memories of conditioned action sequences called programs. In humans, these programs correspond to functional neural circuits (also called pathways). The programs encode memories of long-duration action sequences that remain active to direct behavior in the absence of sensory stimuli. Routine sensory conditions activate *default* program pathways, and novel sensory conditions activate *deliberate* program variations. Some prefrontal programs encode behaviors for daily activities such as cooking, shopping, and bathing. Other programs encode executive function behavior for self-monitoring and self-programming. The Executive Functions determine when and how to replace the automatic, default programs with deliberately planned variations. These executive functions are summarized in TABLE 1.

The main focus of our model is on the definitions of the Executive Function programs, and the four knowledge representations they process. These four representations are: (1) CONDITION structures that represent symbolic descriptions of environmental conditions; (2) GOAL structures that map CONDITIONS into positive and negative reward values; (3) PROGRAM structures that link conditioned action

TABLE 1. The Executive Functions

Function Name	Function Definition	Deficit[a]
Goal Management: Maintain GOALS that map CONDITIONS into reward values		
ADD	Add a new GOAL	Inactivity
REMOVE	Remove an old GOAL	Perseveration
CHANGE	Change reward value associated with GOAL	Perseveration
Simulation Management: Simulate PROGRAMS to predict their effects		
GOAL	Triggers (re)planning when Goals are modified	Unawareness
CONDITION	Triggers replanning when conditions change	Unawareness
EXECUTION	Triggers replanning when execution failures occur	Unawareness
DEADLINE	Triggers replanning as deadline approaches	Unawareness
Error Detection: Analyze SIMULATIONS to detect program errors		
INEFFECTIVE	Routine preconditions fail due to sensory conditions	Unawareness
INTERFERING	Routine succeeds, but causes another program to fail	Distractable
IRRELEVANT	Routine is triggered by sensory conditions and does not fail, but it is unrelated to *active* GOALS	Distractable, stimulus-bound
Error Correction: Replace default PROGRAMS with deliberate variations		
INHIBIT	Override a default *start-condition* that is currently TRUE	Disinhibition
START	Override a default *start-condition* that is currently FALSE	Poor initiation
CONTINUE	Override a default *stop-condition* that is currently TRUE	Poor persistence
STOP	Override a default *stop-condition* that is currently FALSE	Perseveration
CHOOSE	Override a default *choice point selection* in program body	Perseveration
SEQUENCE	Override a default subroutine *order* in program body	Poor sequencing

[a] Indicates the effect if function is impaired.

sequences together; and (4) SIMULATION structures that record the effects of simulating different program variations.

The information processing performed by the Executive Functions can be summarized as follows: First, the Goal Management program generates GOAL structures that identify a person's preferred conditions based on experience. Second, a set of PROGRAMS are learned from experience that represent automatic conditioned action sequences that achieve GOALS in routine situations. These *default* PROGRAMS map CONDITIONS automatically into effector commands in real-time without any deliberation. The main function of the Executive Functions is to monitor the automatic conditioned responses, and to anticipate, detect, and correct any errors that occur due to novel CONDITIONS. The Simulation Management program produces SIMULATION structures that describe the predicted effects of executing any given PROGRAM in the context of current CONDITIONS. The Error Detection program then compares the SIMULATION predictions with the GOALS in order to detect potential errors. If errors are detected, then the Error Correction program overrides the default PROGRAM in order to maximize GOAL achievement.

An important feature of our model is that it is being implemented on top of an AI planning system, called Propel,[3] that provides implemented methods for representing, executing, and simulating PROGRAMS. We have previously used Propel to demonstrate how a single PROGRAM representation can be used to produce both *default* reactions and *deliberate* plans.[3] That system combined default and deliberate modes of action, but it was lacking a theory of how to coordinate the two modes. The executive function programs were designed to provide that capability.

To illustrate the concepts of how the executive functions process the above representations, we will use the following simplified PROGRAM that represents the routine for doing laundry every Thursday. The Do-Laundry program represents a conditional action sequence that will repeatedly wash the clothes, wait 20 minutes, and then dry the clothes, until the laundry basket is empty.

Program Name: Do-Laundry
Start Condition: Today is Thursday and detergent is not empty
Stop Condition: Laundry basket is empty or detergent is empty
Program Steps: Put clothes and detergent in washer
Start washer
Wait 20 minutes
Put clothes in dryer and start dryer

The **Goal Management** program generates and updates the GOAL representations that map CONDITIONS into positive and negative reward values. GOALS can be added, removed, or changed. An initial set of top level GOALS for safety and health are predetermined. New (sub)GOALS are then generated when the Simulation Manager generates SIMULATIONS with hypothetical conditions that are associated with high rewards. Without a well-defined and well-maintained set of GOALS and values, goal-driven behavior is impossible.

The **Simulation Management** program generates and updates the SIMULATION representations. When this program is triggered by one of the four events listed in TABLE 1, it uses Propel's program simulator to predict the effects of a given program in the context of current CONDITIONS. The simulation process is coupled with an AI search method that allows different program variations to be simulated and tested against the GOALS in order to find the most effective behavior. The resulting SIMULATIONS are used for Error Detection and to identify predicted conditions that serve as *plan assumptions* which need to be monitored.

Simulation is triggered by the following events: A GOAL event occurs when the Goal Manager modifies a GOAL structure. Adding new goals will trigger the initial simulation of the default response to the goal. Removing goals or changing their reward value will trigger replanning that involves backtracking through the space of program variations. The CONDITION event triggers replanning if an updated sensory condition conflicts with a predicted condition that was generated by the simulator (a plan assumption). For instance, it may be necessary to delay the start of Do-Laundry if the washing machine breaks on Wednesday, the day before laundry day. The EXECUTION event triggers replanning when a default program fails *during* execution, as when someone drops a coffee mug. Unlike with the CONDITION event, this is the case when program execution has already begun and the motor pathways have already been activated. The DEADLINE event occurs when a GOAL's deadline moves within some threshold temporal distance. This event could trigger replanning using updated sensory CONDITIONS five minutes before execution.

Simulation Management allows the brain to detach mental activity from real-time events in order to reason about SIMULATIONS of the past and the future. This enables the mental independence from sensory CONDITIONS that is required for abstract, nonconcrete thought. Implementation of this component will require resolution of many open issues. One issue involves choosing the best order in which to try different program variations when replanning. Other issues involve deciding how much time to spend planning, and understanding how to simulate actions at an abstract level without simulating every little detail.

The **Error Detection** program analyzes SIMULATIONS to detect the three error patterns described in TABLE 1. INEFFECTIVE routines are detected if the simulation record indicates that a program's preconditions could not be satisfied, for example, if there is no detergent to wash the clothes. This is called a *program failure*. INTERFERING programs are detected when the SIMULATION indicates that multiple PROGRAMS conflict over a shared resource, resulting in at least one program failure. For example, doing laundry may interfere with taking a hot shower if the hot water is limited, or a phone call may distract someone from moving the clothes from the washer to the dryer. IRRELEVANT routines are detected if the SIMULATION does not show any program failures, but it doesn't show any goal achievement either. For instance, taking the garbage out on the regularly scheduled night is irrelevant if it won't be collected due to a holiday. A frontal lobe patient who begins to bake cookies whenever she sees an oven also illustrates the type of deficit that can occur if this function is impaired. When one of these error conditions is detected, then the Error Correction program is activated.

The **Error Correction** program analyzes the SIMULATION and PROGRAM structures in order to generate PROGRAM variations that override inappropriate default programs. Routine PROGRAMS contain default *start* and *stop* conditions that automatically trigger the start and stop of program execution. The first four Error Correction methods in TABLE 1 are INHIBIT, START, CONTINUE, and STOP. These methods correspond to the 2 by 2 matrix produced by overriding the start and stop conditions in the *true* and *false* cases. For example, the start of the above Do-Laundry program can be deliberately postponed from Thursday until Saturday by using INHIBIT on Thursday and START on Saturday. Also, the default stop conditions of Do-Laundry can be overridden by using CONTINUE when the detergent runs out or by using STOP when there is not enough time to wash all the clothes in the basket.

UNDERLYING NEUROPSYCHOLOGICAL THEORIES

Our model combines the following neuropsychological theories, and it extends them by elaborating on the information processing details described above. Luria's early description of the frontal lobes as system for the "programming, regulation, and verification of activity"[4] is perhaps the best one sentence description of prefrontal cortex functionality. However, it is too general to use as a design for computer implementation. We therefore looked for the most detailed descriptions of executive function dimensions we could find, and we selected the models proposed by Sohlberg and Mateer,[5] and by Lezak.[6]

Sohlberg and Mateer developed the Executive Function Behavioral Ratings Scale (EFBRS),[5] to assess behavioral dysfunction after head injury. The EFBRS includes three main executive function components which are further divided into subcomponents. The first component, Selection and Execution of Cognitive Plans, involves the ability to describe goals and procedures, to determine appropriate action sequences, to initiate activity, to repair plans, and to maintain persistent effort until a task is completed. The second component of the EFBRS, Time Management, involves the ability to generate realistic schedules, and to perform the scheduled activities within given time constraints. The third component, Self-regulation, involves using feedback to control behavior and to inhibit inappropriate reactions.

Lezak describes four essential components of executive function.[6] First, Goal Formulation is the ability to generate and select descriptions of desirable future states. Second, Planning involves the selection of steps, elements, and sequences needed to achieve a goal. This requires the ability to recognize and evaluate choices. Third, Carrying Out Activities involves the ability to start, stop, maintain, and switch between planned actions. These subcomponents led directly to several of the Error Correction methods shown in TABLE 1. Fourth, Effective Performance involves the ability to monitor and repair activities.

We began the design of the executive function programs by making a list of the executive function components as described by the EFBRS and by Lezak. In order to facilitate computer implementation, we then reorganized those functions based on the type of information being processed. We tried to capture all of the functionality of these two models in our own. However, due to our functional reorganization, a one-to-one mapping is not always found between their components and our own. Instead, some of their components can be found distributed *across* several of our model components.

The Norman and Shallice model of the frontal lobes as an Supervisory Attentional System (SAS)[7] corresponds strongly to our model's Executive Functions, and is also based (loosely) on an AI information processing model. This model, like our own, proposes two modes of action: automatic *default* responses for routine situations, and *deliberate* planned responses for novel situations. Shallice and Burgess propose that the frontal lobes serve as an SAS that is required to (1) inhibit undesirable automatic responses and (2) generate and execute desirable new responses. The SAS model helped to define the role and function of our executive functions. It also supported our independently developed method for using both default and deliberate action modes. Our work extends the SAS model by providing an implemented PROGRAM representation and by elaborating on exactly how the SAS may detect and correct program errors in novel situations.

Grafman proposes that the prefrontal cortex contains representations called Structured Event Complexes (SECs).[8] SECs encode memories of long-duration action sequences that guide behavior through well-learned activities. SECs correspond strongly to PROGRAMS in our model. Grafman describes SEC *hierarchies*, where the highest SECs are called Managerial Knowledge Units (MKUs) because they manage other SECs. These MKUs correspond to our model's Executive Function PROGRAMS. This SEC-MKU model led us to adopt the idea that the daily activities and the executive functions in our model are all represented as PROGRAMS, rather than requiring a different representation for the executive functions.

Our work extends the SEC model by describing an implemented PROGRAM representation and a planning system that can be used to anticipate, detect, and correct program errors. Also, our Executive Function programs define a specific set of MKUs that have not previously been discussed in detail. Our model predicts that two other representation types, GOALS and SIMULATIONS, are stored in the prefrontal cortex in addition to the SEC-like PROGRAMS. Grafman elaborates on issues we have not addressed such as the effect of different neural activation patterns on SEC development and learning.

Stuss' view of self-awareness[9] is also an important part of our model. Frontal lobe patients often have intact awareness of their sensory environment despite impaired awareness of their interactions with the environment. Stuss proposes that frontal system damage can impair the awareness of one's *Self* as a continuity from the past into the future. This concept of self is represented in our system by the GOALS, which identify a value system that is learned from experience. In our model, self-awareness is the process of relating one's GOALS to external CONDITIONS and SIMULATIONS. This is achieved by the combined functions of our Simulation Management and Error Detection programs.

EVALUATION METHODOLOGY

The model's definitions of the executive functions and the representations they process identify hypothetical neurological functions and connections, and mental representations that can be tested for validity in various ways. Clinical studies can be designed to test for the presence of these model elements. Our plan is to have frontal lobe patients perform daily living tasks in a computer-simulated world. We will then connect our model to the same simulated world and compare the performance of our model with that of the patient. The model will be "lesioned" to produce behavior that is similar to that of the patient. This will allow us to compare the behaviors of the model and patient directly rather than subjectively interpreting the behavior predicted by a verbal model. The predicted deficits produced by these lesions are shown in TABLE 1.

Another benefit of our model is that we can test it on large-scale tasks that last minutes, hours, or even days. Propel's PROGRAM representation is expressive enough that we can represent complex daily living activities such as making dinner. In contrast, many frontal lobe models are based on analysis of simplistic tasks such as the Towers of London (or Hanoi), Block Design, or the Delayed Response Task. We propose that directly measuring the model's performance on large-scale daily activities such as shopping and cooking will be a better measure of the ecological validity of our model.

CONCLUSION

The Propel substrate for our system is currently implemented, providing our basic ability to represent, simulate, and execute Propel programs. The Executive Function programs, however, are still under development. Many difficult technical design and implementation issues remain unresolved. Our current efforts are directed towards extending the system to support the model's full functionality.

We have presented a computer model of prefrontal cortex function that combines several frontal lobe and executive function models based on information processing principles. Before the model is complete, many open research questions will have to be answered from both the neuropsychological and the information processing perspectives. We hope our model definition provides motivation and a common language for future interdisciplinary efforts to improve upon this start.

ACKNOWLEDGMENTS

Thanks to McKay Sohlberg, Tom Boyd, Jordan Grafman, Jeffrey Englander, Richard Delmonico, Peter Robinson, and Steve Farmer for providing many useful comments that have influenced the shape of this work.

REFERENCES

1. LEVINSON, R. 1994. Human frontal lobes and AI planning systems. Proceedings of the Second International Conference on AI Planning Systems. AAAI Press. Menlo Park, CA.
2. LEVINSON, R. 1995. An interdisciplinary theory of autonomous action. 1995. AAAI Stanford Spring Symposium on Extending Theories of Action. AAAI Press. Menlo Park, CA.
3. LEVINSON, R. 1995. A general programming language for unified planning and control. Artif. Intell. **76**.
4. LURIA, A. R. 1973. The Working Brain. Basic Books Inc. New York.
5. SOHLBERG, M. M. & C. MATEER. 1989. Introduction to Cognitive Rehabilitation. Guilford Press. New York.
6. LEZAK, M. 1983. Neuropsychological Assessment. Oxford University Press. New York.
7. SHALLICE, T. & P. BURGESS. 1991. Higher-order cognitive impairments and frontal lobe lesions in man. *In* Frontal Lobe Function and Dysfunction. H. Levin, H. Eisenberg & A. Benton, Eds. Oxford University Press. New York.
8. GRAFMAN, J. 1989. Plans, actions and mental sets: Managerial knowledge units in the frontal lobes. *In* Integrating Theory and Practice in Clinical Neuropsychology. E. Perecman, Ed. Erlbaum Press. Hillsdale, NJ.
9. STUSS, D. 1991. Disturbance of self-awareness after frontal system damage. *In* Awareness of Deficit After Brain Injury. G. Prigatano & D. Schacter, Eds. Oxford University Press. New York.

Symptoms of Depression in Alzheimer's Disease, Frontal Lobe-type Dementia, and Subcortical Dementia

OSCAR L. LOPEZ,[a,b] M. PAZ GONZALEZ,[c]
JAMES T. BECKER,[a,d] CHARLES F. REYNOLDS III,[d]
ABRAHAM SUDILOVSKY,[d] AND STEVEN T. DeKOSKY[d]

Alzheimer's Disease Research Center
Departments of Neurology[a] and Psychiatry[d]
University of Pittsburgh School of Medicine
Pittsburgh, Pennsylvania 15213

[c]Department of Psychiatry
University of Oviedo
Oviedo, Spain

INTRODUCTION

Pathological and neuroimaging data indicate that disruption of the frontal-subcortical circuits is critical to the development of affective and behavioral symptoms in demented and in nondemented individuals. These circuits link the cortex of the frontal lobes with subcortical structures (e.g., basal ganglia, thalamus). These observations suggest that damage to fronto-subcortical circuits may be a common substrate for mood disorders in neurological disease.[1] Although this perspective may explain the presence of symptoms of depression in frontal lobe-type dementia (FLTD) and subcortical dementia (SCD), the possible etiology of depression in Alzheimer's disease (AD) remains unclear. Neuropathological studies in patients with AD with depression have shown significant neuronal loss in the superior dorsal raphe nucleus, substantia nigra, and locus ceruleus.[2] However, single photon emission tomography studies have shown that depressed patients with AD exhibited lower blood flow in the left temporal-parietal regions than those without depression.[3]

In this study, we examine the relationship between frontal-subcortical system dysfunction and depressive symptomatology in dementia. If frontal-subcortical circuits have a role in the etiology of affective disorders in dementia, patients with a predominantly frontal component (e.g., FLTD) will exhibit more affective disorders than patients with a predominantly temporoparietal component (e.g., AD).

[b] Address correspondence to Oscar L. Lopez, M.D., Neuropsychology Research Program, 3600 Forbes Avenue, Suite 502, Pittsburgh, PA 15213.

389

TABLE 1. Demographic and Neuropsychiatric Characteristics of Patients with Frontal Lobe-type Dementia, Alzheimer's Disease and Subcortical Dementia

	FLTD	AD	SCD	AD
Patients (n)	21	21	10	10
Male/female	11/10	12/19	5/5	
Age (years)	65.1 ± 11.4	74.3 ± 5.4[a]	65.9 ± 7.9	69.8 ± 9.3
Education (years)	12.1 ± 3.3	13.3 ± 2.9	13.3 ± 2.9	11.8 ± 2.9
Mini-Mental State	20.5 ± 7.4	19.6 ± 7.1[b]	18.2 ± 6.4	17.5 ± 5.7
Mattis Rating	118.11 ± 15.6	107.4 ± 29.2	100.1 ± 32.1	103.2 ± 22.8
Blessed ADLs	6.1 ± 3.1	5.6 ± 4.3	6.0 ± 4.3	8.1 ± 4.9
NYU	15.6 ± 16.7	14.2 ± 11.5	43.8 ± 26.8[d]	16.6 ± 11.9[e]
HDRS	9.4 ± 5.8	3.5 ± 4.1[c]	10.3 ± 6.8	6.5 ± 3.1

AD versus FLTD: [a]p = .001; [b]p = .004; [c]p = .0001.
FLTD versus SCD: [d]p = .03.
SCD versus AD: [e]p = .04.
Abbreviations: NYU, New York University Scale for parkinsonism; HDRS, Hamilton Depression Rating Scale; ADLs, activities of daily living.

METHODS

The neurological and psychiatric characteristics of 21 patients with FLTD were compared and contrasted with those of 21 patients with AD matched by education level and severity of dementia, as measured by the Mini-Mental State Examination (MMSE). Similarly, the characteristics of 10 patients with SCD (4 with multiple-system atrophy, 3 with progressive supranuclear palsy, and 3 with progressive subcortical gliosis) were compared with 10 matched patients with AD. All AD patients met the NINCDS-ADRDA criteria for probable AD,[4] and FLTD patients exhibited the core diagnostic features for frontotemporal dementia proposed by the Lund-Manchester Groups.[5] The psychiatric evaluations were conducted by board-certified psychiatrists using a semistructured interview[6] with patients and caregivers.

RESULTS

Patients with FLTD were younger, had higher MMSE scores, and had higher Hamilton Depression Rating Scale (HDRS) scores than patients with AD (TABLE 1). Patients with FLTD exhibited more irritability, lability of mood, anxiety, and agitation, and social withdrawal than did patients with (see TABLE 2). Patients with SCD exhibited higher NYU scores than did patients with AD or FLTD. Patients with SCD exhibited more psychomotor retardation than did patients with FLTD.

In order to determine what, if any, factors were associated with the patients' clinical diagnosis, a discriminant function analysis was carried out on the psychiatric symptoms to predict group membership. Anxiety (p = .003), disinhibition (p = .02), social withdrawal (p = .01), and irritability (p = .02) predicted group membership in FLTD; anergia (p = .001), psychomotor retardation (p = .01), and HDRS scores (p = .003) predicted group membership in SCD.

TABLE 2. Psychiatric Symptoms in Patients with Frontal Lobe-type Dementia, Alzheimer's Disease, and Subcortical Dementia

	FLTD (%)	AD (%)	SCD (%)	AD (%)
Patients (n)	21	21	10	10
Major depression	5 (24)	1 (3)	2 (20)	0 (0)
Mood-related signs				
Depressed mood	9 (43)	7 (33)	6 (60)	4 (40)
Lability of mood	6 (29)	0 (0)[a]	2 (20)	3 (30)
Anxiety	9 (43)	1 (5)[a]	4 (40)	1 (10)
Irritability	16 (76)	6 (29)[a]	4 (40)	5 (50)
Behavioral disturbances				
Agitation	10 (48)	0 (0)[a]	4 (40)	1 (10)
Retardation	7 (33)	3 (14)	8 (80)[a]	3 (30)
Loss of interest	16 (76)	10 (48)	5 (50)	8 (80)
Loss of motivation	10 (48)	8 (38)	5 (50)	6 (60)
Bizarre behavior	4 (19)	2 (9.5)	0 (0)	2 (20)
Disinhibition	6 (29)	1 (5)	0 (0)	1 (10)
Social withdrawal	15 (71)	7 (33)[a]	3 (30)	4 (40)
Neurovegetative signs				
Appetite changes				
Increase	3 (14)	0 (0)	1 (10)	0 (0)
Decrease	3 (14)	1 (5)	2 (20)	2 (20)
Sleep changes				
Hypersomnia	1 (5)	3 (14)	1 (10)	2 (20)
Hyposomnia	5 (24)	2 (9.5)	5 (50)	2 (20)
Anergia	15 (71)	7 (33)[a]	9 (90)	4 (40)
Ideation disturbances				
Suicide	4 (19)	1 (5)	3 (30)	2 (20)
Poor self-esteem	2 (9.5)	3 (14)	4 (40)	1 (10)
Anxieties				
General anxiety	4 (19)	0 (0)	1 (10)	1 (10)
Situational anxiety	3 (14)	3 (14)	4 (40)	4 (40)

McNemar's test (binomial distribution): FLTD versus AD, irritability ($p = .006$); anxiety ($p = .007$); agitation ($p = .002$); anergia ($p = .02$); social withdrawal ($p = .02$); lability of mood ($p = .03$).
SCD versus AD: $p > .05$.
Fisher's exact test: FLTD versus SCD, retardation ($p = .02$).
[a] Statistical differences found.

SUMMARY

These findings support the hypothesis that a frontal-subcortical abnormality is necessary to produce symptoms of depression (e.g., mood-related signs, behavioral disturbances, neurovegetative signs) in dementia. Behavioral disturbances (e.g., disinhibition, agitation, social withdrawal) were more likely to occur in FLTD than in AD or SCD.

REFERENCES

1. CUMMINGS, J. L. 1993. Frontal-subcortical circuits and human behavior. Arch. Neurol. 50: 873–880.

2. EMERY, O. V. & T. E. OXMAN. 1992. Update on the dementia spectrum of depression. Am. J. Psychiatry **149:** 305–317.
3. STARKSTEIN, S. E., S. VASQUEZ, R. MIGLIORELLI, A. TESON, G. PETRACCA & R. LEI-GUARDA. 1995. A SPECT study of depression in Alzheimer's disease. Neuropsychiatr. Neuropsychol. Behav. Neurol. **8:** 38–43.
4. McKHANN, G., D. DRACHMAN, M. F. FOLSTEIN, R. KATZMAN, D. PRICE & E. M. STADLAN. 1984. Clinical diagnosis of Alzheimer's disease: Report of the NINCDS-ADRDA Work Group under the auspices of the Department of Health and Human Services Task Force on Alzheimer's disease. Neurology **34:** 939–944.
5. THE LUND AND MANCHESTER GROUPS. 1994. Clinical and neuropathological criteria for frontotemporal dementia. J. Neurol. Neurosurg. Psychiatry **57:** 416–418.
6. MEZZICH, J. E., J. T. DOW & G. A. COTTMAN. 1981. Developing an information system for a comprehensive psychiatric institute. I. Principles, design, and organization. Behav. Res. Methods Instrum. **13:** 459–463.

Target Detection and the Prefrontal Cortex

A PET Scan Study of the P300 Event-Related Potential

R. A. REINSEL, R. A. VESELIS, V. A. FESHCHENKO,
G. R. DI RESTA, O. MAWLAWI, B. BEATTIE, D. SILBERSWEIG,[a]
E. STERN,[a] R. BLASBERG, H. MACAPINLAC, R. FINN,
S. GOLDSMITH, AND S. LARSON

*Departments of Anesthesiology, Radiology/Nuclear Medicine
Service, and Neurology
Memorial Sloan-Kettering Cancer Center
New York, New York 10021*

*[a]Department of Psychiatry
Cornell University Medical College
New York, New York 10021*

INTRODUCTION

Medial and lateral regions of the frontal lobes have been implicated in higher-order attentional processing.[1] The right hemisphere has been found to play a particularly significant role in vigilance or expectancy tasks, independent of stimulus modality or laterality of sensory input.[2] Although visual attention has been well studied,[3] the auditory attentional system has received less scrutiny. One measure often used to study attention to auditory stimuli is the P300 component of the event-related potential (ERP),[4] extracted by signal averaging from the ongoing EEG during performance of the "oddball" stimulus paradigm (see below). Functional PET scanning using radioactively labeled water ($H_2^{15}O$) provides a regional cerebral blood flow (rCBF) index of neuronal activity.[5] In this pilot study, [^{15}O] positron emission tomography (PET) images were obtained during P300 recording and control periods. Statistical parametric mapping (SPM) analysis[6] was used to identify neural processing networks involved in this auditory activation task.

METHODS

Seven normal, healthy, right-handed male volunteers (ages 21–45, mean age 29 years) performed a standard auditory "oddball" task to generate a P300 waveform during simultaneous PET scanning. ERPs were recorded from 19 monopolar scalp electrodes using the NeuroScan system. After artifact rejection, ERPs were averaged over a 1-s epoch with a 100-ms prestimulus baseline. In the P300 (activation) condition, subjects were asked to silently count target high tones (2500 Hz, inci-

TABLE 1. Statistical Maxima (Z-scores) of Regional Increases in Cerebral Blood Flow during P300 Task Performance, Identified by Gyrus and Hemisphere

Gyrus	Side	Brodmann's Area	Maxima (Z-score)	Location (X, Y, Z coordinates)
Precentral	R	6	2.810	48, 2, 28
Superior frontal	R	9	2.696	24, 40, 32
Inferior frontal	R	44	3.184	46, 8, 16
Medial frontal	L	9	3.080	− 34, 40, 28
Superior temporal	L	22	2.632	− 60, − 34, 12

NOTE: X, Y, and Z coordinates refer to three-dimensional spatial coordinates, relative to the anterior commissure, in the Talairach and Tournoux atlas.[7]

dence 20%) on each of three 5-min trials. On control trials, subjects listened to low tones only (1000 Hz), but were instructed to ignore them. Using a PC4600 NeuroPet scanner, six 90-s PET scans were obtained, three P300 scans alternating with three control scans, with 12-min intervals between scans to allow the isotope to be eliminated ([^{15}O] half-life = 2 min). PET images were corrected for head movement and scalp artifact and combined for analysis, normalizing mean global flow to 50 mL/100 g/min. SPM was used to identify regional differences in cerebral blood flow (rCBF) between P300 and control conditions (omnibus p value = 0.01). Significant changes were identified in three-dimensional stereotaxic coordinates[7] and associated with anatomical location and Brodmann's areas (BA) of cortex.

RESULTS

Relative to the control condition, rCBF increased bilaterally in frontal cortex during the P300 recording, with greater activation in the right hemisphere. Significant foci were identified (TABLE 1 and FIG. 1) in the right precentral (BA 4 and 6),

FIGURE 1 (top). Results of the statistical parametric mapping (SPM) analysis of regional changes in cerebral blood flow (CBF) (mean of 7 subjects) during the oddball task are shown as SPM projections of significant foci of activation in sagittal, coronal, and transverse sections. Bright colors indicate areas with relative increases in CBF compared to the control condition at the 0.01 omnibus level of significance.

FIGURE 2 (bottom). Grand average waveforms of the event-related potential (ERP) for target (yellow line) and nontarget (pink line) stimuli are shown for 19 electrodes on the scalp. ERPs were recorded simultaneously with acquisition of PET images. Waveforms were recorded for 100 ms prestimulus and 900 ms poststimulus (vertical white line indicates time of stimulus presentation). P300 amplitude is maximal at central locations. Positive up, negative down.

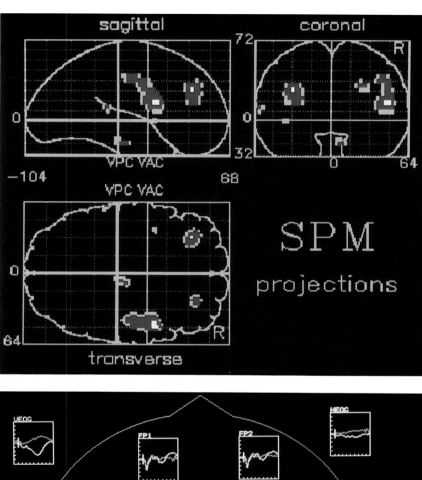

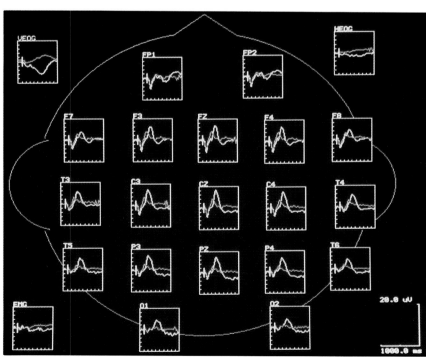

superior frontal (BA 9), medial frontal (BA 9), and inferior frontal gyri (BA 44). In the left hemisphere, the medial frontal gyrus (BA 9 and 46), and the superior temporal gyrus (BA 22) showed increased rCBF compared to control scans. The ERP waveforms were averaged across subjects (FIG. 2) and showed P300 amplitude maximal at Cz (mean amplitude 8.3 μV, mean latency 306 ms). Subjects showed high accuracy in counting the target tones (>95% in all cases).

CONCLUSIONS

Frontal cortex showed bilateral increases in rCBF during the P300 task. This task included target detection, silent counting, and working memory components. Recent research[8] has found dorsolateral prefrontal cortex (BA 9 and 46) to be activated in tasks where information is held in working memory, as with the incremental counting task used in this study. In addition, dorsolateral prefrontal cortex has been implicated in the generation of the P300 response to novel stimuli.[9] The activation of the areas associated with working memory in this standard oddball paradigm suggests that considerable functional overlap may exist between attention and working memory.[10]

The concurrent activation in the prefrontal cortex and the left-sided superior temporal gyrus may reflect top-down attentional modulation of auditory processing. Such top-down modulation has been recently reported in a PET study of visual attention.[11] In addition, studies of the middle latency auditory evoked potential indicate that the dorsolateral prefrontal cortex may play an early (25–35 ms) role in stimulus selection by providing inhibitory modulation of input to primary auditory cortex.[12,13]

The suggested specialized role of the right hemisphere in attentional processing,[14] vigilance,[2] and anticipation of feedback[15] may be reflected in the greater right-sided activation seen in this study. The role of premotor cortex and the right-sided homolog of Broca's area is less clear and remains to be elucidated in further, more specific studies. These preliminary findings also indicate the feasibility of recording EEG and ERPs simultaneously with PET scanning to provide complementary information on brain states during cognitive processing.

REFERENCES

1. POSNER, M. L. & S. E. PETERSEN. 1990. The attention system of the human brain. Annu. Rev. Neurosci. **13:** 25–42.
2. PARDO, J. V., P. T. FOX & M. E. RAICHLE. 1991. Localization of a human system for sustained attention by positron emission tomography. Nature **349:** 61–64.
3. LABERGE, D. 1990. Thalamic and cortical mechanisms of attention suggested by recent positron emission tomographic experiments. J. Cognit. Neurosci. **2:** 358–372.
4. POLICH, J. 1993. P300 in clinical applications: Meaning, method and measurement. In Electroencephalography. 3rd edit. E. Niedermeyer & F. Lopes da Silva, Eds.: 1005–1018. Williams & Wilkins. Baltimore, MD.
5. SILBERSWEIG, D. A., E. STERN, C. D. FRITH, C. CAHILL, L. SCHNORR, S. GROOTOONK, T. SPINKS, J. CLARK, R. FRACKOWIAK & T. JONES. 1993. Detection of thirty-second cognitive activation conditions in single subjects with positron emission tomography:

A new low-dose $H_2{}^{15}O$ regional cerebral blood flow three-dimensional imaging technique. J. Cereb. Blood Flow Metab. **13:** 617–629.

6. FRISTON, K. J., C. D. FRITH, P. F. LIDDLE & R. S. J. FRACKOWIAK. 1991. Comparing functional (PET) images: The assessment of significant change. J. Cereb. Blood Flow Metab. **11:** 690–699.

7. TALAIRACH, J. & P. TOURNOUX. 1988. Co-planar stereotaxic atlas of the human brain (M. Rayport, trans.) Thieme Medical. New York.

8. SMITH, E. E., J. JONIDES & R. KOEPPE. 1996. Dissociating spatial and verbal working memory using PET. Cereb. Cortex **6(1):** In press.

9. YAMAGUCHI, S. & R. T. KNIGHT. 1991. Anterior and posterior association cortex contributions to the somatosensory P300. J. Neurosci. **11:** 2039–2054.

10. BADDELEY, A. D. 1993. Working memory or working attention? *In* Attention: Selection, Awareness and Control: A Tribute to Donald Broadbent. A. Baddeley & L. Weiskrantz, Eds. Oxford University Press. Oxford, UK.

11. CORBETTA, M., F. M. MIEZIN, S. DOBMEYER, G. L. SHULMAN & S. E. PETERSEN. 1990. Attentional modulation of neural processing of shape, color and velocity in humans. Science **248:** 1556–1559.

12. KNIGHT, R. T., D. SCABINI & D. L. WOODS. 1989. Prefrontal cortex gating of auditory transmission in humans. Brain Res. **504:** 338–342.

13. HILLYARD, S. A., G. R. MANGUN, M. G. WOLDORFF & S. J. LUCK. 1995. Neural systems mediating selective attention. *In* The Cognitive Neurosciences. M. S. Gazzaniga, Ed.: 665–681. MIT Press. Cambridge, MA.

14. FOSTER, J. K., G. A. ESTES & D. T. STUSS. 1994. The cognitive neuropsychology of attention: A frontal lobe perspective. Cogn. Neuropsychol. **11:** 133–147.

15. SILBERSTEIN, R. B., M. A. SCHIER, A. PIPINGAS, J. CIORCIARI, S. R. WOOD & D. G. SIMPSON. 1990. Steady-state visually evoked potential topography associated with a visual vigilance task. Brain Topogr. **3:** 337–347.

The Mismatch Negativity to Novel Stimuli Reflects Cognitive Decline[a]

M. M. SCHROEDER,[b] W. RITTER, AND H. G. VAUGHAN, JR.

Departments of Neurology and Neuroscience
Albert Einstein College of Medicine
Bronx, New York 10461

Novel auditory stimuli elicit event-related potential (ERP) components which index frontal lobe function. The P300 response to novel auditory stimuli has a central-frontal topography, and is reduced in amplitude in normal elderly subjects.[1] Patients with frontal lobe lesions have P300 responses to novel stimuli that are delayed and more posterior in topography.[2] The mismatch negativity (MMN) is an automatic response to a change in repetitive auditory stimuli which is thought to index transient auditory memory processes.[3] We expected that the components elicited by novel stimuli would be more sensitive to cognitive decline than those elicited by pitch and duration deviants.

The subjects comprised 14 young persons (mean age, 27.1 years) and 80 elderly persons (mean age, 80.1 years), divided into 3 groups (normal, $n = 35$; low functioning, $n = 32$; and demented, $n = 13$) based on an average of standard scores from three memory tests which were adjusted for age and/or education.

Stimuli were presented at 93 dB SPL and were 100 ms in duration (except for the duration and novel deviants); SOA was 1.1 s. Two stimulus trains were presented, with three tones in each. The first had a standard tone (1000 Hz, 80%), a pitch deviant (1450 Hz, 10%), and a duration deviant (1000 Hz, 10%, 170 ms). The second had the same standard (80%), the same pitch deviant (10%), and novel environmental sounds (10%; average duration 300 ms).

The scalp EEG (bandpass 0.5–100 Hz) was recorded in 32 channels referenced to the nose. Subjects were seated comfortably and were instructed to ignore the stimuli and watch a silent movie. Subjects were told that they would hear novel sounds embedded in trains of tones. Measures of obligatory components (P1 and N1), MMN, and P300 were scored by a program that recorded the latency and amplitude of the largest peak within a broad window around the expected peak. P1 and N1 were measured at Fz and Cz; MMN, at Fz and FC2; and P300 at Fz, Cz, and Pz). The ANOVAs and Tukey post-hoc tests conducted on ERP scores focused on significant age differences (young versus elderly), and differences due to cognitive decline (normal versus demented elderly). The peaks of the obligatory components P1 and N1 showed delays with age, but no amplitude differences. The latency of the MMN to novel stimuli (FIG. 1) was delayed for all elderly groups compared to the young [F(3, 78) = 5.76, $p < .001$]. For all subjects the

[a] This work was supported by National Institutes of Health grant AG03939.

[b] Address correspondence to Dr. Mary M. Schroeder, 915 Rose F. Kennedy Center, Albert Einstein College of Medicine, 1300 Morris Park Avenue, Bronx, NY 10461.

399

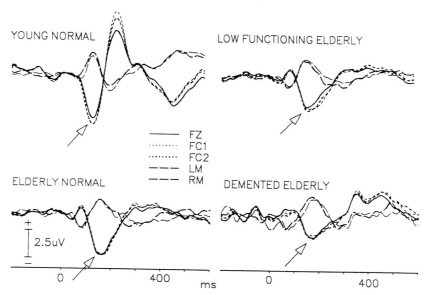

FIGURE 1. The mismatch negativity to novel stimuli is smaller for demented subjects.

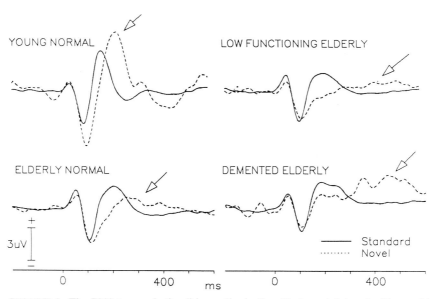

FIGURE 2. The P300 to novel stimuli is smaller in the elderly and delayed with cognitive decline.

amplitude of the MMN was larger over the right hemisphere for the novel and duration, but not the pitch stimuli. The amplitude of the MMN to novel stimuli was smaller for the demented group compared to all three other groups [$F(3, 78) = 3.31, p < .05$]. The duration MMN was significantly smaller in amplitude for the elderly, and the pitch MMN was significantly smaller in amplitude only for the low functioning elderly, compared to the young. The P300 to the novel stimulus was significantly smaller for the normal and low functioning elderly, compared to the young, and paradoxically enhanced for the demented elderly [$F(3, 77) = 6.83, p < .001$]. The latency of the P300 to novel stimuli (FIG. 2) was significantly delayed for the elderly compared to the young, and the P300 for the low functioning elderly was significantly slower than that for the normal elderly [$F(3, 77) = 12.06, p < .0001$].

In summary, only the amplitude of the MMN to the novel stimulus and the latency of the following frontal positivity were sensitive to differences in cognitive function within the elderly group. These two "markers" of cognitive decline may index the timing and efficiency of frontal orienting systems. Because the MMN is recorded optimally when the subject is ignoring the stimuli, the problem of equating groups for task difficulty is eliminated. These markers may be potentially useful in detecting cognitive decline in the elderly.

ACKNOWLEDGMENTS

The novel stimuli were recorded by M. Fabiani and D. Friedman.

REFERENCES

1. KNIGHT, R. T. 1987. Aging decreases auditory event-related potentials to unexpected stimuli in humans. Neurobiol. Aging **8:** 109–113.
2. KNIGHT, R. T. 1984. Decreased response to novel stimuli after prefrontal lesions in man. Electroencephalogr. Clin. Neurophysiol. **59:** 9–20.
3. RITTER, W., D. DEACON, H. GOMES, D. C. JAVITT & H. G. VAUGHAN. 1995. The mismatch negativity of event-related potentials as a probe of transient auditory memory: A review. Ear Hear. **16(1):** 52–67.

Subject Index

A bstraction-Partitioned Evaluator (APE)
MKU comparison with, 273–274
and neuropsychology, 272–274
planning system, 270–272
Acetylcholine, 9
Action disorganization syndrome (ADS)
anoxia and, 332
and executive functions, 325–329
interpretation of
as contention scheduling disorder, 330
as knowledge/memory substrate
disorder, 330–331
as supervisory attention disorder,
329–330
origins of, 331–332
unified hypothesis regarding, 331–332
AD. *See* Alzheimer's disease
ADS. *See* Action disorganization
syndrome
Age-related deficits
in frequencey estimation, 128–129
and frontal dysfunction, 128
in psychomotor tasks, 134
source amnesia, 127–128
in temporal order memory, 124
in verbal fluency tests, 122
on WCST, 122
Aging
and CBF, 28
and cognitive performance, 28
"diffuse" brain disorders and, 25–26
and frontal system changes, 119–121
frontal system deterioration in
and cognitive resources, 138–139
and memory, 137–138
implicit tests of memory in, 133
and memory, 119–121
and recall/recognition, 131
and working-with-memory function, 140
AI. *See* Artificial intelligence
Akinesia, 7, 16
Alcoholism
and cognitive disorders, 27–28
and cortical functional alterations, 32–33
Stroop test with, 35
TMT with, 27
ALS. *See* Amyotrophic lateral sclerosis
Alzheimer's disease (AD)
and ADS, 332
cholinergic input and, 10
depression symptoms in, 389–391
dual-task experiments in
central executive deficit and, 161–163
results of, 164–169
and FLD, 25

and MKUs, 362
temporal order memory in, 124
γ-Aminobutyric acid (GABA), 5, 9
Amnesia. *See also* Source amnesia
frontal form of, 19
in Korsakoff patients, 124, 130, 133, 153
list differentiation performance in,
127–128
metamemory task performance of, 130
temporal order memory in, 123–124
Amyotrophic lateral sclerosis (ALS)
dementia in, 17, 19
MND-type histology in, 19
Analogical transfer in sequence learning
(ATSL)
analogical transfer paradigm, 369–370
model of, 370–371
in PD, 370–371
Anosognosia, 130, 228
Anoxia, and ADS, 332
Anxiety, as PD therapy side effect, 9–10
Apathy, 6–7
as circuit-specific behavior, 10
in FTD, 17
APE. *See* Abstraction-Partitioned
Evaluator
Aphasia
"dynamic aphasia," 20
in FTD, 16
in LA, 15–16
Apraxia. *See* Ideational apraxia
Artificial intelligence (AI)
"intelligent agents" introduction by,
269–270
and models of frontal lobe function, 381
in planning
APE system, 270–274
historical retrospective, 267–269
neuropsychology and, 272–274
ATSL. *See* Analogical transfer in
sequence learning
Attention
anxiety and, 226
concentrating, 197, 199
habituation bias and, 226–227
preparatory, 202–203
redundancy bias and, 226
SAS and, 193–203, 207, 340–341
setting, 203
sharing, 199–200
suppressing, 198, 201
sustaining, 195–197
switching, 201–202
tasks/tests of, 194–195
tests of, 195

Index of Contributors